Contents

Project Team

Health Education Authority

Antony Morgan	**Head of Effectiveness and Monitoring Research**
Mary Hickman	**Senior Research Manager**
Karen Ford	**Research Manager**
Paige Sinkler	**Research Manager**

Office for National Statistics

Tricia Dodd	**Research Director**
Val Mason	**Principal Survey Researcher**
Laura Rainford	**Survey Researcher, HEMS Project Manager**
Michael Staley	**Computing Officer**
Adrian Simpson	**Assistant Computing Officer**
Anne Klepacz	**Field Officer**
Theresa Parker	**Assistant Field Officer**
Richard Price	**Assistant Field Officer**
Nigel Hudson	**Administrative Officer**

HEA to become the new Health Development Agency (HDA)

As the White Paper *Saving Lives: Our Healthier Nation* outlined recently, the Health Education Authority (HEA) will be replaced by the new Health Development Agency (HDA). The existing resources of the HEA will be used to form the basis of the new agency, a special health authority, which will come into being in Spring 2000.

The HDA will work with government, local authorities, the NHS, the voluntary sector, and the public itself. It will be at the heart of co-ordinated strategies to improve the public's health and to reduce health inequalities. The HDA will be the national centre for producing, gathering and disseminating evidence and practical guidelines on the ways to give individuals and communities opportunities to improve their health.

The aim of the HDA, as documented in September 1999, is to contribute to reductions in health inequalities by improving the quality of public health action in England and by promoting a better understanding of both public health and people's own role in improving health. The HDA will seek to measure the success of its own and others' efforts to close the health gap in England.

The HDA has 5 strategic goals:

1. To establish a high quality and credible evidence base for public health action
2. To disseminate the evidence base and to give others easy access to the information about public health and public health action
3. To raise the standards of public health practice
4. To contribute to the development of a broader-based and better co-ordinated public health infrastructure
5. To raise public understanding of public health.

Authors' acknowledgements

We would like to thank everybody who contributed to the Survey and the production of this report. We were supported by our specialist colleagues in ONS who carried out the sampling, fieldwork, computing and coding stages, and by our colleagues who helped us with the administrative duties. We would especially like to thank Ann Bridgwood who was involved in the design of the Survey, Eileen Goddard and Nikki Bennett for their work on developing the report and on the physical activity chapter and Bridget Curry for her contribution during fieldwork and to the diet chapter. Thanks are due to the interviewers who showed commitment and enthusiasm throughout the Survey. We would also like to thank colleagues at the Health Education Authority, especially Paige Sinkler and Karen Ford, for their contribution to the Survey, and to thank Gemma Penn for her background analysis for Chapter 3.

Most importantly, we would like to thank all those people who gave up their time to take part in this Survey, and showed such an interest in its aims.

Notes to tables

1. Where the base number is less than 30, numbers rather than percentages are shown in italics in square brackets.

2. The column percentages may add to 99% or 101% because of rounding.

3. A percentage may be quoted in the text for a single category that is identifiable in the tables only by summing two or more component percentages. In order to avoid rounding errors, particularly as the data were weighted, the percentage has been recalculated for the single category and may therefore differ by one percentage point from the sum of the percentages derived from the tables.

4. The following conventions have been used within tables:

   -   no observations (zero value)
   0   less than 0.5%
   [] numbers on a base of less than 30

5. Unless otherwise stated, changes and differences mentioned in the text have been found to be statistically significant at the 95% confidence level.

6. Values for means, medians, percentiles, standard errors (SE) and confidence intervals are shown to an appropriate number of decimal places.

7. Non-response and missing information: the information from an individual who co-operated in the survey may be incomplete, either because of a partial refusal or because the individual did not understand, did not know the answer or refused to answer a particular question.

   Respondents who did not co-operate at all are omitted from all analysis; those who did not co-operate with a particular section (e.g. the self-completion schedule) are omitted from the analysis of that section. The 'no answers' arising from the omission of particular items have been excluded from the base numbers shown in the tables and from the bases used in percentaging.

Summary of main findings

Background and aims of the survey (Chapter 1)

The 1998 Health Education Monitoring Survey (HEMS) is the third in a series of studies designed to measure a range of health promotion indicators relevant to adults living in private households in England. This survey, and the previous ones in 1995 and 1996, have been designed by the Health Education Authority (HEA) in collaboration with the Social Survey Division (SSD) of the Office for National Statistics (ONS), who were commissioned by the HEA to carry out all these studies.

The HEMS was initially developed within the Government's public health strategy, the Health of the Nation[1]. The design of 1998 survey took into account the subsequent government Green Paper 'Our Healthier Nation'[2], which pointed out the need to look not only at individual behaviour but also at the influences on health of the social environment and of the wider community.

Over the last few years there has been a growing recognition that individually-focussed interventions have a relatively small impact on behaviour change and on health improvement. The individuals influenced by these interventions have tended to be the better off, better motivated and better educated. This has highlighted the need for those working in health promotion to develop a better understanding of the factors that are beyond the control of individual influence on behaviours or health experience.

The 1998 HEMS questionnaire was developed to continue to monitor health and health-related behaviours, but also to increase our understanding of the social environment within which they are expressed. The aim of this report is to explore how people's health and health behaviours relate both to their demographic and socio-economic characteristics and to their social environment. In doing so, we introduce a new set of social indicators to contribute to the debate on the links between social inequalities and health.

The 1998 HEMS report plan (Chapter 2)

The report has five main chapters, covering self-reported health status, smoking, drinking, physical activity and diet. Each chapter investigates a small number of health measures in relation to a range of analysis variables, which describe respondents' personal characteristics and the characteristics of their social environment. A concluding chapter draws together the results of these chapters, showing which of these characteristics were most likely to be independently associated with health status and health behaviour.

The structure of the chapters

The chapters describe each selected health measure, and look at the variation by sex and age. The 1998 results are also placed in the context of the HEMS results from 1995 and 1996.

The health measures are then analysed in relation to two groups of analysis variables which describe the context within which health is experienced. The first group consists of a range of demographic and socio-economic variables, similar to those used in previous HEMS. The second group consists of a new classification of household type and a number of new indicators used to describe people's social environment (including variables of social support, social capital and area deprivation).

Because many of these analysis variables vary in relation to age, age-standardisation has been used in this second stage of analysis to investigate whether the analysis variable has an effect on a health measure which is independent of age.

In the third stage of analysis, logistic regression models are used to assess the independent effects of all the analysis variables on the selected health measures. Logistic regression indicates whether each analysis variable makes a significant contribution to explaining the variation in the health measure, *having held constant all the other analysis variables.* With certain provisos, the method is used to highlight the main factors associated with health and health behaviours.

The health measures investigated

The health measures examined are as follows:

Self-reported health status (Chapter 3)

The proportions of adults who reported having:
- 'less than good' general health,
- a limiting long-standing illness,
- a large amount of stress in the last 12 months.

Smoking (Chapter 4)

The proportions of adults who were:
- current cigarette smokers,
- ex-cigarette smokers, or
- who have never regularly smoked.

Drinking (Chapter 5)

The proportions of adults with usual weekly alcohol consumption of:

- Under one unit, or abstainer, (ie. non- or occasional drinkers)
- 1–21 units for men, and 1–14 units for women,
- 22–35 units for men, and 15–25 units for women,
- 36–50 units for men, and 26–35 units for women,
- 51 or more units for men, and 36 or more units for women.

Physical activity (Chapter 6)

The proportions of adults classified as having:

- a 'sedentary' level of activity, (ie. did 30 minutes or more)
- moderate-intensity activity (less than once a week),
- a 'moderate' level of activity,
- a 'vigorous' level of activity.

Diet (Chapter 7)

The proportions of adults classified as having:

- a 'less healthy diet', or
- a 'more healthy diet' (based on a survey diet score),
- knowledge of what constitutes a healthy diet.

The analysis variables

The health measures are examined in relation to the following analysis variables:

Demographic and socio-economic variables

- Sex
- Age
- Marital status
- Social class
- Gross household income
- Economic activity
- Highest qualification level
- Housing tenure
- Household type

Social environment variables

- Personal support group (- the number of people the respondent could call on at a time of serious personal crisis)
- Community activity (- participation in the last two weeks in adult education, voluntary or community groups or religious activities)
- Satisfaction with amount of control over decisions affecting own life.
- Perceived ability to influence decisions affecting the neighbourhood.
- Neighbourhood social capital score (- derived from answers to six statements about aspects of the respondent's neighbourhood)
- HEMS area deprivation category (- derived for postcodes from 1991 Census rates of unemployment, car ownership, overcrowding and social class)

In addition to the analysis described above, the relationships between the health measures and people's attitudes and

knowledge are described briefly, either within the chapters or in supplementary tables in Part B of the report. Part C of the report presents tables which compare results from HEMS 1995 and 1996 with those for 1998 and tables showing new data for 1998 on:

- Sexual health (16–54 year olds)
- Behaviour in the sun.

Self-reported health status (Chapter 3)

A. General health and limiting long-standing illness

- In 1998, 22% of men and 26% of women reported 'less than good' general health, and 20% of men and 24% of women reported having a limiting long-standing illness.

- As expected, the percentages reporting poorer health increased with age. For example, in the youngest age-group, 14% of men and 22% of women classified their general health as 'less than good', compared with 43% and 50% respectively among those aged 75 and over. Similarly, while only 7% of men and 13% of women aged 16-24 had a limiting long-standing illness, the corresponding percentages among those aged 75 and over were 42% and 54%.

- Only in the youngest age-group were women significantly more likely than men to report 'less than good' general health, and only in the oldest age-group were they more likely than men to report a limiting long-standing illness.

Demographic and socio-economic factors

- Having taken account of age, a number of other demographic and socio-economic characteristics were closely associated with poorer health. Both the proportions reporting 'less than good' health and the proportions having a limiting long-standing illness were relatively greater among men and women in the manual social classes, those with annual household incomes of less than £10,000, those who were economically inactive, those with no educational qualifications, and those in local authority housing. Unemployed women, and men who lived in one-person households were also more likely, than would be expected on the basis of age alone, to report 'less than good' general health, but not limiting long-standing illness.

Social environment factors

- After taking age into account, factors related to the respondents' social environment were also associated with an increased likelihood of reporting poorer health. These factors included having a lack of control over decisions affecting life, a lack of influence over neighbourhood decisions, a low neighbourhood social capital score, living in the more deprived areas, and, especially for men, having no personal support group. Those who had no involvement in community activities were also more likely to report 'less than good' general health (for both sexes) and limiting long-standing illness (for women only).

Factors with independent effects on general health and limiting long-standing illness

- Logistic regression analysis was used to look at the relative importance of the different characteristics. It showed that, after taking into account all the other variables, sex did not have a significant independent effect on either of these health measures. The variables with independent effects on both measures were age, household income, economic activity, housing tenure, household type, satisfaction with control over decisions affecting life, and neighbourhood social capital score. In addition, qualification level and size of personal support group had independent effects but only on reporting 'less than good' health.

B. Stress

- In 1998, 24% of men and 29% of women reported having suffered a 'large amount' of stress in the past 12 months.

- The proportion reporting a large amount of stress was highest in the age-groups between 25-54, peaking among those aged 35-44: about one third in these age-groups reported a large amount of stress, compared with about one fifth in the youngest and oldest groups.

Demographic and socio-economic factors

- Having taken account of age, higher stress levels were associated with a number of other demographic and socio-economic characteristics. Stress was relatively higher among men and women who were widowed, divorced or separated, those in Social Classes I/II, those with annual household incomes of less than £10,000, and those living in local authority housing. Among men, it was also higher among the economically inactive and those living alone. Among women, it was higher among the unemployed and among lone mothers with dependent children.

Social environment factors

- After taking account of age, some of the factors related to the respondents' social environment were also strongly associated with increased stress levels. Levels were particularly high among the small numbers with no personal support group. They were also relatively higher among those with lack of control over decisions affecting their lives, those with a low neighbourhood social capital score, and to a lesser extent those with a lack of influence over neighbourhood decisions.

Factors with independent effects on stress

- Logistic regression analysis was used to look at the relative importance of the different characteristics on reporting a large amount of stress. It showed that, after taking into account all the other variables, many of the analysis variables had significant independent effects on stress levels. These were sex, age, marital status, social class, household income, housing tenure, household type, size of personal support group, control over decisions affecting own life, influence over neighbourhood decisions and neighbourhood social capital score.

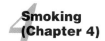

Smoking (Chapter 4)

Smoking status

- Men were more likely than women to smoke cigarettes (29% compared with 26%). Men were also more likely to be heavier smokers (11% smoked 20 cigarettes or more a day, compared with 7% of women).

- Younger people were more likely than older people to be current smokers. For example, 39% of men aged 16–24 were current smokers compared with 13% of men aged 75 or over. The corresponding proportions for women were lower but followed the same pattern, falling from 29% to 9%.

Demographic and socio-economic factors

- Having taken account of age, smoking prevalence was relatively higher among those in Social Classes IV/V, and those with annual household incomes of less than £5,000. It was also relatively higher among single women and lone mothers.

- Conversely, having taken account of age, the likelihood of never having smoked was relatively greater among those with an annual household income of £20,000 or more, those qualified to 'A' level or higher, and those in owner-occupied homes. It was also relatively greater for employed men, men in non-manual social classes, and married or cohabiting women.

Social environment factors

- After taking account of age, factors related to the respondent's social environment, were also strongly related to smoking behaviour. For example, smoking prevalence was relatively higher among those who were not active in their local community, those with lack of control over decisions affecting their lives, those with a low neighbourhood social capital score, and those who lived in more deprived areas. Among men, it was also high among those who had no personal support group.

- Similarly, the likelihood of never having smoked was related to community involvement, control over decisions affecting life, neighbourhood social capital score, and, for women, the HEMS area deprivation measure.

Factors with independent effects on smoking status

- Logistic regression analysis showed that a number of factors had significant independent effects on both of the smoking measures. These were age, marital status, qualification level, tenure, household type, community activity, satisfaction with control over decisions affecting life, neighbourhood social capital score, and the HEMS measure of area deprivation. In addition, social class and influence over neighbourhood decisions were significant for being a smoker, and sex and size of personal support group were associated with never having smoked.

Giving up smoking

- Smokers were asked about their intentions to give up smoking. Those in the middle age-groups (25–54) were more likely than older or younger respondents to say that they would like to give up, though this pattern was more marked among men than women.

- While the heavier smokers were more likely than those who smoked less to say that they would like to give up, it was the lightest smokers who were the most likely to say that they intended to give up smoking within the next month: 15% of those who smoked fewer than 10 cigarettes a day intended to give up within the next month, compared with 7% of those with a higher consumption.

5 Drinking (Chapter 5)

Consumption of alcohol

- Mean weekly alcohol consumption was higher for men (18.4 units) than for women (7.7 units per week).

- The age-groups with the highest mean alcohol consumption were those aged 16–34 among men (just over 22 units per week) and those aged 16–24 among women (just over 13 units).

- Mean weekly alcohol consumption was highest for men in Social Classes IV/V and for women in Social Classes I/II.

Demographic and socio-economic factors

- Having taken account of age, drinking behaviour varied in relation to a number of demographic and socio-economic factors. The likelihood of drinking over 21 units per week for men and over 14 units for women was relatively greater among those with a gross household income of £20,000 or more. The proportions drinking these amounts were also greater for women in Social Classes I/II, women who were single and women with 'A' levels or higher qualifications.

- Conversely, having taken account of age, the likelihood of being a non- or occasional drinker was relatively greater among those who were in Social Classes IV/V, those with a gross household income below £10,000, the economically inactive, those who had no qualifications and women who lived alone.

Social environment factors

- These specific measures of alcohol consumption were associated with only a few of the factors describing people's social environment. After taking account of age, the likelihood of drinking over 21 units per week for men and over 14 units for women was relatively greater for the small numbers of men with no personal support, men who lived alone, women who lived with other adults but no children, and men who were not active in their local community. The likelihood of being a non-or occasional drinker was relatively greater for

those with a personal support group of 1–3 people and for men who were active in the community.

Factors with independent effects on alcohol consumption

- Logistic regression analysis was used to look at the relative importance of the different characteristics. It showed that characteristics of the respondent's social environment, such as whether they were satisfied with the amount of control they had over their own life, and whether their area was classified as deprived, were much less strongly related to drinking behaviour than were social class, income and tenure.

- Significant factors in predicting the odds of drinking more than 21 units per week for men and 14 units for women were: sex, age, income, community activity, size of personal support group and household type.

Attitudes towards drinking

- Those most likely to agree that 'drinking was an important part of having a good social life' and that 'it's OK to get drunk from time to time' were men, younger people, and those who drank more than 21 units per week (men) and 14 units per week (women).

- Those most likely to agree that they felt 'comfortable drinking soft drinks when their friends were drinking alcohol' were women, older people, and those who were non- or occasional drinkers.

6 Physical activity (Chapter 6)

Participation in physical activity

- In 1998, 27% of men and 35% of women aged 16 and over were classified as sedentary – they participated less than once a week in 30 minutes or more of at least moderate-intensity activity.

- Overall, a similar proportion took part in at least moderate-intensity activity on five or more days a week, but the proportions of men and women doing so were almost reversed - 36% of men and 24% of women had done so.

- Only 17% of men and 6% of women took part in vigorous physical activity lasting 20 minutes or more at least three times a week.

Demographic and socio-economic factors

- The characteristic most closely associated with the likelihood of being physically active was the respondent's age, and in all age-groups, women were less likely to be physically active than were men. Thus, for example, 64% of men and 72% of women aged 75 and over were classed as sedentary, compared with 15% of men and 34% of women aged 16–24.

- Having taken account of age, the likelihood of participating in physical activity to either a moderate or a vigorous level was relatively greater among those with higher household incomes, those with educational qualifications, and with indicators of relative affluence, such as being in employment, and not living in local authority housing.

- An exception to this pattern was that, the likelihood of participating in physical activity to one of the recommended levels was *not* higher among those in non-manual social classes: on the whole, the reverse was true, probably because physical activity at work is taken into account. Thus, for example, 44% of men in Social Classes IV/V had participated in at least moderate-intensity activity lasting at least 30 minutes on five or more days a week, compared with 27% of men in Social Classes I/II.

Social environment factors

- In addition, after taking age into account, the likelihood of being classified as sedentary was relatively low for men with a personal support group of 9 or more people, and for lone mothers. It was relatively greater, on the other hand, for those not involved in community activities, for men with a low neighbourhood social capital score, and men living in more deprived areas.

Factors with independent effects on physical activity

- Logistic regression analysis was used to look at the relative importance of the different characteristics. It showed that levels of physical activity were much more strongly related to the demographic and socio-economic variables, than to people's social environment as measured by the survey. Only involvement in community activities was independently related to participation in moderate-intensity physical activity.

- The variables with significant independent effects on the likelihood of being sedentary were age (by far the strongest effect), social class, household income, economic activity, qualification level, household type and involvement in community activities. Two additional variables – sex and marital status – were also associated with the measures of participation to the recommended levels.

Physical activity – attitudes and intentions

- Respondents were asked whether they thought that they were getting enough exercise to keep fit, and whether they would like to take more exercise. On the whole, older people and those who were more physically active were more likely than others to think that they were getting enough exercise. However, as many as two fifths of those classified as sedentary thought that they were getting enough exercise.

- Just over two thirds of both men and women said that they would like to take more exercise. The proportions saying this were highest among men and women under age 55.

- Overall, 28% of respondents said that they intended to start taking more exercise in the next month, and a further 21% that they intended to do so within six months.

Diet (Chapter 7)

Diet quality, and knowledge of a healthy diet

- In 1998, 18% of adults had a 'less healthy diet', and 15% had a 'more healthy diet', based on the survey diet score. Overall, 15% mentioned at least three of the four main components of a healthy diet.

- Among men, 21% reported a 'less healthy diet', compared with 16% of women. Similarly, only 12% of men had a 'more healthy diet', compared with 17% of women. In every sub-group investigated, men were more likely than women to have a 'less healthy diet'.

- Lower proportions of men than women usually ate high-fibre breads (36%, compared with 48%), and fruit or vegetables daily (59% compared with 74%).

- The levels of knowledge about diet differed between the sexes for only one aspect. Men were less likely than women to mention the need to 'eat lots of fruit, vegetables or salad', (62%, compared with 74%). Hence, 14% of men mentioned at least three out of four components of a healthy diet, compared with 16% of women.

- Age was the characteristic most closely associated with diet quality. Those in the younger and older age-groups were more likely than those in the middle age-groups to have a 'less healthy diet'. For example, among those aged 16–24, nearly a third of the men and nearly a quarter of the women, had a 'less healthy diet'. Diet quality improved with increasing age until the 55–64 age-group, but declined in the two oldest age-groups.

- People's knowledge about diet also varied with age, though it was the oldest age-group, rather than youngest, with the lowest levels

Demographic and socio-economic factors

- Having taken age into account, diet quality varied in relation to a wide range of other demographic and socio-economic variables. It decreased with decreasing levels of household income, qualifications, and social class. In addition, it was relatively lower among the widowed divorced and separated, the unemployed, and those in local authority housing. It was also relatively lower among men in privately rented accommodation, among lone mothers and, to a lesser extent, among women who were economically inactive and women living alone.

- Differences in levels of knowledge about diet followed a broadly similar pattern, with a few exceptions. For example, they were not any lower among lone mothers than among women in other household types.

Social environment factors

- Diet quality and knowledge varied only slightly with aspects of people's social environment. They were relatively lower among those with a small personal support group, those not involved in community activities, those who felt that they lacked influence over neighbourhood decisions, those with a low neighbourhood social capital score and those living in more deprived areas.

Factors with independent effects on the dietary indicators

- Logistic regression analysis was used to look at the relative importance of the different factors. Four of the variables – sex, age, income and qualification level - had independent effects on all three of the diet measures. Age had the strongest effects. Most other factors had effects on just one of the diet measures. Two additional variables – tenure and neighbourhood social capital score – were independently associated with having a 'less healthy diet', while community involvement and control over decisions affecting life were associated with having a 'more healthy diet'.

- The social environment variables were slightly more likely to have significant independent effects on knowledge about diet than on diet quality. Three of them – size of personal support group, involvement in community activity and area deprivation category – had independent effects on this measure.

Conclusion (Chapter 8)

Characteristics with independent effects – for all reported health measures

A concluding chapter draws together the results of the preceding five chapters to look at the overall contribution made by different characteristics of individuals and their social environments to variation in health and health behaviours. It also gives a view, with some provisos, on those groups which appear to have 'less healthy' lifestyles, as defined by the survey.

Age was the only characteristic which, after controlling for all the others, had an independent effect on all of the health measures. Of the other demographic variables, household type was independently associated with more of the health measures than were sex or marital status, though sex was associated with at least one of the measures in each of the five broad areas of health.

Of the five variables which describe the socio-economic status of respondents, household income, highest qualification level and tenure had independent effects on more of the health measures than did social class and economic activity. Economic activity had independent (but strong) effects in just two areas –self-reported health and physical activity.

The social environment variables had fewer independent effects on the health measures than the demographic and socio-economic variables. As a group, they were more likely to be independently associated with stress levels and with smoking status, than with the other aspects of health and health behaviour. They featured least in relation to the measures of physical activity and diet quality

The size of the respondent's personal support group and their involvement in community activities were the most likely of these factors to be associated with the health measures. Satisfaction with control over life decisions and 'neighbourhood social capital score' (summarising views and feelings about the neighbourhood) were also important variables.

Subgroups with the highest odds of reporting particular health measures

One of the main aims of HEMS 1998 has been to explore how personal, social and neighbourhood characteristics affect health status and behaviour. The ability to be able to identify particular subgroups who consistently displayed 'less healthy' lifestyles would be useful, but the picture is not altogether clear.

Some characteristics, such age, income and household type are strongly related to health, but the subgroups within these who were most likely to have the less healthy attributes differed for the different aspects of health. However, for other characteristics, particular subgroups did appear consistently across the health measures to be those with the less healthy attributes. These include respondents with no educational qualifications, those with no personal support group, those not involved in community activities, those lacking control over decisions affecting their lives, those with low 'neighbourhood social capital', and to some extent, those in local authority housing.

Notes and references

1   Department of Health. *The Health of the Nation: a strategy for health in England.* HMSO (London 1992)

2   Department of Health. *Saving Lives: Our Healthier Nation.* TSO (London 1999)

Part A – Chapters 1 – 8

1 Aims and background of the survey

1.1 Background to the survey

This 1998 Health Education Monitoring Survey (HEMS) is the third in a series of studies designed to measure a range of health promotion indicators relevant to adults living in private households in England. This survey and previous ones in 1995 and 1996 have been designed by the Health Education Authority (HEA) in collaboration with the Social Survey Division (SSD) of the Office for National Statistics (ONS), who were commissioned by the HEA to carry out all these studies.

To date the HEMS has made an important contribution to the monitoring of factors associated with health and health-related behaviours amongst adults aged 16–74 at a national level. It was initially developed within the Government's public health strategy, the Health of the Nation (HON)[1]. Whilst HON acknowledged the impact of community level factors on the achievement of its health targets, health promotion's contribution was seen very much within the context of the knowledge, attitude and behaviour (KAB) paradigm[2]. Consequently the focus for the 1995 and 1996 surveys was the collection of information to monitor the health-related knowledge, attitudes and behaviours of adults in England. The 1995 and 1996 surveys identified over 30 health promotion indicators which could be used for this purpose[3].

The new government White Paper *Saving Lives: Our Healthier Nation*[4] gives greater recognition to the wider determinants of health. It legitimises the need to look not only at individual behaviour but also at the influences of the social environment and of the wider community on health. The main change in emphasis in the new health strategy is reflected in its two key aims:

- To improve the health of the population as a whole by increasing the length of peoples lives and the number of years people spend free from illness.
- To improve the health of the worst off in society and to narrow the health gap.

Publication of the report of the recent inquiry into inequalities, led by Sir Donald Acheson, has added to the debate on the health inequalities and social inequalities in our society. It had four main recommendations[5]:

- That all policies likely to have a direct or indirect effect on health should be evaluated in terms of their impact on health inequalities and should be formulated in such a way as to reduce such inequalities.
- Mechanisms be established to monitor inequalities in health and evaluate the effectiveness of measures taken to reduce them.
- There needs to be an improvement in the capacity to monitor inequalities in health and their determinants at a national and local level.
- High priority be given to policies aimed at improving health and reducing health inequalities in women of child-bearing age, expectant mothers and young children.

1.2 HEMS and the new public health agenda

Over the last few years there has been growing recognition that individually-focussed behavioural interventions have a relatively small impact on behaviour change and health improvement. The individuals influenced by these interventions have tended to be the better off, better motivated and better educated. This has highlighted the need for those working in health promotion to develop a better understanding of the factors that are beyond the control of individual influence on behaviours or health experience.

Substantial evidence now exists about the effect of social and environmental factors on health. Wealth, occupation, social support, housing and education have all been shown to be related to wide differences in life expectancy, infant mortality and psychosocial well-being, as well as preventative health behaviour. Such health inequalities are also associated with the quality and level of the infrastructure in place within the neighbourhoods in which people live. Studies have shown the adverse effects that poverty and deprivation can have on health and health behaviour[6].

The relative influence of structural factors on health and lifestyle has been the subject of extensive debate in Britain[7,8]. Wilkinson demonstrated the adverse effects on health and well-being of relative inequalities in income within societies and pointed to the benefits of equitable societies with strong social support and cohesion. There is substantial evidence that low social class and poor living conditions adversely influence health and health behaviour. However, it is also known that some poorer communities have fewer health problems than others and one concept put forward to explain this is that of social capital.

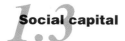

1.3 Social capital

Recent research suggests that social approaches have considerable potential for the improvement of public health but the evidence base is somewhat limited[6]. Researchers have argued that social support and civic engagement build trust in neighbourhoods and in society at large, producing a resource called social capital. This concept of social capital has recently been put forward as a resource for the promotion of health.

Social capital serves as one coherent construct, which will allow us to progress the debate and discussion about social approaches to public health and health promotion. As a construct that emerged from the political science literature, yet which has been applied to the conceptualisation of health related issues and behaviours,[9,10,11] social capital crosses disciplinary boundaries. However, it may underpin the development of new theoretical frameworks for understanding health and health behaviour in individuals and societies as well as the broader social determinants of health.

Although not yet a theory with explanatory power, social capital allows us to examine the processes whereby formal and informal social connections operating through a range of different types of networks can act as a buffer against the worst effects of deprivation. It reinforces partnership and participatory approaches to sustainable development and challenges us to produce new social indicators to capture the benefits of initiatives designed to promote health.

Social capital is conceptualised as a 'community resource' that is created from everyday social interactions and social networks. It is founded on the principles of trust, reciprocity and community participation for mutual benefit[9,12]. Social capital is a multidimensional concept. It may include the collective economic and cultural resources available to a community as well as the level of trust and social support networks[9]. Putnam describes social capital as:

> 'the features of social life - networks, norms and trust - that enables participants to act together more effectively to pursue shared objectives. To the extent that the norms, networks and trust link substantial sectors of the community and span underlying social cleavages - to the extent that social capital is of a bridging sort - then the enhanced co-operation is likely to serve broader interests and to be widely welcomed'[13].

Kawachi et al[14] and Wilkinson suggest that the level of social capital in a community is likely to effect health. Wilkinson [8] demonstrated the adverse effects on health and well-being of relative inequalities in income within societies and pointed to the benefits of equitable societies with strong social support and cohesion.

This work has been influential in the design of the 1998 HEMS study. Further details of the HEA's programme of work on social capital can be found in Appendix B.

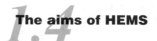

1.4 The aims of HEMS

The theoretical framework for the 1995 and 1996 HEMS was informed by two psychological models of behaviour change. The two models used were the Theory of Planned Behaviour and the Stages of Change Model[15]. The surveys included questions that would make it possible to measure respondents' movement through the different stages of change. These models represent complementary ways to understand health behaviour and its change. The Theory of Planned Behaviour attempts to delineate the factors which influence behaviour, whilst the Stages of Change Model provides an overview of the process of behaviour change itself.

Given the greater recognition now placed on the wider determinants of health, the limitations of these models for predicting behaviour change have been highlighted. However in the absence of any robust alternative models, the 1998 HEMS survey continued to use them as a framework for questionnaire construction but also included measures of social inequality, social support and social capital.

To date much less is known about the contribution of these wider concepts to the health inequalities debate. Therefore, the major challenge for health promotion is how to explain the contribution and influence of these broader determinants of health. The question for health promoters is - how do we promote the health of those most disadvantaged in society, who are also the least responsive to the psychological models of behaviour change? The 1998 survey aimed to contribute to the evidence base in this area.

The 1998 HEMS questionnaire was therefore developed to continue to monitor health and health-related behaviours and additionally to understand the social environment within which they are expressed. This survey offers the opportunity to develop a new set of indicators for health promotion at a national level. The survey report presents information resulting from a series of more detailed analyses than in previous years to understand health and health-related behaviours in the context of other factors. These factors include the respondents' living conditions, their personal circumstances and their social environment.

1.5 The design of the 1998 survey

For the 1998 survey, a probability sample of addresses was selected from the Postcode Address file (PAF). Interviewers contacted each address and identified all residents aged 16 or over. Adults in the household aged 16 and over were listed in order of age, eldest first, and one adult in the household was randomly selected to be interviewed. (In previous HEMS there was an upper age limit of 74 years, so to ensure comparability, trend tables in this report exclude the 1998 respondents aged 75 and over). Full details of the sample and weighting are given in Appendix A.

Interviews were carried out with 5816 adults aged 16 and over in the period May-July 1998. They lasted approximately one hour and in order to collect trend data the questionnaire was similar to that used in 1995 and 1996. However, extra questions were added to explore issues of social capital and social support, as discussed in more detail in Chapter 2. In addition, older respondents were asked questions relating to their specific health needs. The full 1998 questionnaire can be found at Appendix D.

The 1998 questionnaire also included a self-completion module on sexual health for respondents aged 16–54. The interviews were carried out using laptop computers, and for the self-completion module, the interviewers handed the computers to respondents, who keyed in the answers themselves. This included new sexual health questions which have also been asked in a number of European countries as part of a European Commission funded research project.

Notes and references

1. Department of Health. *The Health of the Nation: a strategy for health in England.* HMSO (London: 1992).

2. Buck D, Godfrey C and Morgan A. The contribution of health promotion to meeting health targets: questions of measurement, attribution and responsibility. *Health Promotion International* 12 (1997), 3, 239–250.

3. Morgan A and Ford K. *A series of health promotion monitoring frameworks for use in demonstrating contributions to Health of the Nation targets.* Draft 3 HEA. Unpublished (London: 1998).

4. Department of Health. *Saving Lives: Our Healthier Nation.* TSO (London: 1999).

5. Acheson D *et al*. *Independent Inquiry into Inequalities in Health – Report.* TSO (London: 1998).

6. Gillies P. Effectiveness of alliances and partnerships for health promotion. *Health Promotion International* (1998) vol 13. no 2.

7. Townsend P, Phillimore P and Beattie A. *Health and Deprivation: inequality and the North.* Croom Helm Ltd (London: 1988).

8. Wilkinson RG. *Unhealthy societies: the afflictions of inequalities.* Routledge (London: 1996).

9. Putnam RD. The prosperous community: social capital and public life. *The American Prospect* 13 (Spring 1993), 1–8.

10. Moser C. *Confronting crisis: Comparative Study of Household Responses in Poverty and Vulnerability in Four Poor Urban Communities.* Environmentally Sustainable Investment Studies Monograms Series 3. World Bank (Washington DC: 1996).

11. Higgins D, Gillies PA *et al*. Social capital among community volunteers. The relationship to community-level HIV prevention programmes, Abstract No. WeD3786 *Abstracts of the XI International Conference on AIDS*, 2, 189 July. (Vancouver: 1996).

12. Bullen P and Onyx J. *Measuring social capital in five communities. NSW: an Analysis* CACOM Working Paper Series no.41 (1998).

13. Putnam RD. *Making Democracy Work. Civic Traditions in Modern Italy.* Princeton University Press (New Jersey: 1995).

14. Kawachi I *et al*. Social Capital, Income and Inequality. *American Journal of Public Health* 87 (1997), 1491-98.

15. See Hansbro J, Bridgwood A, with Morgan A and Hickman M. *Health in England 1996: what people know, what people think, what people do.* HMSO (London: 1997).

2 The 1998 HEMS report plan

The aim of this report, as described in Chapter 1, is to explore how people's health and health behaviours relate to their demographic and socio-economic characteristics and to their social environment. In doing so, we introduce a new set of social indicators to contribute to the debate on the links between social inequalities and health.

However, we recognise the limitations of a quantitative health and lifestyle survey to investigate these links for the following reasons:

- The limitations in the ability of cross-sectional surveys to prove causal links are well known.

- The questions that were used in the survey to measure the concepts relating to people's social environment are as yet imperfect and have been little tested. More work needs to be done at a qualitative level to refine the measures. (See also Appendix B).

- A quantitative survey such as HEMS has only a limited space for asking questions of this type if it is to continue with its primary function - to monitor health behaviours.

2.1 Outline of analysis used in each chapter

For each chapter a number of health measures are analysed in relation to two groups of analysis variables which describe the context within which health is experienced. The first group consists of a range of demographic and socio-economic variables, similar to those used in previous HEMS. The second group consists of a new classification of household type and a number of new indicators used to describe people's social environment (including variables of social support, social capital and area deprivation). These two groups of analysis variables are listed in Figure 2.1. The second group is described in detail in Section 2.4. **(Figure 2.1)**

There are four stages in each chapter.

- The first stage of each chapter describes the selected health measure, and explores the variation by sex and age. The 1998 results are also placed in the context of the previous HEMS reports of 1995 and 1996.

- In the second stage of analysis for each chapter, the selected health measures are analysed in relation to the two groups of analysis variables:

- The demographic and socio-economic variables, used in the analysis of previous HEMS surveys

- Household type and the new variables relating to the social environment

Because many of the analysis variables vary in relation to age, age-standardisation has been used in this second stage of analysis. Thus as well as showing the proportions of each subgroup reporting a health measure, age-standardised data are shown. The age-standardised figure is the percentage that would be 'expected' given the age composition of the particular subgroup, and this can be compared with the actual or 'observed' proportion. The method helps to investigate whether the analysis variable has an effect on a health measure, which is independent of age.

A detailed explanation of age-standardisation is given in Appendix C.

- In the third stage of analysis, logistic regression models are used to assess the independent effects of all the explanatory variables on the selected health measure. Logistic regression indicates whether each analysis variable makes a significant contribution to explaining variation in the health measures, having held constant all the other analysis variables under consideration.

A detailed explanation of logistic regression is given in Appendix C.

- As a final stage in the analysis, for the health measures in Chapters 4, 5 and 6, the relationships between the health measures and people's attitudes and knowledge are briefly described.

A concluding chapter draws together the results of Chapters 3 to 7. In addition to the tables within the chapters, supplementary tables relating to each health topic are included in Part B of the report. These include trend data, and data which, while key to the HEMS series of surveys, are outside the main focus of the chapters.

2.2 Health measures investigated in this report

The following health measures are examined:

Self-reported health status (Chapter 3)
The proportions of adults who reported having:

- 'less than good' health,
- having a limiting long-standing illness,
- having a large amount of stress.

Figure 2.1   The analysis variables used in HEMS 1998 report

Group 1 - Demographic and socio-economic variables (used in previous HEMS reports)	Group 2 - Household type and social environment variables (new variables for HEMS 1998 report)

Sex
Men
Women

Age
16-24
25-34
35-44
45-54
55-64
65-74
75 and over

Marital status
Single
Married/cohabitating
Widowed, divorced, separated

Social class (based on own current or last job)
I & II
III (Non-manual)
III (Manual)
IV & V

Gross household income (annual)
£20,000 or more
£10,000 - £19,999
£5,000 - £9,999
Under £5,000

Economic activity
Employed
Unemployed
Economically inactive

Highest qualification level
'A' Level or above
GCSE A-G or below
No qualifications

Housing tenure
Owner-occupier
Rents from local authority
Rents privately

Household type
One person household
Living with others (no dependent children)
Living with others (with dependent children)
Lone adult (with dependent children)

Personal support group
9 or more people
4-8 people
1-3 people
No support

Community activity
Some community activity
No community activity

Whether agrees that 'I am satisfied with the amount of control I have over decisions that affect my life'
Agree
Neither agree nor disagree
Disagree

Whether agrees that 'I can influence decisions that affect my neighbourhood'
Agree
Neither agree nor disagree
Disagree

Neighbourhood social capital score
Very high
High
Medium
Low

Area deprivation category
1 More affluent
2
3
4
5 More deprived

Smoking (Chapter 4)
The proportions of adults who were:

- current cigarette smokers,
- ex-cigarette smokers, or
- who have never regularly smoked.

Drinking (Chapter 5)
The proportions of adults whose usual weekly consumption of alcohol (in units) was:

- Under one unit, or abstainer (i.e non-or occasional drinkers),
- 1–21 units for men, and 1–14 units for women,
- 22–35 units for men, and 15–25 units for women,
- 36–50 units for men, and 26–35 units for women,
- 51 or more units for men, and 36 or more units for women.

Physical activity (Chapter 6)
The proportions of adults classified as having:

- a 'sedentary' level of activity,
- a 'moderate' level of activity,
- a 'vigorous' level of activity.

Diet (Chapter 7)
The proportions of adults classified as having:

- a 'less healthy' diet, or
- a 'more healthy' diet (based on a survey diet score),
- knowledge of what constitutes a healthy diet.

2.3 Demographic and socio-economic variables used in this report

As in previous HEMS health measures will be analysed in relation to the following variables:

- Sex and age
- Marital status
- Social class
- Gross household income
- Economic activity
- Highest qualification level
- Housing tenure

Table 2.1 shows the distribution of these variables by sex and age. **(Table 2.1)**

2.4 Household type and social environment variables used in this report

Questions, which looked at aspects of the social environment, have been used on a previous HEA Health and Lifestyle Survey[1]. These were used in HEMS for the first time in 1998. Questions were developed in particular to measure personal support and the various constructs of social capital. Measures of area deprivation were also included in HEMS for the first time. Household type has always been collected on the HEMS but was used as an analysis variable for the first time in 1998. Therefore, whilst not strictly a new variable it will be discussed with the other new variables in this report. These new variables are discussed in more detail below, and the variations by sex and age, shown in Table 2.2, are also described.

2.4.1 Household type

This variable was divided into four categories; living in a one-person household, living with other adults (with no dependent children), living with other adults (and dependent children) and a lone adult with dependent children (termed 'lone parent'). Among men and women, 11% of men and 17% of women lived in a one-person household. The likelihood of living in a one-person household increased with age, from 2% of men and 4% of women aged 16–24, rising to 28% of men and 58% of women aged 75 and over. There was very little difference by sex in the proportions living in households with other adults, with or without children. However, the lone parents were almost exclusively women: 5% of all women were in this group. As would be expected, these women were concentrated into the younger age-groups: 6% were aged 16–24, 12% were aged 25–34 and 8% were aged 35–44. Among men, 1% of those aged 35–44 lived alone with dependent children. **(Table 2.2)**

2.4.2 Personal support group

Respondents were asked 'If you had a personal crisis, how many people do you feel you could turn to for help and comfort'. Answers were recorded verbatim and then grouped into categories ranging from 'none' to 'nine or more'.

There was very little difference by age or sex in the levels of support respondents felt they could call on. Only 2% of men and 1% of women felt that there was no-one that they could turn to for help and comfort in a crisis. **(Table 2.2)**

2.4.3 Constructs of social capital

Community involvement

Space constraints meant that it was not possible to measure the construct of civic engagement in detail. We therefore decided to look at one part of it (involvement in community activity). Respondents were asked whether they had done any of the following three activities in the past two weeks:

- Attended an adult education or night class course
- Participated in a voluntary group or local community group
- Participated in community or religious activities

The community activity variable identified two groups of respondents: those who had taken part in at least one of these activities and those who had been involved in no community activity.

In all age-groups women were more likely than men to have been involved in some community activity. For example, 23% of men and 33% of women overall were involved in some community activity. The proportion who were active increased with age for women up to ages 65–74, but not for men: 25% of women aged 16–24 had some involvement, rising to 39% of those aged 65–74. Even women aged 75 and over had more community involvement (31% were involved) than men in any age-group. **(Table 2.2)**

Satisfaction with decisions affecting life, and influence in neighbourhood decisions

Respondents were asked how much they agreed with the statements:

- 'I am satisfied with the amount of control I have over decisions that affect my life.'
- 'I can influence decisions that affect my neighbourhood.'

Overall, 75% of men and 80% of women agreed with first statement, those in the youngest and oldest age-groups being the most likely to agree. For example, 83% of men and women aged 16-24 agreed with the statement, compared with 72% of men and 77% of women aged 35-44. Women aged 55 and over were significantly more likely to agree with the statement than men in similar age-groups.

When asked about their influence over decisions that affected their neighbourhood, both men and women were more likely to disagree than to agree and this applied to all age-groups. Overall, 51% of men and 49% of women felt that they could not influence the decisions that affected their neighbourhood, whereas 22% and 24%, respectively, felt that they could. The remainder were undecided. **(Table 2.2)**

Neighbourhood social capital

The HEMS questionnaire asked respondents about six aspects of neighbourhood social capital. Respondents were asked to say 'Yes' or 'No' to each of the following:

Would you say this neighbourhood …
- … is a place you enjoy living in?
- … is a place where you personally feel safe?
- … is a place where the neighbours look after each other?
- … has good facilities for young children?
- … has good local transport?
- … has good leisure facilities for people like yourself?

From answers to these six questions a neighbourhood social capital score was calculated (see Appendix C for details). It is those with a low score who are of particular interest to this study. Overall 27% of men and women had a low neighbourhood social capital score and it was those in the youngest age-group who were most likely to have a low neighbourhood social capital score. For example, 33% of men and 38% of women aged 16–24 had a low neighbourhood social capital score, compared with 21% of men and 24% of women aged 65–74. **(Table 2.2)**

2.4.4 Area deprivation measures

For the first time in 1998, the HEMS analysis has investigated two systems of classifying the areas in which respondents lived. The aim in doing so was twofold – to see the extent to which factors such as these appear to be related to the likelihood of an individual having health problems, and if they were, to assess their importance relative to the characteristics of the individuals themselves.

Preliminary analysis on HEMS used two measures of area characteristics – the HEMS index of area deprivation and the ACORN index.

The HEMS area deprivation score was based on the work of Carstairs[2]. It was created using 1991 Census small area statistics for England. Like the Carstairs index, it was derived from measures of overcrowding, male unemployment, social class and car ownership.

The calculation of the HEMS deprivation score differs from the Carstairs index in two respects. First, HEMS used 1991 Census small area statistics for postcode sectors whereas the Carstairs index for England and Wales is based on 1981 ward-level data. Second, the HEMS score does not include an adjustment to the overcrowding measure, which was needed by Carstairs to compare England and Wales with Scotland.

The HEMS deprivation index is divided into five categories, with '1' being the most affluent and '5' the least affluent. On this index, 20% of men and 19% of women lived in the most affluent areas and 14% of men and 15% of women lived in the least affluent areas. There were no large variations by age. A full discussion of the derivation of the HEMS index is in Appendix C. **(Table 2.3)**

The ACORN classificatory system was also investigated for the HEMS study[3]. ACORN (A Classification of Residential Neighbourhoods) is based on Census data at Enumeration District (ED) level. Using links to the postcodes of the addresses sampled in the survey, respondents are classified according to the ACORN categorisation developed by CACI Limited. ACORN was derived using 79 variables from the 1991 Census, including (among others) age, marital status, ethnic group, long-term illness, household size, household tenure, unemployment, occupation and car ownership.

ACORN can be collapsed into six categories describing areas as: thriving, expanding, rising, settling, aspiring and striving. Overall, 29% of men and 28% of women lived in thriving areas, compared with 18% of men and women who lived in striving areas. **(Table 2.3)**

This initial analysis found that the HEMS deprivation index had a greater descriptive power for these data than the ACORN index. The analysis using the ACORN system is not therefore presented in this report.

Notes and references

1. Health Education Authority. *Health and Lifestyles: A Survey of the UK Population, Part 1*. Health Education Authority (London: 1995).

2. Carstairs V. and Morris R. *Deprivation and health in Scotland*. Aberdeen University Press (1991).

3. *ACORN User Guide*. CACI Limited: (London: 1993).

Table 2.1 Demographic and socio-economic characteristics by age and sex
Adults aged 16 and over

Age	16-24	25-34	35-44	45-54	55-64	65-74	75 and over	Total
Characteristics	%	%	%	%	%	%	%	%
Marital status								
Men								
Single	88	26	11	6	6	5	3	23
Married or cohabiting	12	72	82	86	81	80	68	69
Widowed, divorced, separated	0	3	7	8	12	15	30	8
Women								
Single	81	23	7	4	3	5	6	19
Married or cohabiting	18	70	79	82	74	56	29	61
Widowed, divorced, separated	1	7	14	13	23	39	65	20
Social class*								
Men								
I & II	13	40	44	45	39	37	34	38
III (Non-manual)	23	13	12	10	7	9	11	12
III (Manual)	26	32	30	31	33	39	30	31
IV & V	38	15	14	13	21	15	25	19
Women								
I & II	13	34	32	30	27	19	19	26
III (Non-manual)	45	35	34	38	30	35	33	36
III (Manual)	11	8	6	7	10	11	11	9
IV & V	31	22	29	25	33	35	36	29
Household income								
Men								
£20,000 or more	58	69	66	61	40	18	10	53
£10,000 - £19,999	25	23	24	28	36	34	28	28
£5,000 - £9,999	14	5	7	7	18	42	48	15
Under £5,000	3	2	2	5	7	6	14	4
Women								
£20,000 or more	46	53	55	58	33	7	7	41
£10,000 - £19,999	27	27	25	24	34	24	15	26
£5,000 - £9,999	12	12	14	13	24	48	45	21
Under £5,000	16	9	6	5	10	20	33	12
Economic activity								
Men								
Employed	67	93	90	86	59	10	-	69
Unemployed	8	3	4	4	2	-	-	4
Economically inactive	25	4	6	10	39	90	100	28
Women								
Employed	70	78	81	82	71	-	-	60
Unemployed	5	4	3	3	1	-	-	3
Economically inactive	25	18	16	16	28	100	100	37

Table 2.1 - *continued*
Adults aged 16 and over

Age	16-24	25-34	35-44	45-54	55-64	65-74	75 and over	Total
Characteristics	%	%	%	%	%	%	%	%
Highest qualification level								
Men								
'A'Level or above	36	50	56	48	34	23	18	42
GCSE A-G or below	50	41	31	34	34	30	32	37
No qualifications	14	8	13	18	32	47	49	21
Women								
'A'Level or above	30	42	36	28	23	14	12	28
GCSE A-G or below	56	48	48	43	35	30	23	42
No qualifications	14	10	16	29	43	56	66	30
Housing tenure								
Men								
Owner-occupier	67	71	81	85	78	78	67	76
Rents from local authority	15	12	11	7	14	16	23	13
Rents privately	18	17	8	8	8	6	10	11
Women								
Owner-occupier	63	67	75	81	78	68	62	71
Rents from local authority	16	17	13	12	16	21	24	16
Rents privately	21	16	12	7	6	11	14	13
Men								
Base = 100%†	*193*	*420*	*448*	*412*	*375*	*333*	*233*	*2414*
Women								
Base = 100%†	*233*	*607*	*551*	*428*	*360*	*402*	*412*	*2993*

* Members of the armed forces, persons in inadequately described occupations and persons who had never worked are not shown as separate categories but are included in the figures for all persons.

† Bases are taken from gross household income - bases may vary slightly for other items.

Table 2.2 Household type and the characteristics of the respondents' social environment by age and sex
Adults aged 16 and over

Age	16-24	25-34	35-44	45-54	55-64	65-74	75 and over	Total
Characteristics	%	%	%	%	%	%	%	%
Household type								
Men								
One person household	2	11	10	9	12	17	28	11
Living with others (no dependent children)	72	44	26	62	82	83	72	58
Living with others (with dependent children)	25	44	62	29	6	1	-	30
Lone adult (with dependent children)	0	0	1	0	0	-	-	0
Women								
One person household	4	7	4	8	18	38	58	17
Living with others (no dependent children)	56	28	24	71	79	62	41	50
Living with others (with dependent children)	34	52	63	19	2	-	1	29
Lone adult (with dependent children)	6	12	8	1	0	0	-	5
Personal support group								
Men								
9 or more people	29	24	22	22	26	26	17	24
4-8 people	43	46	44	45	43	38	49	44
1-3 people	28	28	32	31	28	35	32	30
No support	1	2	2	2	3	1	2	2
Women								
9 or more people	19	19	23	26	28	26	14	22
4-8 people	54	47	47	49	45	46	42	47
1-3 people	27	34	29	24	26	28	43	30
No support	0	0	1	1	2	1	1	1
Community activity								
Men								
Some community activity	22	18	25	24	23	24	24	23
No community activity	78	82	75	76	77	76	76	77
Women								
Some community activity	25	29	38	32	33	39	31	33
No community activity	75	71	62	68	67	61	69	67
Whether agrees is satisfied with the amount of control over decisions that affect own life								
Men								
Agree	83	74	72	71	70	79	82	75
Neither agree nor disagree	6	10	12	11	10	8	9	10
Disagree	11	16	16	18	20	14	8	16
Women								
Agree	83	77	77	76	81	87	82	80
Neither agree nor disagree	8	10	12	8	8	6	10	9
Disagree	9	13	12	16	11	7	8	11

Table 2.2 - *continued*
Adults aged 16 and over

Age	16-24	25-34	35-44	45-54	55-64	65-74	75 and over	Total
Characteristics	%	%	%	%	%	%	%	%
Whether agrees can influence decisions that affect own neighbourhood								
Men								
Agree	14	20	24	25	22	26	29	22
Neither agree nor disagree	34	32	30	27	21	17	21	27
Disagree	52	49	46	49	57	57	50	51
Women								
Agree	16	24	25	31	26	26	22	24
Neither agree nor disagree	30	30	30	24	22	22	21	26
Disagree	54	47	45	45	52	52	58	49
Neighbourhood social capital score								
Men								
Very High	12	18	20	14	20	19	20	17
High	24	30	27	31	25	35	31	29
Medium	31	26	28	30	24	25	28	28
Low	33	26	26	25	31	21	21	27
Women								
Very High	9	20	21	16	19	20	19	18
High	20	27	30	29	28	27	31	28
Medium	33	29	24	25	28	29	26	28
Low	38	24	25	30	25	24	24	27
Men								
*Base = 100%**	232	429	463	430	384	348	246	2532
Women								
*Base = 100%**	270	628	567	457	403	444	444	3213

* Bases are taken from whether agrees with the statement 'I can influence decisions that affect my neighbourhood' - bases may vary slightly for other items.

Table 2.3 HEMS area deprivation categories, and ACORN categories by age and sex
Adults aged 16 and over

Age	16-24	25-34	35-44	45-54	55-64	65-74	75 and over	Total
Characteristics	%	%	%	%	%	%	%	%
HEMS area deprivation categories								
Men								
1 More affluent	25	15	20	21	24	20	24	20
2	15	18	19	20	17	19	15	18
3	22	28	26	24	27	26	27	26
4	21	26	21	20	16	24	22	22
5 More deprived	17	13	14	14	16	12	12	14
Women								
1 More affluent	13	12	18	24	25	23	20	19
2	19	20	23	22	17	17	17	20
3	25	24	21	28	23	29	26	25
4	27	23	21	17	20	19	22	21
5 More deprived	15	21	16	9	14	12	14	15
ACORN categories								
Men								
A - Thriving	31	24	25	30	36	31	33	29
B - Expanding	9	12	16	9	8	8	4	10
C - Rising	4	9	8	7	6	7	4	7
D - Settling	26	26	22	29	21	25	27	25
E - Aspiring	12	9	13	10	12	12	12	11
F - Striving	18	20	17	16	16	18	19	18
Women								
A - Thriving	23	18	28	36	34	30	33	28
B - Expanding	12	14	14	14	7	8	3	11
C - Rising	9	8	7	5	3	4	7	6
D - Settling	23	24	24	22	28	27	26	25
E - Aspiring	13	13	11	9	11	12	10	11
F - Striving	20	22	17	15	17	19	21	18
Men								
*Base = 100%**	233	433	468	433	391	350	254	2562
Women								
*Base = 100%**	272	631	572	464	406	447	462	3254

* Bases are taken from the HEMS area deprivation variable - bases may vary slightly for other items.

3 Self-reported health status

Summary of main findings

General health and limiting long-standing illness

■ In 1998, 22% of men and 26% of women reported 'less than good' general health, and 20% of men and 24% of women reported having a limiting long-standing illness. (Sections 3.3.1 and 3.4.1).

■ As expected, the percentages reporting poorer health increased with age. For example, in the youngest age-group, 14% of men and 22% of women classified their general health as 'less than good', compared with 43% and 50% respectively among those aged 75 and over. Similarly, while only 7% of men and 13% of women aged 16–24 had a limiting long-standing illness, the corresponding percentages among those aged 75 and over were 42% and 54%. (Sections 3.3.1 and 3.4.1).

■ Only in the youngest age-group were women significantly more likely than men to report 'less than good' general health, and only in the oldest age-group were they more likely than men to report a limiting long-standing illness. (Section 3.3.1 and 3.4.1).

■ Having taken account of age, a number of other demographic and socio-economic characteristics were closely associated with poorer health. Both the proportions reporting 'less than good' health and the proportions having a limiting long-standing illness were relatively greater among men and women in the manual social classes, those with annual household incomes of less than £10,000, those who were economically inactive, those with no educational qualifications, those in local authority housing. Unemployed women and men who lived in one-person households were also more likely, than would be expected on the basis of age alone, to report 'less than good' general health, but not limiting long-standing illness. (Sections 3.3.1 and 3.4.1).

■ After taking age into account, factors related to the respondents' social environment were also associated with an increased likelihood of reporting poorer health. These factors included having lack of control over decisions affecting life, lack of influence over neighbourhood decisions, low neighbourhood social capital, living in more deprived areas, and, especially for men, having no personal support group (or a small group of 1–3 people). Those who had no involvement in community activities were also more likely to report 'less than good' general health (for both sexes) and limiting long-standing illness (for women only). (Sections 3.3.2 and 3.4.2).

continued

■ Logistic regression analysis was used to look at the relative importance of the different characteristics. It showed that, after taking into account all the other variables, sex did not have a significant independent effect on either of these health measures. The variables with independent effects on both measures were age, household income, economic activity, housing tenure, household type, satisfaction with control over decisions affecting life, and level of neighbourhood social capital. In addition, qualification level and size of personal support group had independent effects but only on reporting 'less than good' health. (Section 3.6).

Stress

■ In 1998, 24% of men and 29% of women reported having suffered a 'large amount' of stress in the past 12 months. (Section 3.5.1).

■ The proportion reporting a large amount of stress was highest in the age-groups between 25–54, peaking among those aged 35–44: about one third in these age-groups reported a large amount of stress, compared with about one fifth in the youngest and oldest groups. (Section 3.5.1).

■ Having taken account of age, higher stress levels were associated with a number of other demographic and socio-economic characteristics. Stress was relatively higher among men and women who were widowed, divorced or separated, those in Social Classes I / II, those with annual household incomes of less than £10,000, and those in local authority housing. Among men, it was also higher among the economically inactive and those living alone. Among women, it was higher among the unemployed and among lone mothers with dependent children. (Section 3.5.1).

■ After taking account of age, some of the factors related to the respondents' social environment were also strongly associated with increased stress levels. Levels were particularly high among the small numbers with no personal support group. They were also relatively higher among men and women with support groups of 1–3 people, those with lack of control over decisions affecting their lives, those with low neighbourhood social capital, and to a lesser extent those who lacked influence over neighbourhood decisions. (Section 3.5.2).

■ Logistic regression analysis was used to look at the relative importance of the different characteristics on reporting a large amount of stress. It showed that, after taking into account all the other variables, as many as eleven of the analysis variables had significant independent effects on stress levels. These were sex, age, marital status, social class, household income, housing tenure, household type, size of personal support group, control over decisions affecting own life, influence over neighbourhood decisions and neighbourhood social capital. (Section 3.6).

3.1 Introduction and background

This chapter will examine three measures of self-reported health status; perceptions of health in general, limiting long standing illness and levels of stress. Health is an abstract and multi-dimensional concept, which is difficult to define. Blaxter[1] argues that much of modern medicine is based on a biomedical model, which defines disease as 'deviations of measurable biological variables from the norm, or the presence of defined and categorised forms of pathology'. The World Health Organization (WHO) offers a much wider definition of health as a 'state of complete physical, social and mental well-being and not merely an absence of disease or infirmity.[2]

Neither objective nor subjective accounts of health are sufficient on their own. On the one hand, individuals may misinterpret, be misinformed or unaware of their biomedical condition; on the other, they have information about their symptoms and feeling states which only they can give. In a survey of this kind it is not possible to collect objective measures of health and it therefore relies on the subjective views of respondents about their own health. However, it has been shown that subjective assessments of health are related to objective measures such as standardised mortality ratios, doctor diagnoses and use of services.

All three measures used in this survey have been validated in a number of ways:

General health

Self-reported general health has been shown to be a strong predictor of mortality; it is also associated with the use of health services.[3] Several studies have confirmed the validity of this measure; there is a high level of agreement between studies based on self-reporting and on medical examinations[4].

Limiting long-standing illness

Associations between self-reported illness and standardised mortality ratios have also been demonstrated.[5] Commentators note that discrepancies do not necessarily indicate that data from self-reported sources are inaccurate. Informants may not have brought a condition to the attention of a doctor, medical records could be inaccurate[6], doctors may not have informed patients of their diagnosis, and lay descriptions may differ from those given by doctors[7].

Stress

Stress has been identified as a major contributory factor to both mental and physical health;[8] more specifically, several studies have shown that psychological factors are implicated in the development of cardiovascular disease.[9]

The structure of the chapter

This chapter will begin by describing prevalence levels in each of the three self-reported health measures used: 'less than good' general health, limiting long-standing illness and stress. For each of the three health measures under discussion it will investigate the effects on them of the respondent's age, sex, marital status, employment status, social class (derived from his or her current or most recent occupation), household income and tenure, and educational attainment measures. It will then describe the relationship between self-reported health and a range of variables new to HEMS 1998 which represent the social environment and household type. The variables, which are described in detail in Chapter 2, are as follows:

- Household type.
- Personal support group – that is, the number of people the respondent could call on at a time of serious personal crisis.
- Community activity – that is, participation in the last two weeks in adult education, voluntary or community groups or religious activities.
- Satisfaction with amount of control over decisions affecting own life.
- Perceived ability to influence decisions affecting the neighbourhood.
- Neighbourhood social capital score – derived from level of respondents' agreement with statements about their neighbourhood (see Appendix C).
- Area deprivation category – based on the HEMS area deprivation score for postcode sectors, which takes into account the 1991 Census rates of unemployment, car ownership, overcrowding and social class (see Appendix C).

Finally, the chapter will describe the results of logistic regressions, undertaken to investigate the independent effects of individual variables whilst keeping others constant.

Age-standardisation has also been carried out on the data. Thus, as well as the measured percentage for a particular sub-group, Tables 3.5 to 3.17 also show the percentage that would be 'expected', given the age composition of each subgroup. The ratio of these two percentages indicates whether the observed percentage is higher (if it is greater than 100) or lower (if it is less than 100) than would be expected on the basis of age alone. The tables also indicate if the ratio of observed to expected values is significantly different from 100. If it does differ significantly, this suggests that the observed variation is not explained by age alone. For further details on age-standardisation, see Appendix C of this report.

3.2 Measurement of health status in HEMS

As in previous surveys the measurement of health status was achieved using three well-tested measures. Cognitive work carried out at the pilot stage of the 1997 HEMS survey looked at respondents' understanding of these three self-reported measures of health.[10] At the end of the pilot interview a sub-sample of respondents were asked some additional questions. This part of the interview was carried out using a qualitative research methodology. Respondents were asked to explain their frame of reference for answering each of the health questions discussed above. Responses to this section of the study were recorded onto tape, transcribed and analysed, using qualitative analysis techniques. The cognitive understanding of these questions is discussed below.

'Less than good' general health

The first measure discussed is that of 'less than good' general health. Respondents were asked

'How is your health in general? Would you say it was very good, good, fair, bad or very bad?'

For the purposes of this discussion, those who reported fair, bad or very bad general health were classified as having 'less than good' general health and this was used as the outcome of interest.

In the cognitive study, respondents felt that good general health was an absence of ill-health and that it was associated with how fit they thought they were. They related it to the amount of exercise they took and the type of diet they followed. Some respondents compared their health to members of the family and friends of a similar age but whose health was less good. Very good general health was perceived as not only physical but also mental health, that had to be maintained with a lot of exercise. Good health was seen as 'normal' health and was linked to fitness. Having slight health problems such as a cold did not prevent respondents from seeing themselves as having good general health. Respondents saw having 'less than good' health as a cause for concern, especially if they felt that their health was very bad.

Limiting long-standing illness

The second health measure used was limiting, long-standing illness. For this respondents were asked

'Do you have any long-standing illness, disability or infirmity? By long-standing I mean anything that has troubled you over a period of time or that is likely to affect you over a period of time'.

If they responded positively to this question they were asked whether the illness or disability limited their activities in any way[11]. For the purposes of these analyses 'limiting long-standing illness' refers to a combination of these two questions; those who said they had a long-standing illness and who felt that this limited their activities in some way.

In the cognitive study, the limiting long-standing illness and disability questions were understood in two ways. Respondents explained long-standing illness as something that would affect them for a long time, although the actual times specified varied widely. However, disability was understood as a restriction on normal life, which applied to both physical and mental disabilities. A disability was not believed to be curable.

Stress

The third variable discussed is a self-reported measure of stress. Respondents were asked to describe the amount of stress or pressure they had experienced in the past 12 months. The categories given were; completely free of stress, small amount of stress, moderate amount of stress and large amount of stress. It is those with a large amount of stress that are discussed in this chapter.

Most respondents to the cognitive study described pressure as either being imposed on you by others or self-imposed. For many it came from deadlines at work or from having more and more work to do. Respondents did not see pressure as constant but as coming and going as deadlines were met or problems solved. Some thought that pressure was positive and helped them to concentrate. Stress was seen as being caused by pressure; it was understood as the feelings experienced when under pressure. It was felt to come from inside and to affect people mentally and physically. Generally respondents to the cognitive study saw a small amount of stress as positive because it helped them to work harder. However, large amounts of stress were considered to be harmful and bad for health.

3.3 'Less than good' general health

3.3.1 'Less than good' general health in relation to demographic and socio-economic variables

Age and sex
In the 1998 HEMS, 22% of men and 26% of women aged 16 and over reported their general health to be 'less than good'. The percentages reporting 'less than good' health increased with age. For example, in the youngest age-group, 14% of men and 22% of women classified their general health as 'less than good', compared with 43% and 50% respectively among those aged 75 and over.

Only in the youngest age-group were women significantly more likely than men to report 'less than good' general health. (**Figure 3.1 and Table 3.1**)

Figure 3.1 Self-reported health status by age and sex: adults aged 16 and over

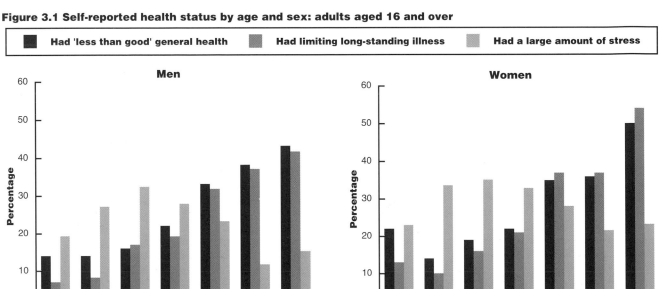

Base numbers are given in Table 3.1 to 3.3.

In 1998, adults aged 75 and over were included in HEMS for the first time. Provided that this age-group is excluded from the 1998 data, the results can be compared with those for 1995 and 1996. In 1998, the percentage of people reporting 'less than good' general health was very similar to that reported in previous HEMS reports. (**Table 3.4**)

Marital status

On the whole, the widowed, divorced or separated were more likely than those in other marital status groups to report 'less than good' general health. Around two-fifths of those who were widowed, divorced or separated reported 'less than good' general health, compared with a fifth of those who were married or cohabiting. Even allowing for differences in the age composition of the marital status groups (for example, single men tend to be younger, on average), there were wide differences between the marital status groups. (**Table 3.5**)

Social class

Men and women in the manual social classes were more likely than the non-manual social classes to report 'less than good' general health. For example, 29% of men and 33% of women in Social Classes IV / V reported 'less than good' general health, compared with 17% of men and women in Social Classes I / II. Even allowing for the differences in the age composition of the social classes (for example, those in Social Classes I / II tend to be concentrated in the middle age groups), there were differences in self-reported general health by social class. (**Table 3.6**)

Gross household income

Men and women in the two lowest income groups were more likely than respondents in the higher income groups to report 'less than good' general health. Among those in households with a gross income of less than £5,000, 51% of men and 41% of women reported 'less than good' general health, and in the next highest income group (£5,000 to £9,999), 44% of men and 38% of women did so. This compared with 11% of men and 14% of women living in households with an income of £20,000 or more. Even allowing for the differences in the age composition of the household income groups (for example, those in the lower income groups tend to be older, on average), this association remained. (**Table 3.7**)

Economic activity

Unemployed and economically inactive men and women were more likely than were working respondents to report 'less than good' general health. For example, 45% of men and 38% of women who were economically inactive reported 'less than good' general health compared with 13% of men and 18% of women in full-time employment. After controlling for age, economically inactive people and unemployed women remained more likely than expected on the basis of age to report 'less than good' general health. (**Table 3.8**)

Highest qualification level

Men and women with no qualifications were almost twice as likely as were those with some qualifications to report 'less than good' general health. Two-fifths of those without qualifications reported 'less than good' general health, compared with around a sixth of those with 'A' level or higher qualifications.

Those without qualifications were more likely than expected on the basis of age alone to report 'less than good' general health, and those with 'A' level or higher qualifications were less likely to do so. (**Table 3.9**)

Housing tenure

Those in local authority housing were twice as likely to report 'less than good' general health as were those who were in owner-occupied accommodation. For example, 41% of men and women whose accommodation was rented from the local authority reported 'less than good' general health, compared with 19% of men and 22% of women who lived in owner-occupied housing. This association remained after age had been taken into account. (**Table 3.10**)

3.3.2 'Less than good' general health in relation to household type and the social environment

Household type

Men and women who lived alone were more likely than those in any other type of household to report 'less than good' general health. For example, 35% of men and 41% of women in one-person households reported 'less than good' general health, compared with 17% of men and 16% of women who lived with other adults and dependent children. This association was explained by age for women, though not for men.

Two groups were slightly less likely than would be expected, given their ages, to report 'less than good health': women who lived with others and dependent children and men who lived with others but no dependent children. (**Table 3.11**)

Personal support group

Not having a personal support group was associated with 'less than good' general health for both men and women. For example, 48% of men and 35% of women with no personal support reported 'less than good' general health compared with 19% of men and 22% of women who could call on a personal support group of 4–8 people. However, because of the small number of women with no personal support, the differences were only statistically significant for men. The association for men remained even after taking account of age. (**Table 3.12**)

Community activity

After controlling for age, men and women who had been involved in activity in the community were less likely than those not involved in activity to report 'less than good' general health: 17% of men and 22% of women who were active in their community did so, compared with 24% of men and 28% of women who were not active. (**Table 3.13**)

Satisfaction with control over decisions that affect life

Those who were satisfied with the amount of 'control they had over decisions affecting their life' (referred to hereafter as 'control'), were much less likely than either those who were dissatisfied or those who were neither satisfied nor dissatisfied with their 'control' to report 'less than good' general health. For example, 21% of men and 24% of women who were satisfied with the 'control' they had over their lives reported 'less than good' general health, compared with 26% of men and 33% of women who were dissatisfied with their 'control'. This association was true for women but not for men when age was taken into account. (**Table 3.14**)

Influence over decisions that affect neighbourhood

Men and women who agreed that they could 'influence decisions that affected their neighbourhood' (referred to hereafter as 'influence'), were less likely than those who felt they had no 'influence' to report 'less than good' general health. Those who had no opinion about their 'influence' were the least likely to report 'less than good' general health. For example, 25% of men and 29% of women who disagreed with the statement on 'influence' reported 'less than good' general health, compared with 22% of men and 24% of women who agreed and 17% of men and 21% of women who neither agreed nor disagreed. After taking age into account, those who were dissatisfied were more likely than expected, given their ages, to report 'less than good' general health. (Table 3.15)

Neighbourhood social capital score

Those who had a low neighbourhood social capital score were more likely than those with a very high score to report 'less than good' general health (30% of men and 31% of women with a low score, compared with 16% of men and 20% of women with a very high neighbourhood social capital score). This relationship remained even when age was taken into account. (Table 3.16)

Area deprivation category

Men and women who lived in the more deprived areas were more likely to report 'less than good' general health than those who lived in the more affluent areas. For example, 31% of men and 32% of women who lived in the more deprived areas reported 'less than good' general health, compared with 17% of men and 22% of women who lived in the more affluent areas. This association remained when age was taken into account. (Table 3.17)

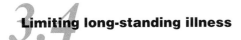

3.4 Limiting long-standing illness

3.4.1 Limiting long-standing illness in relation to demographic and socio-economic variables

Age and sex

In the 1998 HEMS, 20% of men and 24% of women aged 16 and over reported having a limiting long-standing illness. As with 'less than good' general health, the proportions reporting a limiting long-standing illness increased with age: 7% of men and 13% of women aged 16–24 did so, compared with 42% of men and 54% of women aged 75 and over. Only in the oldest age-group were women more likely than men to report having a limiting long-standing illness. (Figure 3.1 and Table 3.2)

Comparing the data for 1995 and 1996 with 1998 shows that the proportions of those aged 16–74 who had a limiting long-standing illness were very similar in all three years. (Table 3.4)

Marital status

Men and women who were widowed, divorced or separated were more likely than other marital status groups to have a limiting long-standing illness. For example, 33% of men and 42% of women who were widowed, divorced or separated had a limiting long-standing illness, compared with 12% of men and 17% of women who were single. However, after controlling for age, only the association for widowed, divorced or separated women remained significant. (Table 3.5)

Social class

Men and women in the manual social classes were more likely than those whose social class was non-manual to have a limiting long-standing illness. For example, 25% of men and 29% of women in Social Classes IV / V had a limiting long-standing illness. This compared with 17% of men and 19% of women in

Social Classes I / II. These differences were greater than would be expected on the basis of age alone. (Table 3.6)

Gross household income

Men and women in low-income households were more likely to have a limiting long-standing illness. For example, 45% of men and 37% of women with a gross household income of less than £5,000 and 44% of men and 39% of women with a household income of between £5,000 and £9,999 had a limiting long-standing illness. However, among men and women who lived in households with a gross income of £20,000 or more this was true for 11% of men and 14% of women. Even allowing for the differences in the age composition of the groups (those in the lower income groups tend to be older, on average), there were still wide differences between the household income groups. (Table 3.7)

Economic activity

Economically inactive men and women were more likely to have a limiting long-standing illness than either employed or unemployed respondents. However, it must be remembered that some people may have been economically inactive because of ill-health, although it is not possible to identify this group in the data. Among the economically inactive, 42% of men and 40% of women had a limiting long-standing illness, compared with 11% of men and 15% of women who were employed. After allowing for age, the economically inactive were more likely, and the employed were less likely than expected, given their ages, to report having a limiting long-standing illness. (Table 3.8)

Highest qualification level

Men and women with no qualifications were more likely than respondents with some qualifications to have a limiting long-standing illness. For example, 37% of men and women with no qualifications had a limiting long-standing illness, compared with 13% of men and 17% of women with 'A' levels or higher qualifications. When the ages of those with no qualifications were taken into account (they tend to be older than others), they were more likely than would be expected from their ages to report a limiting long-standing illness. (Table 3.9)

Housing tenure

Respondents in local authority accommodation were more likely than those in owner-occupied housing to have a limiting long-standing illness. For example, 37% of men and 36% of women who were in local authority accommodation had a limiting long-standing illness, compared with 17% of men and 22% of women who were in owner-occupied housing. This association remained even when age was taken into account. (Table 3.10)

3.4.2 Limiting long-standing illness in relation to household type and the social environment

Household type

Before controlling for age, those who lived alone were more likely than those who lived with others (with or without dependent children) to report a limiting long-standing illness. This was even more marked for women than for men. For example, 29% of men and 41% of women who lived alone reported a limiting long-standing illness, compared with 14% of men and 11% of women who were living with other adults, and dependent children. However, after allowing for the differences in the age composition of the household types, (older people being more likely to live in one-person households) those who lived alone were not more likely to report a limiting long-standing illness. (Table 3.11)

Personal support group

Those respondents who either had no personal support group or a very small support group (1–3 people) were more likely than those with a personal support group of 4–8 people to have a limiting long-standing illness. For example, 31% of men and 45% of women with no personal support group and 24% of men and 26% of women with a personal support group of 1–3 people had a limiting long-standing illness. This compares with 17% of men and 22% of women with a personal support group of 4–8 people. However, only men with a support group of 1–3 people remained more likely than expected on the basis of age to report a limiting long-standing illness. (**Table 3.12**)

Community activity

There was no relationship between community activity and limiting long-standing illness for men. However, among women, those who were involved in some community activity were slightly less likely than those with no community involvement to have a limiting long-standing illness. Twenty-five percent of women who were not involved in any community activity reported having a limiting long-standing illness, compared with 22% who had been involved in some activity in the community. This relationship remained when age was taken into account. However, these differences are quite small and it is not possible to say which affects the other, whether it is the limiting long-standing illness that hinders the community activity or vice versa. (**Table 3.13**)

Satisfaction with control over decisions that affect life

Men and women who were satisfied with the amount of control they had over decisions affecting their life (referred to hereafter as 'control'), were less likely than men and women who were dissatisfied with their 'control' to have a limiting long-standing illness. For example, 18% of men and 23% of women who were satisfied with their 'control' had a limiting long-standing illness, compared with 24% of men and 28% of women who were not satisfied with their 'control'. This relationship remained when age was taken into account. (**Table 3.14**)

Influence over decisions that affect neighbourhood

Respondents who felt that they could influence decisions that affected their neighbourhood (referred to hereafter as 'influence'), were less likely than those who did not feel that they had this 'influence' to report a limiting long-standing illness. For example, 19% of men and 22% of women who felt they had 'influence' reported having a limiting long-standing illness, compared with 23% of men and 27% of women who did not feel they had any 'influence'. However, for men it was those who were unable to decide about their 'influence' who reported the lowest levels of limiting long-standing illness (13%). After controlling for age, those who disagreed that they had 'influence' remained more likely than others to report a limiting long-standing illness. (**Table 3.15**)

Neighbourhood social capital score

The proportions reporting a limiting long-standing illness increased as neighbourhood social capital score decreased. For example, 24% of men and 28% of women with a low neighbourhood social capital score reported a limiting long-standing illness, compared with 14% of men and 19% of women with a very high neighbourhood social capital score. This association remained significant even after taking age into account. (**Table 3.16**)

Area deprivation category

Those who were living in more deprived areas were more likely than those living in more affluent areas to have a limiting long-standing illness. For example, 27% of men and 30% of women who lived in the more deprived areas reported a limiting long-standing illness, compared with 16% of men and 23% of women who lived in the more affluent areas. After controlling for age, those who lived in the more deprived area types remained most likely to report a long-standing illness. (**Table 3.17**)

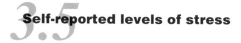

3.5 Self-reported levels of stress

3.5.1 Self-reported stress in relation to demographic and socio-economic variables

Age and sex

Twenty-four percent of men and 29% of women aged 16 and over had suffered from a large amount of stress over the past twelve months, whilst 8% of men and 6% of women said that they had been completely free of stress in that period.

While in all age-groups, men were less likely than women to report having had a large amount of stress over the past twelve months, some of the differences were small and not statistically significant, given the sample sizes. For both men and women, levels of stress rose until age 35–44 and then began to decline. For example, 19% of men and 23% of women aged 16–24 reported a large amount of stress over the past twelve months, compared with 32% of men and 35% of women aged 35–44. The percentage reporting a large amount of stress then fell to 15% of men and 23% of women aged 75 and over. (**Figure 3.1 and Table 3.3**)

A comparison of the 1998 data with those available from earlier HEMS, suggests that reported levels of stress for those aged 16–74 rose steeply between 1995 and 1996, especially for women, but at present appears to have stabilised at around 1996 levels. For example, 21% of respondents reported a high level of stress in 1995, rising to 28% in 1996 and 27% in 1998. (**Table 3.4**)

Marital status

On the whole, widowed, divorced or separated men and women were more likely than those in other marital status groups to have had a large amount of stress in the past twelve months. For example, 33% of men and 34% of women who were widowed, divorced or separated had a large amount of stress in the past twelve months, compared with 24% of men and 28% of women who were married or cohabiting. After controlling for age, this association remained significant. Becoming widowed, divorced or separated are all stressful life events but the data do not allow us to differentiate between those to whom this happened within the last 12 months and those to whom it happened a long while ago. (**Table 3.5**)

Social class

Men and women in Social Classes I / II were more likely than those in manual social classes to have had a large amount of stress in the past twelve months. For example, 28% of men and 35% of women in Social Classes I / II had a large amount of stress in the past twelve months, compared with 23% of men and 28% of women in Social Classes IV / V. After controlling for age, those in Social Classes I / II remained most likely to report a large amount of stress.

This agrees with results of work by Cooper et al,[12] who found that men in Social Class II reported the highest levels of stress, which consistently decreased in the manual social classes. However, other studies have produced different results. Marmot et al,[13] for example, found that those in the lower social classes suffer higher levels of stress than do those in the higher social classes. The difference may be explained by the methodology – the HEMS asked only one self-reported stress question, whilst the Marmot study used scales devised to measure stress levels in far greater detail. **(Table 3.6)**

Gross household income

On the whole, respondents in low-income households were slightly more likely than respondents in high-income households to have had a large amount of stress in the past twelve months. For example, 32% of men and women in households with a gross income of less than £5,000 reported a large amount of stress over the previous 12 months. This compared with 27% of men and 28% of women with a household income of more than £20,000 per annum. Men in the second lowest and women in the two lowest income bands were more likely than expected on the basis of their ages alone to report a large amount of stress. **(Table 3.7)**

Economic activity

Unemployed men and women were more likely than either those currently employed or the economically inactive to have had a large amount of stress in the past twelve months. For example, 34% of men and 44% of women who were unemployed had a large amount of stress in the past twelve months, compared with 22% of men and 27% of women who were economically inactive. However, when the age structure of the groups was taken into account, only economically inactive men and unemployed women were significantly more likely to report a large amount of stress, than would be predicted by age alone. **(Table 3.8)**

Housing tenure

Those in local authority accommodation were more likely than other tenure groups to have had a large amount of stress in the past twelve months. For example, 30% of men and 34% of women in local authority accommodation had a large amount of stress in the past twelve months, compared with 23% of men and 27% of women in owner-occupied housing. This relationship remained when age was taken into account. **(Table 3.10)**

3.5.2 Self-reported stress in relation to household type and the social environment

Household type

Men who lived alone reported higher levels of stress than men who lived in other household types. For example, 30% of men who lived in a one-person household reported a large amount of stress over the previous 12 months. This compared with 21% of men who lived with other adults only and 27% of men who lived in a household containing both other adults and dependent children. After controlling for age, men who lived in one-person households remained more likely than expected on the basis of age alone to report a large amount of stress.

For women the pattern was different. After taking account of their ages, lone mothers were the group most likely to report high levels of stress in the past 12 months. Almost half (47%) of lone mothers reported high levels of stress, compared with around a third of women in other household types. **(Table 3.11)**

Personal support group

Men and women with no personal support were over twice as likely as those with a support group of 4–8 people to report high levels of stress. For example, 46% of men and 63% of women with no personal support group reported high levels of stress, compared with 22% of men and 26% of women with a support group of 4–8 people. Stress levels were also relatively high for those with a support group of 1–3 people. After allowing for the differences in the age composition of the groups (those with low personal support tend to be older), there were still significant differences in the proportions reporting a large amount of stress by size of personal support group. **(Table 3.12)**

Satisfaction with control over decisions that affect life

Respondents who were satisfied with the amount of control they had over decisions affecting their life (referred to hereafter as 'control'), were much less likely than those who were dissatisfied with their 'control' to report high levels of stress. For example, 20% of men and 25% of women who were happy with their 'control' reported a high level of stress over the previous 12 months, compared with 39% of men and 50% of women who were dissatisfied with their 'control'. Women who were neither satisfied nor dissatisfied with their 'control' also reported high stress levels (38%). This association remained even after taking into account the age structure of the groups. **(Table 3.14)**

Influence over decisions that affect neighbourhood

On the whole, men and women who felt that they could influence decisions that affected their life (referred to hereafter as 'influence'), were less likely to report high levels of stress (22% of men and 28% of women compared with 27% of men and 33% of women who did not feel they had any 'influence'). After taking account of age, those who felt that they did not have any 'influence' remained most likely to report a large amount of stress. **(Table 3.15)**

Neighbourhood social capital score

Men and women with a low neighbourhood social capital score were more likely than others to report a high level of stress. Around a third of those with a low neighbourhood social capital score reported a high level of stress, compared with one fifth of men (18%) and a quarter of women with a very high neighbourhood social capital score. This pattern held after age had been taken into account. **(Table 3.16)**

Assessing the relative importance of different characteristics associated with people's self-reported health

The previous sections have shown that a number of variables are associated with people's self-reported health status. This section uses logistic regression to look at the relative importance of the different factors.

Odds ratios and logistic regression

Logistic regression is a multivariate technique which can be used to predict the odds of a behaviour occurring for people with different combinations of the characteristics. Odds are the ratio of the probability that an event will occur (for example, reporting 'less than good' general health) to the probability that an event will not occur. This technique is valuable because it indicates whether each analysis variable makes a significant contribution to explaining the variation in the outcome variable (the health status in question), having held all of the other analysis variables under consideration constant.

Two sets of logistic regressions relating to the health status measures were carried out. The first included only the demographic and socio-economic variables discussed for each health status, and the second included the new variables. Once Model 2 had been run to identify significant variables it was re-run to obtain relative odds for only those variables which had been significant (that is, those which had an independent association with the health status).

The results of the logistic regression analysis are shown in Tables 3.18 and 3.19. The columns headed 'multiplying factors' can be thought of as 'weights'. For example, they represent the factor by which the odds of someone reporting 'less than good' general health increase with the characteristic shown compared with a reference category. For each variable, the reference category (shown with a value of 1.00) was taken to be the first category. The baseline odds shown at the top of each table represent the average odds for the respondents with all of the reference categories shown[14]. For each category of the variable, a 95% confidence interval is also shown. If the interval contains the value 1.00, then the odds ratio is likely to be significantly different from the reference category. Undue weight should not be given to the significance or otherwise of particular categories, as this depends to some extent of which was chosen as the reference category. A more detailed explanation of logistic regression is given in Appendix C.

Logistic regression model including the demographic and socio-economic variables – Model 1

Table 3.18 shows the first logistic regression model, for the three measures of self-reported health status. Figure 3.2 gives a summary, indicating which of the variables had significant independent effects in this model.

Four of the variables – age, household income, economic activity and housing tenure – had independent effects on all three of the self-reported health measures. In addition, highest qualification was related to having 'less than good' general health, and sex, marital status and social class were all related to the likelihood of having a large amount of stress.

The model confirms the pattern of the results discussed above for the individual health measures. The groups with the lowest odds of reporting these aspects of poorer health were the higher income groups, the employed and the better qualified.

Holding all other variables constant, the odds of those in the lowest income groups having 'less than good' general health was nearly twice as great as those for respondents with a household income of £20,000 or more. Similarly, the odds for the economically inactive were over twice as high as for those who were employed, and the odds for respondents who lived in local authority accommodation were higher than for those who lived in owner-occupied or privately rented housing. Those aged 55–64 had higher odds than other age-groups in this model. The odds of reporting 'less than good' general health also decreased as the level of qualifications rose so that those with no qualifications had the highest odds for this variable (1.75).

In the model for reporting a limiting long-standing illness, the economically inactive had odds which were over three times higher (3.43) than for the employed. Those who lived in local authority accommodation had higher odds than those in other housing types, and those in a household with an income of £5,000–9,999 had the highest odds (2.25) for the income variable. The odds for reporting a limiting long-standing illness were also relatively greater for those aged 55–64.

In the model for reporting a large amount of stress, holding all the other variables constant, women had higher odds than men, the widowed, divorced or separated had higher odds than other marital status groups, and the unemployed higher odds than the employed or economically inactive. Those in Social Classes I / II had the highest odds among the different social classes. The pattern of odds in this model increased with age until age 35–44 and from then declined in each subsequent age-group. **(Table 3.18)**

Figure 3.2 Logistic regression Model 1 for self-reported health status - variables with significant independent effects

	General health 'less than good'	Limiting long-standing illness	Large amount of stress
Demographic and socio-economic variables:			
Sex	-	-	*
Age	*	*	*
Marital status	-	-	*
Social class	-	-	*
Gross household income	*	*	*
Economic activity	*	*	*
Highest qualification level	*	-	-
Housing tenure	*	*	*

*Has an independent effect

- Has no independent effect

Logistic regression model including all the analysis variables – Model 2

Table 3.19 shows the second logistic regression model. It includes all the variables from Model 1 plus household type and the social environment variables. Figure 3.3 shows the variables which had an independent effect in Model 2.

Six of the variables – age, household income, housing tenure, household type, satisfaction with 'control' over life and neighbourhood social capital score had independent effects on all three of the health status measures.

Interestingly, after controlling all the other variables, the odds of reporting poorer health ('less than good' general health or a limiting long-standing illness) did not increase with age beyond the age-group 55–64. The odds fell among those aged 65–74, and rose again among those aged 75 and over but not to the levels in the 55–64 age-group. This pattern would suggest that other variables play an increased part in determining the poorer reported health status found among older people.

Again the socio-economic groups with the lower odds of reporting poorer health were the higher income groups, the employed, those not in local authority housing and, for general health status, the better qualified. However, household type and several of the social environment variables also had an effect on self-reported health.

Holding all other variables constant, the odds of reporting 'less than good' general health or a limiting long-standing illness were relatively greater among those who lived alone and those who lived with other adults but with no dependent children. Similarly,

they were relatively greater for those who felt they had no 'control' over decisions affecting their lives and those with a low neighbourhood social capital score. The size of personal support group also had an independent effect on the odds of reporting 'less than good' general health, such that those with no support had the highest odds for this variable.

In the model for reporting large amounts of stress, after taking into account all the other variables, as many as eleven of the analysis variables had significant independent effects on stress levels. These were sex, age, marital status, social class, household income, housing tenure, household type, size of personal support group, 'control' over decisions affecting own life, 'influence' over neighbourhood decisions and neighbourhood social capital. In this model, the effects of some of the social environment variables were particularly large. For example, those who were not satisfied with the amount of 'control' had odds which were over twice as high as the odds for those who were satisfied with their 'control'. Similarly, those with no personal support group had higher odds of reporting stress (2.63) than those with a support group of 4 – 8 people (0.77). **(Table 3.19)**

Notes and references

1.   Blaxter M. *Health and Lifestyles*. Routledge (London: 1990).

2.   This five-fold definition is recommended by the World Health Organisation Regional Office for Europe. It is used by a number of UK surveys, including the Health Survey for England and the ONS Psychiatric Morbidity Surveys. It is also used by a number of European countries.

Figure 3.3 Logistic regression Model 2 for self-reported health measures - variables with significant independent effects

	General health 'less than good'	Limiting long-standing illness	Large amount of stress
Demographic and socio-economic variables:			
Sex	-	-	*
Age	*	*	*
Marital status	-	-	*
Social class	-	-	*
Gross household income	*	*	*
Economic activity	*	*	-
Highest qualification level	*	-	-
Housing tenure	*	*	*
Household type	*	*	*
Social environment variables:			
Personal support group	*	-	*
Community activity	-	-	-
Satisfaction with control over own life decisions	*	*	*
Influence over decisions affecting neighbourhood	-	-	*
Neighbourhood social capital score	*	*	*
Area deprivation category	-	-	-

* Has an independent effect

- Has no independent effect

3.   Blaxter M. Self-definition of health status and consulting rates in primary care. *Quarterly Journal of Social Affairs (1987)*, 1, 131–171; Bennett N *et al. Health Survey for England 1993.* HMSO (London: 1995).

4.   Blaxter M. Self-reported health. In *The Health and Lifestyles Survey.* Health Promotion Research Trust (London: 1987).

5.   *General Household Survey 1972.* HMSO (London: 1975).

6.   Bridgwood A, Malbon G, Lader D and Matheson J. *Health in England 1995: what people know, what people think, what people do.* HMSO (London: 1996).

7.   White A, Nicolaas G, Foster K, Browne F and Carey S. *Health Survey for England.* HMSO (London: 1993).

8.   Goldberg E L and Brenitz S (eds). *Handbook of stress.* Free Press (New York: 1993).

9.   Fredikson M. Psychophysiological and biochemical indices in 'stress' research; applications and pathophysiology. In Turpin G (ed) *Handbook of clinical psychophysiology.* Wiley and Sons (1989). Cited in Colhoun H *et al. Health Survey for England 1994.* HMSO (London: 1996).

10.   Mortimer L. (1997) *Cognitive question-testing for the Health Education Monitoring Survey (HEMS)* Report for the HEA (Unpublished)

11.   They were also asked what was wrong with them, The responses to this third question were recorded verbatim by the interviewer but will not be discussed further in this report.

12.   Cooper H, Arber S, Fee L and Ginn J. *The influence of social support and social capital on health.* HEA (London: 1999).

13.   Marmot M, Davey Smith G. Health inequalities among British civil servants: the Whitehall II study, by M.G. Marmot *et al* in *Lancet* (1991), June 8, 1387–1393.

14.   For example, in Model 1, the odds of reporting 'less than good' general health for people with different characteristics can be calculated by multiplying the baseline odds shown at the top of the table by the appropriate factors. So, for example, a person aged 16–24, whose household has an income of less than £5,000, who is economically inactive , has no educational qualifications and is in local authority housing would have odds calculated as shown below:

0.089 x 1.00 x 1.94 x 2.60 x 1.75 x 1.16 = 0.91

This would give odds of 0.91 to 1 that a person with these characteristics would report 'less than good' general health.

Table 3.1   Self-reported general health by age and sex

Adults aged 16 and over

Age	16-24	25-34	35-44	45-54	55-64	65-74	75 and over	Total
Self-reported general health	%	%	%	%	%	%	%	%
Men								
Very good	32	41	39	42	32	30	20	36
Good	54	45	45	36	36	31	37	42
Fair	12	12	12	15	21	28	31	16
Bad	2 ⌉14	2 ⌉14	4 ⌉16	5 ⌉22	8 ⌉33	8 ⌉38	7 ⌉43	4 ⌉22
Very bad	-	0	0	2	3	2	5	2
Base = 100%	*233*	*433*	*467*	*433*	*391*	*350*	*254*	*2561*
Women								
Very good	28	43	39	36	31	25	18	33
Good	50	43	42	42	35	40	32	41
Fair	20	11	16	16	26	26	34	20
Bad	2 ⌉22	2 ⌉14	2 ⌉19	5 ⌉22	7 ⌉35	7 ⌉36	12 ⌉50	5 ⌉26
Very bad	-	1	1	1	2	2	4	1
Base = 100%	*272*	*630*	*571*	*464*	*406*	*444*	*460*	*3247*
All								
Very good	30	42	39	39	31	27	19	34
Good	52	44	43	39	35	36	34	41
Fair	16	12	14	15	24	27	33	18
Bad	2 ⌉18	2 ⌉14	3 ⌉18	5 ⌉22	8 ⌉34	8 ⌉37	10 ⌉47	4 ⌉24
Very bad	0	1	1	1	2	2	4	1
Base = 100%	*505*	*1063*	*1038*	*897*	*797*	*794*	*714*	*5808*

Table 3.2   Self-reported long-standing illness by age and sex

Adults aged 16 and over

Age	16-24	25-34	35-44	45-54	55-64	65-74	75 and over	Total
Self-reported long-standing illness	%	%	%	%	%	%	%	%
Men								
Has limiting long-standing illness	7	8	17	19	32	37	42	20
Has non-limiting long-standing illness	11	12	13	16	19	18	18	15
No long-standing illness	82	80	70	65	50	44	40	66
Base = 100%	*233*	*433*	*467*	*433*	*390*	*350*	*254*	*2560*
Women								
Has limiting long-standing illness	13	10	16	21	37	37	54	24
Has non-limiting long-standing illness	13	15	14	17	18	21	16	16
No long-standing illness	74	75	69	62	46	42	30	60
Base = 100%	*272*	*630*	*572*	*463*	*406*	*446*	*460*	*3249*
All								
Has limiting long-standing illness	10	9	17	20	34	37	49	22
Has non-limiting long-standing illness	12	14	14	17	18	20	17	15
No long-standing illness	78	77	70	63	48	43	34	63
Base = 100%	*505*	*1063*	*1039*	*896*	*796*	*796*	*714*	*5809*

Table 3.3 Self-reported stress by age and sex

Adults aged 16 and over

Age	16-24	25-34	35-44	45-54	55-64	65-74	75 and over	Total
Self-reported stress	%	%	%	%	%	%	%	%
Men								
Completely free of stress	7	4	2	4	12	20	26	8
Small amount of stress	36	27	20	28	33	38	36	30
Moderate amount of stress	38	42	45	40	32	30	22	38
Large amount of stress	19	27	32	28	23	12	15	24
Don't know	-	-	0	-	0	1	2	0
Base = 100%	*233*	*433*	*466*	*433*	*390*	*350*	*254*	*2559*
Women								
Completely free of stress	2	4	3	3	8	14	16	6
Small amount of stress	34	27	22	24	29	36	31	28
Moderate amount of stress	40	35	40	41	35	29	28	36
Large amount of stress	23	34	35	33	28	22	23	29
Don't know	-	0	-	-	-	0	1	0
Base = 100%	*272*	*631*	*571*	*464*	*406*	*447*	*460*	*3251*
All								
Completely free of stress	5	4	3	4	10	16	20	7
Small amount of stress	36	27	21	26	31	37	33	29
Moderate amount of stress	39	39	42	40	34	29	26	37
Large amount of stress	21	30	34	30	26	17	20	27
Don't know	-	0	0	-	0	0	1	0
Base = 100%	*505*	*1064*	*1037*	*897*	*796*	*797*	*714*	*5810*

Table 3.4 Self-reported health status by year and sex
Adults aged 16-74

Year	Men 1995	Men 1996	Men 1998	Women 1995	Women 1996	Women 1998	All 1995	All 1996	All 1998
Self-reported health status	%	%	%	%	%	%	%	%	%
General health									
Very good	36	37	37	35	36	35	36	37	36
Good	42	43	42	42	42	42	42	43	42
Fair	17	15	16	18	17	18	18	16	17
Bad	3 ⎤22	3 ⎤20	4 ⎤21	4 ⎤23	4 ⎤22	4 ⎤23	4 ⎤22	4 ⎤21	4 ⎤22
Very bad	1 ⎦	1 ⎦	1 ⎦	1 ⎦	1 ⎦	1 ⎦	1 ⎦	1 ⎦	1 ⎦
Base = 100%	*2121*	*2038*	*2305*	*2548*	*2598*	*2791*	*4669*	*4636*	*5096*
Long-standing illness									
Has limiting long-standing illness	18	18	18	20	21	21	19	19	20
Has non-limiting long-standing illness	15	18	14	17	16	16	16	17	15
No long-standing illness	67	65	68	64	63	63	65	64	65
Base = 100%	*2120*	*2041*	*2306*	*2546*	*2600*	*2789*	*4666*	*4641*	*5095*
Stress									
Completely free of stress	11	7	7	7	5	5	9	6	6
Small amount of stress	36	31	29	33	26	28	35	29	28
Moderate amount of stress	34	38	39	36	36	37	35	37	38
Large amount of stress	18	24	25	23	32	30	21	28	27
Don't know	0	0	0	0	0	0	0	0	0
Base = 100%	*2121*	*2041*	*2307*	*2548*	*2598*	*2787*	*4669*	*4639*	*5094*

Table 3.5 Self-reported health status by marital status and sex
Adults aged 16 and over

Self-reported health status	Less than good general health Observed %*	Expected %†	Obs/exp (%)†	Limiting longstanding illness Observed %*	Expected %†	Obs/exp (%)†	Large amount of stress Observed %*	Expected %†	Obs/exp (%)†	Base = 100%
Marital status										
Men										
Single	**19**	16	120**	**12**	11	117	**23**	23	103	*504*
Married/cohabiting	**22**	24	92**	**20**	21	94**	**24**	25	94**	*1637*
Widowed/divorced/ separated	**38**	30	125**	**33**	29	117	**33**	22	151**	*418*
Total	**22**	22	100	**20**	20	100	**24**	24	100	*2559*
Women										
Single	**23**	21	111	**17**	16	106	**26**	27	99	*554*
Married/cohabiting	**22**	24	89**	**21**	23	91**	**28**	31	92**	*1668*
Widowed/divorced/ separated	**41**	35	117**	**42**	36	115**	**34**	27	127**	*1029*
Total	**26**	26	100	**24**	24	100	**29**	29	100	*3251*

* The percentages refer to the proportions of the subgroups reporting each health status, so do not add to 100.

† See Appendix C for a full explanation of age-standardisation.

** Age-standardised ratio is significantly different from 100, at the 95% level.

Table 3.6 Self-reported health status by social class based on own current or last job and sex
Adults aged 16 and over

Self-reported health status	Less than good general health			Limiting longstanding illness			Large amount of stress			Base = 100% ††
	Observed %*	Expected %†	Obs/exp (%)†	Observed %*	Expected %†	Obs/exp (%)†	Observed %*	Expected %†	Obs/exp (%)†	
Social class										
Men										
I & II	17	23	75**	17	20	84**	28	25	112**	948
III (Non-manual)	19	20	94	17	17	95	26	24	107	274
III (Manual)	26	23	113**	22	21	106	20	24	83**	792
IV & V	29	22	131**	25	20	126**	23	23	100	467
Total	22	22	100	20	20	100	24	24	100	2481
Women										
I & II	17	24	71**	19	22	86**	35	31	116**	830
III (Non-manual)	24	25	96	22	23	93	27	29	92	1063
III (Manual)	31	27	115	31	26	120	25	28	88	292
IV & V	33	27	123**	29	26	112**	28	29	98	930
Total	26	26	100	24	24	100	29	29	100	3115

*   The percentages refer to the proportions of the subgroups reporting each health status, so do not add to 100.
†   See Appendix C for a full explanation of age-standardisation.
** Age-standardised ratio is significantly different from 100, at the 95% level.
†† Members of the Armed Forces, persons in inadequately described occupations and persons who have never worked are excluded from this analysis and from the bases shown.

Table 3.7 Self-reported health status by gross household income and sex
Adults aged 16 and over

Self-reported health status	Less than good general health			Limiting longstanding illness			Large amount of stress			Base = 100%
	Observed %*	Expected %†	Obs/exp (%)†	Observed %*	Expected %†	Obs/exp (%)†	Observed %*	Expected %†	Obs/exp (%)†	
Gross household income										
Men										
£20,000 or more	11	19	61**	11	16	70**	27	26	103	1093
£10,000-£19,999	26	23	111	18	21	85**	18	24	75**	683
£5,000-£9,999	44	30	147**	44	28	161**	25	20	126**	441
Under £5,000	51	27	186**	45	25	180**	32	22	145	197
Total	22	22	100	19	19	100	24	24	100	2414
Women										
£20,000 or more	14	21	68**	14	18	76**	28	32	90**	982
£10,000-£19,999	25	24	102	22	23	93	26	30	89	726
£5,000-£9,999	38	31	120**	39	32	123**	34	27	125**	740
Under £5,000	41	32	131**	37	31	118**	32	27	121**	544
Total	25	25	100	24	24	100	30	30	100	2992

*   The percentages refer to the proportions of the subgroups reporting each health status, so do not add to 100.
†   See Appendix C for a full explanation of age-standardisation.
** Age-standardised ratio is significantly different from 100, at the 95% level.

Table 3.8 Self-reported health status by economic activity and sex
Adults aged 16 and over

Self-reported health status	Less than good general health			Limiting longstanding illness			Large amount of stress			Base = 100%
	Observed %*	Expected %†	Obs/exp (%)†	Observed %*	Expected %†	Obs/exp (%)†	Observed %*	Expected %†	Obs/exp (%)†	
Economic activity status										
Men										
Employed	**13**	19	72**	**11**	15	69**	**25**	27	93**	*1571*
Unemployed	**22**	17	125	**13**	13	96	**34**	26	131	*91*
Economically inactive	**45**	33	138**	**42**	30	140**	**22**	18	121**	*890*
Total	**22**	22	100	**19**	19	100	**24**	24	100	*2552*
Women										
Employed	**18**	21	86**	**15**	18	80**	**30**	31	95**	*1786*
Unemployed	**34**	19	172**	**17**	16	113	**44**	31	144**	*81*
Economically inactive	**38**	34	112**	**40**	35	117**	**27**	26	106	*1381*
Total	**26**	26	100	**24**	24	100	**29**	29	100	*3248*

* The percentages refer to the proportions of the subgroups reporting each health status, so do not add to 100.

† See Appendix C for a full explanation of age-standardisation.

** Age-standardised ratio is significantly different from 100, at the 95% level.

Table 3.9 Self-reported health status by highest qualification level and sex
Adults aged 16 and over

Self-reported health status	Less than good general health			Limiting longstanding illness			Large amount of stress			Base = 100%
	Observed %*	Expected %†	Obs/exp (%)†	Observed %*	Expected %†	Obs/exp (%)†	Observed %*	Expected %†	Obs/exp (%)†	
Highest qualification level										
Men										
'A' Level or above	**14**	20	68**	**13**	17	78**	**27**	26	103	*1007*
GCSE A-G or below	**22**	21	101	**16**	18	91	**22**	24	91	*908*
No qualifications	**41**	29	143**	**37**	26	139**	**23**	21	109	*639*
Total	**22**	22	100	**19**	19	100	**24**	24	100	*2554*
Women										
'A' Level or above	**16**	22	72**	**17**	20	88	**31**	31	102	*897*
GCSE A-G or below	**22**	23	92	**20**	21	95	**29**	30	98	*1279*
No qualifications	**41**	32	126**	**37**	33	111**	**27**	27	101	*1066*
Total	**26**	26	100	**24**	24	100	**29**	29	100	*3242*

* The percentages refer to the proportions of the subgroups reporting each health status, so do not add to 100.

† See Appendix C for a full explanation of age-standardisation.

** Age-standardised ratio is significantly different from 100, at the 95% level.

Table 3.10 Self-reported health status by housing tenure and sex
Adults aged 16 and over

Self-reported health status	Less than good general health			Limiting longstanding illness			Large amount of stress			Base = 100%
	Observed %*	Expected %†	Obs/exp (%)†	Observed %*	Expected %†	Obs/exp (%)†	Observed %*	Expected %†	Obs/exp (%)†	
Housing tenure										
Men										
Owner-occupier	19	23	85**	17	20	86**	23	25	95**	1890
Rents from local authority	41	24	170**	37	21	176**	30	23	132**	367
Rents privately	24	20	121	16	16	101	24	24	100	297
Total	22	22	100	19	19	100	24	24	100	2554
Women										
Owner-occupier	22	26	85**	22	24	90**	27	29	92**	2169
Rents from local authority	41	28	148**	36	26	135**	34	28	121**	620
Rents privately	29	25	118	24	23	108	34	29	117	458
Total	26	26	100	24	24	100	29	29	100	3247

* The percentages refer to the proportions of the subgroups reporting each health status, so do not add to 100.

† See Appendix C for a full explanation of age-standardisation.

** Age-standardised ratio is significantly different from 100, at the 95% level.

Table 3.11 Self-reported health status by household type and sex
Adults aged 16 and over

Self-reported health status	Less than good general health			Limiting longstanding illness			Large amount of stress			Base = 100%
	Observed %*	Expected %†	Obs/exp (%)†	Observed %*	Expected %†	Obs/exp (%)†	Observed %*	Expected %†	Obs/exp (%)†	
Household type										
Men										
One person household	35	26	132**	29	24	120	30	23	131**	595
Living with others (no dependent children)	23	25	92**	21	22	96	21	22	96	1308
Living with others (with dependent children)	17	17	103	14	14	97	27	28	96	635
Lone adult (with dependent children)	[7]	-	-	[4]	-	-	[13]	-	-	21
Total	22	22	100	20	20	100	24	24	100	2559
Women										
One person household	41	42	98	41	47	87**	32	33	97	965
Living with others (no dependent children)	27	28	98	27	26	103	27	28	94	1243
Living with others (with dependent children)	16	18	87**	11	15	73**	29	32	89**	764
Lone adult (with dependent children)	22	17	125	18	14	138	47	32	146**	279
Total	26	26	100	24	24	100	29	29	100	3251

*   The percentages refer to the proportions of the subgroups reporting each health status, so do not add to 100.

†   See Appendix C for a full explanation of age-standardisation.

** Age-standardised ratio is significantly different from 100, at the 95% level.

Table 3.12 Self-reported health status by size of personal support group and sex
Adults aged 16 and over

Self-reported health status	Less than good general health			Limiting longstanding illness			Large amount of stress			Base = 100%
	Observed %*	Expected %†	Obs/exp (%)†	Observed %*	Expected %†	Obs/exp (%)†	Observed %*	Expected %†	Obs/exp (%)†	
Personal support group										
Men										
9 or more people	21	22	96	17	19	91	22	24	93	580
4 - 8 people	19	22	87**	17	19	90	22	24	90**	1104
1 - 3 people	26	23	114**	24	20	118**	28	24	115**	806
No support	48	24	205**	31	21	145	46	25	186**	55
Total	22	22	100	19	19	100	24	24	100	2545
Women										
9 or more people	28	26	108	25	24	103	30	30	102	692
4 - 8 people	22	25	87**	22	24	94	26	29	87**	1518
1 - 3 people	30	27	114**	26	25	105	34	29	116**	996
No support	35	27	125	45	26	173	63	30	207**	35
Total	26	26	100	24	24	100	29	29	100	3241

* The percentages refer to the proportions of the subgroups reporting each health status, so do not add to 100.
† See Appendix C for a full explanation of age-standardisation.
** Age-standardised ratio is significantly different from 100, at the 95% level.

Table 3.13 Self-reported health status by community activity and sex
Adults aged 16 and over

Self-reported health status	Less than good general health			Limiting longstanding illness			Large amount of stress			Base = 100%
	Observed %*	Expected %†	Obs/exp (%)†	Observed %*	Expected %†	Obs/exp (%)†	Observed %*	Expected %†	Obs/exp (%)†	
Community activity										
Men										
Some community activity	17	23	76**	18	20	87	24	24	97	577
No community activity	24	22	107**	20	19	104	25	24	101	1982
Total	22	22	100	19	19	100	24	24	100	2559
Women										
Some community activity	22	26	84**	22	25	90**	27	29	93	1088
No community activity	28	26	108**	25	24	105**	30	29	104	2163
Total	26	26	100	24	24	100	29	29	100	3251

* The percentages refer to the proportions of the subgroups reporting each health status, so do not add to 100.
† See Appendix C for a full explanation of age-standardisation.
** Age-standardised ratio is significantly different from 100, at the 95% level.

Table 3.14 Self-reported health status by whether agrees with the statement 'I am satisfied with the amount of control I have over decisions that affect my life' and sex
Adults aged 16 and over

Self-reported health status	Less than good general health			Limiting longstanding illness			Large amount of stress			Base = 100%
	Observed %*	Expected %†	Obs/exp (%)†	Observed %*	Expected %†	Obs/exp (%)†	Observed %*	Expected %†	Obs/exp (%)†	
Whether agrees is satisfied with the amount of control over decisions that affect own life										
Men										
Agree	21	22	92**	18	19	93**	20	24	85**	1895
Neither agree nor disagree	30	22	135**	22	19	112	32	25	125	252
Disagree	26	22	116	24	19	125**	39	25	155**	397
Total	22	22	100	19	19	100	24	24	100	2544
Women										
Agree	24	26	93**	23	24	95**	25	29	88**	2566
Neither agree nor disagree	30	25	120	28	23	119	38	30	127**	294
Disagree	33	24	139**	28	22	124**	50	30	164**	369
Total	26	26	100	24	24	100	29	29	100	3229

*   The percentages refer to the proportions of the subgroups reporting each health status, so do not add to 100.
†   See Appendix C for a full explanation of age-standardisation.
** Age-standardised ratio is significantly different from 100, at the 95% level.

Table 3.15 Self-reported health status by whether agrees with the statement 'I can influence decisions that affect my neighbourhood' and sex
Adults aged 16 and over

Self-reported health status	Less than good general health			Limiting longstanding illness			Large amount of stress			Base = 100%
	Observed %*	Expected %†	Obs/exp (%)†	Observed %*	Expected %†	Obs/exp (%)†	Observed %*	Expected %†	Obs/exp (%)†	
Whether can influence decisions that affect own neighbourhood										
Men										
Agree	22	23	95	19	21	93	22	24	91	584
Neither agree nor disagree	17	20	84**	13	17	76**	21	25	85**	653
Disagree	25	23	110**	23	20	115**	27	24	112**	1295
Total	22	22	100	19	19	100	24	24	100	2532
Women										
Agree	24	26	93	22	24	88**	28	30	95	775
Neither agree nor disagree	21	24	86**	22	22	96	24	30	81**	819
Disagree	29	26	110**	27	25	107**	33	29	113**	1619
Total	26	26	100	24	24	100	29	29	100	3213

*   The percentages refer to the proportions of the subgroups reporting each health status, so do not add to 100.
†   See Appendix C for a full explanation of age-standardisation.
** Age-standardised ratio is significantly different from 100, at the 95% level.

Table 3.16 Self-reported health status by neighbourhood social capital score and sex
Adults aged 16 and over

Self-reported health status	Less than good general health			Limiting longstanding illness			Large amount of stress			Base = 100%
	Observed %*	Expected %†	Obs/exp (%)†	Observed %*	Expected %†	Obs/exp (%)†	Observed %*	Expected %†	Obs/exp (%)†	
Neighbourhood social capital score										
Men										
Very high	16	23	71**	14	20	69**	18	24	75**	450
High	18	23	81**	17	20	85**	20	24	84**	739
Medium	23	22	103	21	19	111	24	24	99	694
Low	30	22	140**	24	19	128**	33	24	134**	663
Total	22	22	100	19	19	100	24	24	100	2546
Women										
Very high	20	26	77**	19	25	75**	24	30	80**	578
High	24	26	94	24	25	96	28	29	95	903
Medium	26	26	102	25	24	104	29	29	102	889
Low	31	25	120**	28	23	119**	34	29	117**	869
Total	26	26	100	24	24	100	29	29	100	3239

*   The percentages refer to the proportions of the subgroups reporting each health status, so do not add to 100."

†   See Appendix C for a full explanation of age-standardisation.

** Age-standardised ratio is significantly different from 100, at the 95% level.

Table 3.17 Self-reported health status by area deprivation category and sex
Adults aged 16 and over

Self-reported health status	Less than good general health			Limiting longstanding illness			Large amount of stress			Base = 100%
	Observed %*	Expected %†	Obs/exp (%)†	Observed %*	Expected %†	Obs/exp (%)†	Observed %*	Expected %†	Obs/exp (%)†	
Area deprivation category										
Men										
1 More Affluent	17	23	72**	16	20	80**	27	24	112	491
2	21	22	95	18	20	94	24	25	96	461
3	21	23	93	17	20	88	23	24	92	653
4	25	22	113	21	19	111	22	24	90	564
5 More Deprived	31	22	142**	27	19	143**	29	24	118	390
Total	22	22	100	20	20	100	24	24	100	2559
Women										
1 More Affluent	22	28	79**	23	27	88	27	29	94	569
2	22	25	90	21	23	90	27	30	92	636
3	25	26	97	23	25	92	28	29	96	806
4	29	26	114**	26	24	110	32	29	110	726
5 More Deprived	32	25	128**	30	23	132**	33	30	113	514
Total	26	26	100	24	24	100	29	29	100	3251

*   The percentages refer to the proportions of the subgroups reporting each health status, so do not add to 100.

†   See Appendix C for a full explanation of age-standardisation.

** Age-standardised ratio is significantly different from 100, at the 95% level.

Table 3.18   Logistic regression for self-reported health status variables - model 1
Adults aged 16 and over

Characteristics	Number of cases	General health less than good — Multiplying factors (0.089)	General health less than good — 95% Confidence intervals	Limiting long-standing illness — Multiplying factors (0.079)	Limiting long-standing illness — 95% Confidence intervals	Large amount of stress — Multiplying factors (0.346)	Large amount of stress — 95% Confidence intervals
Sex							
Male (R)	2352	-	- -	-	- -	1.00	
Female	2874	-	- -	-	- -	1.28 *	1.12 - 1.47
Age							
16-24 (R)	346	1.00		1.00		1.00	
25-34	1001	0.83	0.59 - 1.17	0.69	0.46 - 1.02	1.34	1.00 - 1.80
35-44	987	1.12	0.80 - 1.57	1.47 *	1.01 - 2.14	1.57 *	1.16 - 2.13
45-54	834	1.44 *	1.02 - 2.02	2.08 *	1.43 - 3.03	1.41 *	1.03 - 1.93
55-64	729	1.78 *	1.27 - 2.51	2.68 *	1.84 - 3.89	0.90	0.65 - 1.26
65-74	719	0.95	0.66 - 1.38	1.26	0.84 - 1.88	0.40 *	0.27 - 0.59
75 and over	613	1.17	0.80 - 1.72	1.65 *	1.10 - 2.47	0.42 *	0.28 - 0.61
Marital status							
Single(R)	851	-	- -	-	- -	1.00	
Married/cohabiting	3088	-	- -	-	- -	0.93	0.76 - 1.13
Widowed, divorced, separated	1287	-	- -	-	- -	1.51 *	1.21 - 1.89
Social class							
I&II (R)	1698	-	- -	-	- -	1.00	
IIINM	1236	-	- -	-	- -	0.71 *	0.59 - 0.84
IIM	1014	-	- -	-	- -	0.63 *	0.52 - 0.77
IV&V	1278	-	- -	-	- -	0.69	0.58 - 0.83
Gross household income							
£20,000 or more (R)	2031	1.00		1.00		1.00	
£10,000 - £19,999	1370	1.56 *	1.29 - 1.90	1.19	0.98 - 1.46	0.84	0.71 - 1.00
£5,000 - £9,999	1138	2.03 *	1.62 - 2.54	2.25 *	1.81 - 2.80	1.41 *	1.13 - 1.75
Under £5,000	690	1.94 *	1.49 - 2.51	1.81 *	1.40 - 2.34	1.12 *	0.85 - 1.47
Economic activity							
Employed (R)	3161	1.00		1.00		1.00	
Unemployed	148	1.42	0.96 - 2.09	1.04	0.67 - 1.63	1.42	0.99 - 2.03
Economically inactive	1920	2.60 *	2.13 - 3.18	3.43 *	2.80 - 4.21	1.23 *	1.01 - 1.51
Highest qualification level							
'A'Level or above (R)	1786	1.00		-	- -	-	- -
GCSE A-G or below	1959	1.28 *	1.07 - 1.53	-	- -	-	- -
No qualifications	1484	1.75 *	1.44 - 2.13	-	- -	-	- -
Housing tenure							
Owner-occupier (R)	3672	1.00		1.00		1.00	
Rents local authority	899	1.63 *	1.36 - 1.96	1.53 *	1.26 - 1.84	1.36 *	1.13 - 1.64
Rents privately	658	1.16	0.94 - 1.43	1.13	0.90 - 1.41	1.18	0.97 - 1.44
Number of cases in the model		5229		5230		5226	

* Significant at the 95% level.
(R) reference category

Table 3.19 Logistic regression for self-reported health status variables - model 2
Adults aged 16 and over

Characteristics	Number of cases	General health less than good		Limiting long-standing illness		Large amount of stress	
Baseline odds		0.066		0.045		0.344	
		Multiplying factors	95% Confidence intervals	Multiplying factors	95% Confidence intervals	Multiplying factors	95% Confidence intervals
Sex							
Male (R)	2312	-	- -	-	- -	1.00	
Female	2833	-	- -	-	- -	1.41 *	1.22 - 1.63
Age							
16-24 (R)	422	1.00		1.00		1.00	
25-34	1016	1.01	0.73 - 1.40	1.01	0.69 - 1.48	1.17	0.86 - 1.60
35-44	989	1.43 *	1.03 - 1.97	2.20 *	1.53 - 3.16	1.43 *	1.03 - 1.97
45-54	835	1.58 *	1.14 - 2.19	2.48 *	1.74 - 3.55	1.15	0.82 - 1.62
55-64	721	1.91 *	1.37 - 2.65	2.99 *	2.08 - 4.28	0.70	0.49 - 1.01
65-74	721	1.07	0.75 - 1.53	1.42	0.97 - 2.08	0.40 *	0.27 - 0.58
75 and over	623	1.31	0.91 - 1.89	1.87 *	1.27 - 2.76	0.41 *	0.28 - 0.61
Marital status							
Single(R)	837	-	- -	-	- -	1.00	
Married/cohabiting	3052	-	- -	-	- -	1.33	1.00 - 1.77
Widowed, divorced, separated	1256	-	- -	-	- -	1.46 *	1.15 - 1.85
Social class							
I&II (R)	1679	-	- -	-	- -	1.00	
IIINM	1220	-	- -	-	- -	0.70 *	0.59 - 0.84
IIM	996	-	- -	-	- -	0.60 *	0.49 - 0.74
IV&V	1250	-	- -	-	- -	0.67 *	0.56 - 0.81
Gross household income							
£20,000 or more (R)	2063	1.00		1.00		1.00	
£10,000 - £19,999	1399	1.56 *	1.28 - 1.90	1.17	0.96 - 1.44	0.81 *	0.68 - 0.97
£5,000 - £9,999	1149	2.11 *	1.68 - 2.67	2.35 *	1.87 - 2.94	1.41 *	1.13 - 1.76
Under £5,000	716	1.95 *	1.46 - 2.61	1.91 *	1.44 - 2.54	0.96	0.72 - 1.27
Economic activity							
Employed (R)	3154	1.00		1.00		-	- -
Unemployed	160	1.13	0.76 - 1.66	0.84	0.53 - 1.32	-	- -
Economically inactive	2013	2.48 *	2.04 - 3.02	3.50 *	2.86 - 4.27	-	- -
Highest qualification level							
'A'Level or above (R)	1811	1.00		-	- -	-	- -
GCSE A-G or below	1997	1.36 *	1.13 - 1.63	-	- -	-	- -
No qualifications	1519	1.85 *	1.52 - 2.26	-	- -	-	- -
Housing tenure							
Owner-occupier (R)	3725	1.00		1.00		1.00	
Rents local authority	913	1.54 *	1.28 - 1.85	1.46 *	1.21 - 1.77	1.31 *	1.08 - 1.60
Rents privately	689	1.12	0.91 - 1.38	1.07	0.86 - 1.33	1.14	0.93 - 1.40
Household type							
One person household (R)	1425	1.00		1.00		1.00	
Living with others (no dependent children)	2292	0.91	0.77 - 1.09	1.02	0.85 - 1.21	0.69 *	0.51 - 0.92
Living with others (with dependent children)	1318	0.73 *	0.57 - 0.93	0.68 *	0.52 - 0.88	0.54 *	0.39 - 0.75
Lone parent	292	0.53 *	0.37 - 0.76	0.53 *	0.36 - 0.78	1.04	1.04 - 1.41

continued

Table 3.19 - *continued*
Adults aged 16 and over

Characteristics	Number of cases	General health less than good (Baseline odds 0.066)		Limiting long-standing illness (Baseline odds 0.045)		Large amount of stress (Baseline odds 0.344)	
		Multiplying factors	95% Confidence intervals	Multiplying factors	95% Confidence intervals	Multiplying factors	95% Confidence intervals
Personal support group							
9 or more people (R)	1165	1.00		-	- -	1.00	
4-8 people	2430	0.81 *	0.67 - 0.96	-	- -	0.77 *	0.65 - 0.91
1-3 people	1652	1.03	0.86 - 1.24	-	- -	1.08	0.90 - 1.29
No support	80	1.65	0.99 - 2.74	-	- -	2.63 *	1.58 - 4.38
Whether satisfied with amount of control over decisions that affect life							
Agree (R)	4111	1.00		1.00		1.00	
Neither agree nor disagree	501	1.59 *	1.27 - 1.98	1.45 *	1.15 - 1.83	1.67 *	1.36 - 2.05
Disagree	715	1.53 *	1.26 - 1.86	1.51 *	1.24 - 1.84	2.36 *	1.97 - 2.81
Whether can influence decisions that affect neighbourhood							
Agree (R)	1241	-	- -	-	- -	1.00	
Neither agree nor disagree	1311	-	- -	-	- -	0.94	0.78 - 1.14
Disagree	2593	-	- -	-	- -	1.17	0.99 - 1.37
Neighbourhood social capital score							
Very High (R)	947	1.00		1.00		1.00	
High	1514	1.15	0.93 - 1.43	1.34 *	1.08 - 1.68	1.05 *	0.86 - 1.28
Medium	1467	1.34 *	1.08 - 1.66	1.49 *	1.19 - 1.85	1.13	0.92 - 1.38
Low	1399	1.66 *	1.34 - 2.06	1.70 *	1.36 - 2.12	1.41 *	1.15 - 1.73
Number of cases in the model		5327		5350		5145	

* Significant at the 95% level.
(R) reference category

Smoking

Summary of main findings

- Men were more likely than women to smoke cigarettes (29% compared with 26%). As a proportion of all respondents, men were also the more likely to be heavier smokers (11% smoked 20 or more a day, compared with 7% of women). (Section 4.3).

- Younger people were more likely than older people to be current smokers. For example, 39% of men aged 16-24 were current smokers compared with 13% of men aged 75 or over. The corresponding proportions for women were lower but followed the same pattern, falling from 29% to 9%. (Section 4.3).

- Having taken account of age, smoking prevalence was relatively higher among those in Social Classes IV / V, and those with annual household incomes of less than £5,000. It was also relatively higher among single women and lone mothers. (Section 4.4).

- Conversely, having taken account of age, the likelihood of never having smoked was relatively greater among those with annual household incomes of £20,000 or more, those qualified to 'A' level or higher, and those in owner-occupied homes. It was also relatively greater for employed men (compared with men in other economic status groups), men in non-manual social classes, and married or cohabiting women. (Section 4.4).

- After taking account of age, factors related to the respondent's social environment, were also strongly related to smoking behaviour. For example, smoking prevalence was relatively higher among those who were not active in their local community, those with lack of control over decisions affecting their lives, those with a low neighbourhood social capital score, and those who lived in more deprived areas. Among men, it was also high among those who had no personal support group. (Section 4.5).

- Similarly, the likelihood of never having smoked was related to community involvement, control over decisions affecting life, neighbourhood social capital score, and, for women, area deprivation. (Section 4.5).

- Logistic regression analysis showed that a number of factors had significant independent effects on both of the smoking measures. These were age, marital status, qualification level, tenure, household type, community activity, satisfaction with control over decisions affecting life, neighbourhood social capital score, and

continued

area deprivation. In addition, social class and influence over neighbourhood decisions were significant for being a smoker, and sex and size of personal support group were associated with never having smoked. (Section 4.6).

■ Smokers were asked about their intentions to give up smoking. Those in the middle age-groups were more likely than older or younger respondents to say that they would like to give up, though this pattern was more marked among men than women. (Section 4.7).

■ While the heavier smokers were more likely than those who smoked less to say that they would like to give up, it was the lightest smokers who were the most likely to say that they intended to give up smoking within the next month: 15% of those who smoked fewer than 10 cigarettes a day intended to give up within the next month, compared with 7% of those with higher consumption. (Section 4.7).

4.1 Cigarette smoking and health

Cigarette smoking is the main cause of disease leading to early death in England and it is estimated that it caused over 120,000 deaths in the UK in 1995[1]. Smoking is associated with several types of disease, including cancers of the lung, upper respiratory site, stomach, bladder and kidney. Other diseases caused by smoking are heart disease, circulatory diseases, respiratory disorders such as pneumonia, and digestive disorders such as ulcer of the stomach. Smokers have higher death rates than people who have never smoked, both overall and for each of the many smoking-related diseases. Smokers therefore have a high risk of dying prematurely as a result of their habit. For a person who smokes, stopping would be more effective than any other change in behaviour in reducing the risk of premature death[2].

The current government strategy for reducing the number of deaths from smoking has been set out in two White Papers - *Smoking Kills: A White Paper on Tobacco* in 1998 and *Saving Lives: Our Healthier Nation* in 1999[3,4]. The first paper set out targets to reduce adult smoking and women's smoking during pregnancy, as well as smoking amongst young people. It also set out measures to achieve these targets which included ending tobacco advertising and providing new services to help people give up. Building upon the earlier Green Paper (*Our Healthier Nation*), *Saving Lives: Our Healthier Nation* outlined four main priority areas for improvement in health - cancer, coronary heart disease and strokes, accidents, and mental illness[5].

Previous HEMS reports have briefly described some of the characteristics of adults which are associated with smoking behaviour. These included demographic and socio-economic characteristics such as marital status, employment status, social class, and qualification level. This chapter focuses on results from the 1998 HEMS and looks at smoking in relation to a wider range of factors, including household type and the social environment. It also looks briefly at smoker's intentions in 1998 to give up smoking.

4.2 Measurement of smoking behaviour

The HEMS measures smoking prevalence in a similar way to the General Household Survey (GHS) and the Health Survey for England (HSE). Respondents are asked whether they have ever smoked. If they have, they are asked whether they smoke at all nowadays and, if so, how many cigarettes they smoke on weekdays and at weekends. This chapter will look briefly at cigarette consumption but will mainly focus on smoking status and the percentages of adults who were:

- current smokers,
- ex-smokers, or
- who had never (i.e. never or only occasionally) smoked.

4.3 Cigarette smoking status in relation to sex and age

Sex

Men were more likely than women to be current cigarette smokers (29% compared with 26%). They were also more likely than women to be heavier smokers (11% of men smoked 20 or more a day compared with 7% of women). A lower proportion of men than women said that they had never smoked, that is that they had never or only occasionally smoked: just over two fifths of men said they had never smoked compared with over half of women. (**Table 4.1**)

Age

For both sexes, the proportion of current smokers was generally lower among the older age-groups. For example, 39% of men

Figure 4.1 Cigarette smoking status by age and sex: adults aged 16 and over

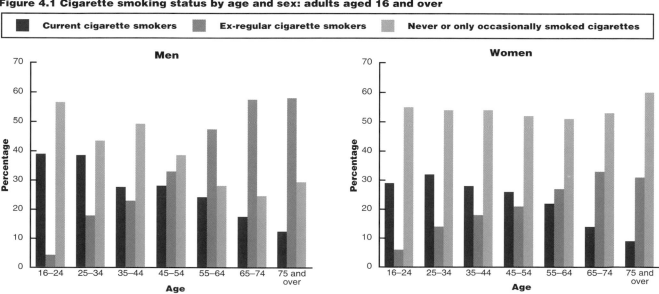

Base numbers are given in Table 4.1.

aged 16–24 were current smokers compared with 13% of men aged 75 or over. The corresponding proportions for women were lower but followed the same pattern, falling from 29% to 9%. However, part of the fall in the proportions of current smokers in older age-groups will be attributed to higher mortality rates due to smoking, as well as a move towards giving up as smoking has affected health.

Not surprisingly, older people were more likely than younger people to be ex-cigarette smokers. In the older age-groups (those aged 65 and over), around three-fifths of men and a third of women were ex-smokers of cigarettes. This compares with less than one tenth of those aged 16–24 (4% of men and 6% of women) and a quarter of those aged 35–44 (23% of men and 18% of women).

For women, there was very little difference by age in the proportions who had never regularly smoked. However, for men, the proportions tended to be lower in the older age-groups; 57% of men aged 16-24 had never regularly smoked compared with 30% of men aged 75 and over. (**Figure 4.1 and Table 4.1**)

Trends by sex and age

In 1998, the HEMS included for the first time people aged 75 and over. Provided that people in this age-group are excluded from the 1998 data, we can compare smoking prevalence for all three years of the survey (1995, 1996 and 1998). Table 4.2 shows that there is no significant difference between smoking prevalence over the three years. (**Table 4.2**)

4.4 Cigarette smoking status in relation to other demographic and socio-economic characteristics of individuals

Age-standardisation

As with previous HEMS surveys, in 1998, smoking behaviour was also explored in relation to a number of other characteristics – for example, marital status, employment status, social class, income, and qualification level. However, each of these variables is also related to the respondent's age (for example, higher proportions of younger respondents would be single, and of older respondents married or widowed). Therefore, it is helpful to take account of this by age-standardising the data.

Tables 4.3 – 4.15 present age-standardised data and show the actual, or 'observed', percentages as well as the percentage that would be expected, given the age composition of the subgroup. The ratio of these two percentages indicates whether the observed percentage is higher (if it is greater than 100) or lower (if it is less than 100) than would be expected on the basis of age alone. The tables also indicate if the ratio of observed to expected values is significantly different from 100. If it does differ significantly this suggests that the observed variation is not explained by age alone. For further details on age-standardisation see Appendix C in this report.

Marital status

For both sexes, smoking prevalence was highest among single people (38% were current smokers). However, for men, this was largely explained by age - single men being younger and more

likely to smoke than older men. For both men and women, the prevalence among the widowed, divorced and separated was also higher than would be expected given their age alone. Prevalence was lowest among married people. For example, among men, a quarter of those who were married or cohabiting were smokers compared with over a third of non-married men. Taking into account the age structure of the groups, married people of both sexes were significantly less likely to smoke than would be predicted by their age alone.

Single people were least likely to be ex-cigarette smokers (9% of single men and 10% of single women, compared with 36% of men and 21% of women who were married or cohabiting, and similar or higher proportions of those who were widowed, divorced or separated). Among women, this difference could be explained by the age structure of the group, but among men even taking account of the fact that single men tend to be younger than married men, there were still significant differences in the proportion of ex-smokers by marital status.

Among men, the highest percentage of those who had never smoked were single but this was mainly explained by the age composition of this group. Among women, however, taking into account the age structure of the groups, a higher proportion of married or cohabiting and a lower proportion of widowed, divorced or separated respondents had never regularly smoked than would be predicted by the age structure alone. (**Table 4.3**)

Social class

In line with other research, the HEMS 1998 survey confirmed that smoking prevalence was lowest among those in the professional groups and highest among those in manual social classes.[6] For both men and women, those classified in Social Classes I/II were least likely to be current smokers (21% of men and 20% of women, compared with at least 31% of men and women in other social classes). Among women, prevalence in Social Class III (non-manual) was also relatively low with only 22% being current smokers.

For men only, the non-manual social classes were the most likely to have never regularly smoked: at least 45% had never smoked compared with 35% or fewer of manual social classes. After taking into account the age structure of the different groups, there were still significant differences in smoking behaviour between people from different social classes. (**Table 4.4**)

Gross household income

Smoking prevalence decreased as gross household income increased. The highest prevalence was among men and women with a gross household income of under £5,000 (48% of men and 32% of women). This income group were also the least likely to have never regularly smoked. Conversely, men and women in the highest income band were least likely to smoke and most likely to have never smoked. All of these differences between income bands were significant even after age distributions were taken into account. (**Table 4.5**)

Economic activity

Smoking prevalence varied with economic activity. Overall, the highest proportions of current smokers were among the unemployed and the lowest among the economically inactive. However, because of the small numbers of unemployed in the sample, these differences were only statistically significant for unemployed men (45% of unemployed men smoked compared with 30% of the men who were working). This pattern largely reflects the age of the groups - for example, the economically inactive tend to be older and older people are less likely to be current smokers. However, even when the age structure of the groups was taken into account, employed men were significantly less likely to smoke and more likely to have never smoked, than would be predicted by age alone. (Table 4.6)

Highest qualification level

The general pattern for both sexes was of increasing smoking prevalence as qualification level decreased. Respondents who were qualified to 'A' level standard or above were least likely to be current smokers, with just over a fifth smoking, and most likely to have never smoked. This association remained even after age was taken into account. Those without qualifications were most likely to be ex-smokers but this was mainly due to age - given that older people have fewer qualifications. (Table 4.7)

Housing tenure

Those who lived in owner-occupied accommodation were less likely than those in rented accommodation (particularly local authority housing) to be current smokers. A quarter of men and one fifth of women who lived in owner-occupied housing were current smokers, around half the proportion of those in rented accommodation. This association remained even after age was taken into account. Those who lived in privately rented housing were least likely to be ex-smokers. However, given that people in this type of housing are usually younger rather than older, the difference was mainly a result of age.

Respondents who lived in owner-occupied housing were the most likely to have never regularly smoked cigarettes, with 44% of men and 60% of women never having smoked compared with 26% of men and 38% of women who lived in local authority housing. Even after allowing for the age structure of the groups, there were still significant differences in the proportions who had never regularly smoked by tenure. (Table 4.8)

4.5 Cigarette smoking status in relation to household type and social environment

Previous HEMS reports have mainly concentrated on the demographic and socio-economic variables outlined in Section 4.4, above. However, with the 1998 HEMS, additional information was collected on the social environment, and in addition a new analysis variable was created - household type. In this section, the links between these variables and smoking behaviour are investigated. The new variables, described in detail in Chapter 2, were as follows:

- Household type.
- Personal support group - that is, the number of people the respondent could call on at a time of serious personal crisis.
- Community activity - that is, participation in the last two weeks in adult education, voluntary or community groups or religious activities.
- Satisfaction with amount of control over decisions affecting own life.

- Perceived ability to influence decisions affecting the neighbourhood.
- Neighbourhood social capital score - derived from level of respondents' agreement with statements about their neighbourhood (see Appendix C).
- Area deprivation category - based on the HEMS area deprivation score for postcode sectors, which takes into account the 1991 Census rates of unemployment, car ownership, overcrowding and social class (see Appendix C).

These factors were just as strongly related to smoking behaviour as were those discussed earlier, such as social class, income, qualifications and tenure. There were associations with many of the variables, especially community activity, whether the respondent agreed that 'I am satisfied with the amount of control I have over decisions that affect my life', neighbourhood social capital score, and area deprivation category, and, for women, household type.

Household type

Among women, lone mothers were the household type most likely to smoke and least likely to have never smoked and this was regardless of age patterns. Over half of them smoked, almost twice the proportion for the next highest group of women (those who lived with one or more adults and dependent children). Dorsett and Marsh (1998) explain the high prevalence of smoking among lone parents as being associated with hardship and its attendant characteristics: social or private tenancy; unemployment; receipt of benefits; and leaving school early and without qualifications.[7] Although, smoking prevalence among male lone parents was high, the sample of respondents was too small to draw any conclusions, as the differences for men were not statistically significant. (Table 4.9)

Personal support group

For both men and women, there were very few significant differences by size of personal support group. However, although the sample numbers were very small, half of men who said that they could not call upon anyone in a crisis were current cigarette smokers. Even after taking age into account, this was significantly higher than among men with other sizes of support group. (Table 4.10)

Community activity

Smoking prevalence was lower among those who were active in their local community than among those who were not active. Less than a fifth of these respondents were smokers, compared with around a third of respondents who were not active in their community, and this was significant even after the age structure of the groups had been taken into account. Respondents who were active in the community were also most likely to have never smoked, with 53% of men and 61% of women who were active having never smoked, compared with 38% of men and 50% of women who were not active in their community.

Similarly, never having smoked was associated with involvement in the local community. Those who were involved were more likely than expected on the basis of age alone to have never smoked. (Table 4.11)

Control over decisions that affect own life

Respondents were asked whether they agreed or disagreed with the following statement:

'I am satisfied with the amount of control I have over decisions that affect my life'.

After taking account of age, those who disagreed with the statement were more likely to be smokers than those who agreed (over a third compared with around a quarter of those who agreed). **(Table 4.12)**

Neighbourhood social capital score

Respondents with a low neighbourhood social capital score were more likely than other respondents to be current smokers (39% of men and 33% of women compared with at least 29% of men and 26% of women with a higher score). There was a clear pattern of smoking prevalence falling steadily as the neighbourhood social capital score increased, although this was more marked for women with only 18% of women with a very high neighbourhood social capital score being current smokers. This pattern held even after the age structure of the groups had been taken into account. These results for women are consistent with those shown by Cooper et al[8] who in analysing the Health and Lifestyles Survey, found that smoking among women was similarly associated with a neighbourhood social capital score derived for that survey. The HEMS results suggest that there may also be an association for men but to a lesser extent. **(Table 4.14)**

Area deprivation category

Smoking prevalence increased with area deprivation, and respondents living in the more deprived area types were most likely to be current smokers. This pattern was especially noticeable for women, with a third of women in the two most deprived area types being current smokers compared with a quarter or fewer of those in more affluent areas. Even after allowing for the age structure of the respondents who lived in the five area types, there were wide differences by area type. **(Table 4.15)**

4.6 Assessing the relative importance of different characteristics associated with cigarette smoking status

The previous sections have shown that a number of variables are associated with the likelihood of a person being a smoker but, of course, many of these factors will be inter-related. This section uses logistic regressions to look at the relative importance of the different factors associated with being a current cigarette smoker, and with never having smoked.

Odds ratios and logistic regression

Logistic regression is a multivariate technique which can be used to predict the odds of a behaviour occurring for people with different combinations of the characteristics. Odds are the ratio of the probability that an event will occur (for example, being a smoker) to the probability that an event will not occur. This technique shows the effect of each of the independent variables on the dependent variable (the health behaviour in question), while holding all of the others constant.

The columns headed 'multiplying factors' can be thought of as 'weights'; they represent the factor by which the odds of someone being a current smoker or never having smoked increase with the attribute shown compared with a reference category. For each variable, the reference category (shown with a value of 1.00) was taken to be the first category for each attribute. The baseline odds shown at the top of each table represent the average odds for the respondents with all of the reference categories shown.[9] For each category of the variable, a 95% confidence interval is also shown. If the interval contains the value 1.00, then that odds ratio is not significantly different from the reference category. Undue weight should not be given to the significance or otherwise of particular categories, as this depends to some extent on which was chosen as the reference category. A more detailed explanation of logistic regression is given in Appendix C.

Two sets of logistic regressions were carried out, the first included the variables discussed in Section 4.4, and the second included the new variables discussed in Section 4.5. Once Model 2 had been run to identify significant variables it was re-run to obtain relative odds for only those variables which had been significant (that is, those which had an independent association with smoking behaviour)[10].

Logistic regression model including the demographic and socio-economic variables - Model 1

Table 4.16 shows the first logistic regression model, with the two dependent variables being current smoking and never having smoked. Figure 4.2 shows which demographic and socio-economic variables had independent effects in Model 1.

All the variables except economic activity had an independent effect on the likelihood of being a current smoker, and all except economic activity and household income on the likelihood of never having smoked. Looking first at the model for being a current smoker, having controlled for all the other variables, men had higher odds than women and the widowed, divorced and separated had higher odds than single or married people. The pattern of odds for being a current smoker decreased with age and increased with increasing social class and household income. Those with 'A' level or higher qualifications had lower odds than

Figure 4.2 Logistic regression Model 1 for cigarette smoking - variables with significant independent effects

	Current cigarette smoker	Never smoked cigarettes
Demographic and socio-economic variables:		
Sex	*	*
Age	*	*
Marital status	*	*
Social class	*	*
Gross household income	*	-
Economic activity	-	-
Highest qualification level	*	*
Housing tenure	*	*

* Has an independent effect

- Has no independent effect

those with fewer qualifications of being a current smoker. The odds for those living in privately rented or local authority housing were almost twice as high as for those living in owner occupied accommodation. These results were all consistent with the analysis shown in Section 4.4.

As might be expected, the pattern of odds of being a current smoker, for these variables, was the converse of those for never having smoked. The slight exceptions to this were for age and marital status. The pattern of odds by age for never having smoked cigarettes was not as linear as for the model for current smokers. Among the age-groups, the highest odds were for those aged 75 and over but also for those aged 35–44, whereas the lowest were for respondents aged 55–64. In addition, single, rather than married, respondents were the most likely to have never smoked. (**Table 4.16**)

Logistic regression model including all the analysis variables – Model 2

Model 2 included the additional variables discussed in Section 4.5. Full details of the logistic regression analysis are shown in Table 4.17. The variables which had significant independent effects are shown in Figure 4.3.

The retention by the model of many of the variables from Section 4.5 reflects how strongly some of these variables were associated with smoking behaviour. In addition to the other variables which were not significant for current smoking, after the new variables were added, sex was dropped from Model 2. This suggests that some of the new variables may be correlated with sex. For

example, Section 4.5 showed that household type, neighbourhood social capital score and area deprivation were more strongly related to smoking behaviour for women than for men. Furthermore, in Model 2, income was no longer independently associated with being a current smoker. Further testing of Model 2 suggested that this was because of the inclusion of area deprivation, and that area deprivation was acting as a proxy for income.

Looking first at the model for being a current smoker, the pattern of odds for the demographic and socio-economic variables was similar to Model 1. A possible exception was marital status, where married or cohabiting people were least likely to be current smokers but also slightly less likely than the widowed, divorced, or separated to have never smoked. Having controlled for all the other variables, in model 2, for categories of the household type variable, lone parents had the highest odds of being current smokers (1.42) and those who lived in a household with other adults and children had the lowest odds (0.86). Respondents who were not active in the community had odds of being current smokers which were almost twice as high as for respondents who were active in the community. Respondents who felt that they did not have control over the decisions which affected their lives had the highest odds of being current smokers for this variable (1.49). On the other hand, people who were undecided whether they could influence decisions that affected their neighbourhood also had the lowest odds of being current smokers. The odds of being a current smoker increased with decreasing neighbourhood social capital score. Those who lived in more affluent area types had lower odds of being current smokers than those who lived in more deprived area types.

Again, as would be expected, for those variables which were common to both the smoking measures, the pattern of odds were the converse of each other. However, two variables were significant for never having smoked but not for being a current smoker. These were sex and personal support group. Holding other variables constant, the odds for women never having smoked were almost twice as high as those for men. Respondents with a personal support group of one to three people had the highest odds of never having smoked (1.29), for this variable. (Table 4.17)

Figure 4.3 Logistic regression Model 2 for cigarette smoking - variables with significant independent effects

	Current cigarette smoker	Never smoked cigarettes
Demographic and socio-economic variables:		
Sex	-	*
Age	*	*
Marital status	*	*
Social class	*	-
Gross household income	-	-
Economic activity	-	-
Highest qualification level	*	*
Housing tenure	*	*
Household type	*	*
Social environment variables:		
Personal support group	-	*
Community activity	*	*
Satisfaction with control over own life decisions	*	*
Influence over decisions affecting neighbourhood	*	-
Neighbourhood social capital score	*	*
Area deprivation category	*	*

* Has an independent effect

\- Has no independent effect

4.7 Wanting to give up and intentions to give up smoking

Respondents were asked whether they would like to give up smoking altogether. They were also asked to say which of the following statements applied to them:

- I intend to give up smoking within the next month.
- I intend to give up smoking within the next six months.
- I intend to give up smoking within the next year.
- I intend to give up smoking but not in the next year.
- I am unlikely to give up smoking.

This section explores the intentions towards giving up smoking by sex, age and the number of cigarettes currently smoked. However, this brief exploration does not touch upon the wider analysis variables used earlier in this chapter. Further analysis could investigate the relationship between giving up and intentions to give up smoking by the wider range of factors.

Wanting to give up smoking, and age

The proportion of smokers saying they would like to give up smoking was higher in the middle age-groups than in the very oldest or youngest age-groups. However, only among men were the differences by age statistically significant. This was mainly because of the small numbers of women smokers in each age-group. As discussed in previous HEMS reports, this pattern might be due to younger people feeling that they have time to give up and older smokers being the ones who have already tried and failed to give up. **(Table 4.18)**

Wanting to give up and the number of cigarettes smoked

Smokers who consumed more than 10 cigarettes a day were more likely than others to say that they wanted to give up smoking. Almost three-quarters of respondents who smoked this amount said that they would like to give up compared with less than two-thirds of those who smoked fewer cigarettes. **(Table 4.19)**

Intentions to give up, by age

For both sexes, the proportions saying that they intended to give up smoking in the next month or next six months was lowest among the older age-groups. The highest proportions saying that they intended to give up smoking in the next month were smokers aged under 35. However, the differences between other age-groups were not statistically significant and there were no further significant differences for the other intention statements. **(Table 4.20)**

Intentions to give up and the number of cigarettes smoked

The lightest smokers were the most likely to say that they intended to give up within the next month (15% of those who smoked fewer than 10 cigarettes a day compared with 7% of those with a higher consumption). Women who smoked 20 or more cigarettes per day were least likely to say that they planned to give up within the next six months (8% compared with at least 16% of those who smoked fewer cigarettes). Over half of those who smoked 20 or more cigarettes a day said that they were unlikely to give up smoking (50% of men and 58% of women). **(Table 4.21)**

Comparing Tables 4.19 and 4.21 shows that the heaviest smokers say that they wish to give up smoking but when asked about intentions say that they are unlikely to give up. This suggests that respondents may be being realistic about their intentions to give up smoking. If the two variables are compared, just over a quarter (27%) of respondents who said that they wanted to give up also said that they were unlikely to give up. The majority of those who did not want to give up said that they were unlikely to do so in the next year or at all (93%). The 1997 follow-up survey for HEMS showed how important wanting to give up smoking was. Smokers who in 1996 had said that they would like to give up were more likely than those who had no intentions to quit to have attempted to have given up smoking by the time of the follow-up survey[11]. **(Table 4.22)**

Notes and references

1. Callum C. *The UK smoking epidemic: deaths in 1995.* Health Education Authority (1998).

2. British Medical Association. *The BMA guide to living with risk.* Penguin (Harmondsworth: 1990).

3. Department of Health. *Smoking Kills: A white paper on tobacco.* TSO (London: 1998).

4. Department of Health. Saving Lives: *Our healthier nation.* TSO (London: 1999).

5. Department of Health. *Our Healthier Nation.* TSO (London: 1998).

6. *See* for example, Thomas M, Walker A, Wilmot A and Bennett N. *Living in Britain: results from the 1996 General Household Survey.* TSO (London: 1998).

7. Dorsett R and Marsh A. *The health trap: poverty, smoking and lone parenthood.* HEA/PSI (1998).

8. Cooper H, Arber S, Fee L, and Ginn J. *The influence of social support and social capital on health.* Health Education Authority (1999).

9. For example in Model 1, the odds of being a current cigarette smoker for people with different characteristics can be calculated by multiplying the baseline odds shown at the top of the table by the appropriate factors. So, for example, a single male aged 16–24, working in Social Class III (Non-Manual), and who has an income of between £10,000 and £19,999 and has 'A' Levels and is privately renting would have odds calculated as shown below:

    0.41 x 1.00 x 1.00 x 1.00 x 1.01 x 1.24 x 1.00 x 1.84 = 0.94.

    This would give odds of 0.94 to one that a person with these characteristics would be a current cigarette smoker.

10. Where a variable has missing values, for example social class, this adds to the missing cases in the overall model. Excluding the non-significant variables reduces the total missing cases thereby improving the precision of the multiplying factors.

11. Bridgwood A, Rainford L, Walker A with Hickman M and Morgan A. *All change? The Health Education Monitoring Survey one year on.* TSO (London: 1998).

Table 4.1   Cigarette smoking status by age and sex
Adults aged 16 and over

Age	16-24	25-34	35-44	45-54	55-64	65-74	75 and over	Total
Smoking status	%	%	%	%	%	%	%	%
Men								
Current cigarette smokers:								
Less than 10 a day	19	9	5	4	6	4	3	8
10, less than 20 a day	14	17	9	10	8	6	6	11
20 or more per day	6	13	13	14	10	7	3	11
Total current cigarette smokers*	39	39	28	28	24	18	13	29
Ex-regular cigarette smokers	4	18	23	33	48	58	58	30
Never or only occasionally smoked cigarettes	57	44	49	39	28	25	30	41
Base = 100%	*233*	*432*	*464*	*432*	*389*	*350*	*254*	*2554*
Women								
Current cigarette smokers:								
Less than 10 a day	17	12	8	6	6	4	4	8
10, less than 20 a day	18	12	9	11	10	6	4	10
20 or more per day	4	8	11	10	6	4	2	7
Total current cigarette smokers*	29	32	28	26	22	14	9	26
Ex-regular cigarette smokers	6	14	18	21	27	33	31	20
Never or only occasionally smoked cigarettes	55	54	54	52	51	53	60	54
Base = 100%	*272*	*631*	*572*	*463*	*406*	*447*	*458*	*3249*
All								
Current cigarette smokers:								
Less than 10 a day	18	11	6	5	6	4	3	8
10, less than 20 a day	16	14	9	10	9	6	5	11
20 or more per day	5	10	12	12	8	5	2	9
Total current cigarette smokers *	39	35	28	27	23	16	10	27
Ex-regular cigarette smokers	5	16	20	27	37	44	41	25
Never or only occasionally smoked cigarettes	56	48	52	46	40	40	49	48
Base = 100%	*505*	*1063*	*1036*	*895*	*795*	*797*	*712*	*5803*

* Includes those for whom number of cigarettes was not known.

Table 4.2   Cigarette smoking status by year and sex
Adults aged 16-74

Year	1995	1996	1998
Smoking status	%	%	%
Men			
Current cigarette smokers:			
Less than 10 a day	8	8	8
10, less than 20 a day	11	12	11
20 or more per day	11	11	11
Total current cigarette smokers*	31	31	30
Ex-regular cigarette smokers	28	28	28
Never or only occasionally smoked cigarettes	42	41	42
Base = 100%	*2117*	*2042*	*2300*
Women			
Current cigarette smokers:			
Less than 10 a day	9	9	9
10, less than 20 a day	11	12	11
20 or more per day	8	7	7
Total current cigarette smokers*	27	29	27
Ex-regular cigarette smokers	19	20	19
Never or only occasionally smoked cigarettes	53	52	53
Base = 100%	*2548*	*2600*	*2791*
All			
Current cigarette smokers:			
Less than 10 a day	9	9	8
10, less than 20 a day	11	12	11
20 or more per day	9	9	9
Total current cigarette smokers*	29	30	28
Ex-regular cigarette smokers	23	24	24
Never or only occasionally smoked cigarettes	47	46	48
Base = 100%	*4665*	*4642*	*5091*

* Includes those for whom number of cigarettes was not known.

Table 4.3 Cigarette smoking status by marital status and sex
Adults aged 16 and over

Cigarette smoking status	Current cigarette smoker			Ex-cigarette smoker			Never smoked			Base = 100%
	Observed %*	Expected %†	Obs/exp (%)†	Observed %*	Expected %†	Obs/exp (%)†	Observed %*	Expected %†	Obs/exp (%)†	
Marital status										
Men										
Single	38	36	104	9	14	67**	53	50	106	502
Married/cohabiting	26	28	93**	36	33	107**	38	39	99	1636
Widowed/divorced/ separated	35	23	155**	36	43	83**	29	34	85	416
Total	29	29	100	30	30	100	41	41	100	2554
Women										
Single	38	34	111**	10	11	87	52	54	96	554
Married/cohabiting	22	26	86**	21	21	102	56	53	106**	1668
Widowed/divorced/ separated	26	18	142**	27	27	100	48	55	86**	1027
Total	26	26	100	20	20	100	54	54	100	3249

* The percentages refer to the proportions of the subgroups reporting each smoking status, so do not add to 100.

† See Appendix C for a full explanation of age-standardisation.

** Age-standardised ratio is significantly different from 100, at the 95% level.

Table 4.4 Cigarette smoking status by social class on own current or last job and sex
Adults aged 16 and over

Cigarette smoking status	Current cigarette smoker			Ex-cigarette smoker			Never smoked			Base = 100%††
	Observed %*	Expected %†	Obs/exp (%)†	Observed %*	Expected %†	Obs/exp (%)†	Observed %*	Expected %†	Obs/exp (%)†	
Social class										
Men										
I & II	21	28	73**	34	32	107	45	39	114**	948
III (Non-manual)	31	32	98	22	26	85	47	42	111	274
III (Manual)	34	29	118**	32	32	100	34	39	87**	792
IV & V	38	31	125**	26	29	93	35	41	86**	466
Total	29	29	100	31	31	100	40	40	100	2480
Women										
I & II	20	26	75**	21	21	101	60	53	112**	830
III (Non-manual)	22	27	85**	22	20	106	56	53	105	1063
III (Manual)	31	25	124	19	22	87	50	53	94	292
IV & V	34	25	136**	21	22	97	45	53	84**	931
Total	26	26	100	21	21	100	53	53	100	3116

* The percentages refer to the proportions of subgroups reporting each level of smoking status, so do not add to 100.

† See Appendix C for a full explanation of age-standardisation.

** Age-standardised ratio is significantly different from 100, at the 95% level.

†† Members of the Armed Forces, persons in inadequately described occupations and persons who have never worked are excluded from this analysis and from the bases shown.

Table 4.5   Cigarette smoking status by gross household income and sex
Adults aged 16 and over

Cigarette smoking status	Current cigarette smoker			Ex-cigarette smoker			Never smoked			Base = 100%
	Observed %*	Expected %†	Obs/exp (%)†	Observed %*	Expected %†	Obs/exp (%)†	Observed %*	Expected %†	Obs/exp (%)†	
Gross household income										
Men										
£20,000 or more	26	32	83**	28	25	110**	46	43	107**	1093
£10,000-£19,999	31	28	108	30	33	94	39	39	99	683
£5,000-£9,999	31	23	132**	40	42	95	29	34	84**	440
Under £5,000	48	25	190**	29	39	75**	22	36	63**	197
Total	29	29	100	30	30	100	40	40	100	2413
Women										
£20,000 or more	21	28	73**	20	18	111**	60	54	111**	982
£10,000-£19,999	27	26	104	20	20	101	52	53	98	726
£5,000-£9,999	28	21	135**	22	25	89	49	54	91**	740
Under £5,000	32	22	150**	22	23	91	46	55	84**	545
Total	25	25	100	21	21	100	54	54	100	2993

*   The percentages refer to the proportions of the subgroups reporting each smoking status, so do not add to 100.

†   See Appendix C for a full explanation of age-standardisation.

**   Age-standardised ratio is significantly different from 100, at the 95% level.

Table 4.6   Cigarette smoking status by economic activity and sex
Adults aged 16 and over

Cigarette smoking status	Current cigarette smoker			Ex-cigarette smoker			Never smoked			Base = 100%
	Observed %*	Expected %†	Obs/exp (%)†	Observed %*	Expected %†	Obs/exp (%)†	Observed %*	Expected %†	Obs/exp (%)†	
Economic activity status										
Men										
Employed	30	32	96**	24	24	101	45	44	103**	1571
Unemployed	45	33	134	17	19	91	38	47	80	91
Economically inactive	24	22	110	44	45	99	31	33	95	889
Total	29	29	100	30	30	100	41	41	100	2551
Women										
Employed	28	29	97	18	17	107**	53	53	100	1786
Unemployed	40	32	125	6	15	38**	54	54	102	81
Economically inactive	20	19	106	24	26	95	55	55	100	1380
Total	26	26	100	20	20	100	54	54	100	3247

*   The percentages refer to the proportions of the subgroups reporting each smoking status, so do not add to 100.

†   See Appendix C for a full explanation of age-standardisation.

**   Age-standardised ratio is significantly different from 100, at the 95% level.

Table 4.7   Cigarette smoking status by highest qualification level and sex
Adults aged 16 and over

Cigarette smoking status	Current cigarette smoker			Ex-cigarette smoker			Never smoked			Base = 100%
	Observed %*	Expected %†	Obs/exp (%)†	Observed %*	Expected %†	Obs/exp (%)†	Observed %*	Expected %†	Obs/exp (%)†	
Highest qualification level										
Men										
'A' Level or above	23	30	77**	27	27	102	49	43	116**	1007
GCSE A-G or below	32	30	105	29	27	105	39	42	93**	908
No qualifications	36	25	147**	36	40	92	27	36	77**	639
Total	29	29	100	30	30	100	41	41	100	2554
Women										
'A' Level or above	22	28	77**	17	18	96	61	54	114**	897
GCSE A-G or below	27	28	97	19	18	103	54	54	101	1279
No qualifications	28	20	137**	25	25	100	47	54	86**	1067
Total	26	26	100	20	20	100	54	54	100	3243

*   The percentages refer to the proportions of the subgroups reporting each smoking status, so do not add to 100.

†   See Appendix C for a full explanation of age-standardisation.

**   Age-standardised ratio is significantly different from 100, at the 95% level.

Table 4.8   Cigarette smoking status by housing tenure and sex
Adults aged 16 and over

Cigarette smoking status	Current cigarette smoker			Ex-cigarette smoker			Never smoked			Base = 100%
	Observed %*	Expected %†	Obs/exp (%)†	Observed %*	Expected %†	Obs/exp (%)†	Observed %*	Expected %†	Obs/exp (%)†	
Housing tenure										
Men										
Owner-occupier	25	29	86**	31	30	101	44	41	109**	1889
Rents from local authority	45	28	160**	29	32	93	26	40	63**	365
Rents privately	41	32	129**	24	24	98	35	44	80**	295
Total	29	29	100	30	30	100	41	41	100	2549
Women										
Owner-occupier	20	26	77**	21	21	100	60	54	111**	2168
Rents from local authority	40	24	163**	22	21	106	38	54	70**	620
Rents privately	41	27	148**	16	18	89	43	54	79**	457
Total	26	26	100	20	20	100	54	54	100	3245

*   The percentages refer to the proportions of the subgroups reporting each smoking status, so do not add to 100.

†   See Appendix C for a full explanation of age-standardisation.

**   Age-standardised ratio is significantly different from 100, at the 95% level.

Table 4.9 Cigarette smoking status by household type and sex
Adults aged 16 and over

Cigarette smoking status	Current cigarette smoker			Ex-cigarette smoker			Never smoked			Base = 100%
	Observed %*	Expected %†	Obs/exp (%)†	Observed %*	Expected %†	Obs/exp (%)†	Observed %*	Expected %†	Obs/exp (%)†	
Household type										
Men										
One person household	34	26	132**	30	37	79**	36	37	98	591
Living with others (no dependent children)	29	28	102	32	33	99	39	39	100	1308
Living with others (with dependent children)	28	32	87**	25	22	117**	47	46	102	634
Lone adult (with dependent children)	[11]	-	-	[2]	-	-	[8]	-	-	21
Total	29	29	100	30	30	100	41	41	100	2554
Women										
One person household	22	21	103	28	35	79**	50	70	72**	963
Living with others (no dependent children)	22	25	90**	22	22	100	56	53	105**	1242
Living with others (with dependent children)	29	31	93	15	15	100	56	54	104	764
Lone adult (with dependent children)	56	32	177**	14	15	93	31	54	57**	280
Total	26	26	100	20	20	100	54	54	100	3249

*   The percentages refer to the proportions of the subgroups reporting each smoking status, so do not add to 100.

†   See Appendix C for a full explanation of age-standardisation.

** Age-standardised ratio is significantly different from 100, at the 95% level.

Table 4.10 Cigarette smoking status by size of personal support group and sex
Adults aged 16 and over

Cigarette smoking status	Current cigarette smoker			Ex-cigarette smoker			Never smoked			Base = 100%
	Observed %*	Expected %†	Obs/exp (%)†	Observed %*	Expected %†	Obs/exp (%)†	Observed %*	Expected %†	Obs/exp (%)†	
Personal support group										
Men										
9 or more people	30	30	99	30	29	105	40	41	97	579
4 - 8 people	27	29	93	31	29	104	42	41	102	1104
1 - 3 people	31	29	106	29	31	93	41	41	101	804
No support	50	28	177**	16	32	54**	33	40	82	55
Total	29	29	100	30	30	100	41	41	100	2542
Women										
9 or more people	28	26	108	22	21	104	51	54	95	692
4 - 8 people	24	26	93	21	20	104	55	54	102	1518
1 - 3 people	26	25	105	19	21	91	55	54	101	996
No support	29	24	116	23	23	98	48	53	94	35
Total	26	26	100	20	20	100	54	54	100	3241

* The percentages refer to the proportions of the subgroups reporting each smoking status, so do not add to 100.

† See Appendix C for a full explanation of age-standardisation.

** Age-standardised ratio is significantly different from 100, at the 95% level.

Table 4.11 Cigarette smoking status by community activity and sex
Adults aged 16 and over

Cigarette smoking status	Current cigarette smoker			Ex-cigarette smoker			Never smoked			Base = 100%
	Observed %*	Expected %†	Obs/exp (%)†	Observed %*	Expected %†	Obs/exp (%)†	Observed %*	Expected %†	Obs/exp (%)†	
Community activity										
Men										
Some community activity	17	29	58**	30	31	99	53	41	130**	576
No community activity	33	29	112**	30	30	100	38	41	91**	1978
Total	29	29	100	30	30	100	41	41	100	2554
Women										
Some community activity	18	25	73**	21	21	98	61	54	113**	1089
No community activity	29	26	113**	20	20	101	50	54	94**	2160
Total	26	26	100	20	20	100	54	54	100	3249

* The percentages refer to the proportions of the subgroups reporting each smoking status, so do not add to 100.

† See Appendix C for a full explanation of age-standardisation.

** Age-standardised ratio is significantly different from 100, at the 95% level.

Table 4.12 Cigarette smoking status by whether agrees with the statement 'I am satisfied with the amount of control I have over decisions that affect my life' and sex

Adults aged 16 and over

Cigarette smoking status	Current cigarette smoker			Ex-cigarette smoker			Never smoked			Base = 100%
	Observed %*	Expected %†	Obs/exp (%)†	Observed %*	Expected %†	Obs/exp (%)†	Observed %*	Expected %†	Obs/exp (%)†	
Whether satisfied with amount of control over decisions that affect life										
Men										
Agree	27	29	93**	29	30	99	44	41	106**	1894
Neither agree nor disagree	33	29	113	32	30	109	35	41	85	251
Disagree	37	29	127**	29	30	97	33	40	83**	397
Total	29	29	100	30	30	100	41	41	100	2542
Women										
Agree	24	26	94**	20	20	100	56	54	103**	2567
Neither agree nor disagree	27	26	103	21	20	104	52	54	97	294
Disagree	38	26	141**	20	20	100	43	54	80**	368
Total	26	26	100	20	20	100	54	54	100	3229

* The percentages refer to the proportions of the subgroups reporting each smoking status, so do not add to 100.

† See Appendix C for a full explanation of age-standardisation.

** Age-standardised ratio is significantly different from 100, at the 95% level.

Table 4.13 Cigarette smoking status by whether agrees with the statement 'I can influence decisions that affect my neighbourhood' and sex

Adults aged 16 and over

Cigarette smoking status	Current cigarette smoker			Ex-cigarette smoker			Never smoked			Base = 100%
	Observed %*	Expected %†	Obs/exp (%)†	Observed %*	Expected %†	Obs/exp (%)†	Observed %*	Expected %†	Obs/exp (%)†	
Whether can influence decisions that affect neighbourhood										
Men										
Agree	29	28	103	31	32	95	41	40	102	584
Neither agree nor disagree	24	31	78**	29	26	109	48	43	110**	652
Disagree	32	29	111**	30	30	98	38	41	93**	1294
Total	29	29	100	30	30	100	41	41	100	2530
Women										
Agree	24	25	96	22	21	104	54	54	100	775
Neither agree nor disagree	24	27	88**	19	19	97	58	54	107**	819
Disagree	28	25	109**	20	21	100	52	54	96**	1618
Total	26	26	100	20	20	100	54	54	100	3212

* The percentages refer to the proportions of the subgroups reporting each smoking status, so do not add to 100.

† See Appendix C for a full explanation of age-standardisation.

** Age-standardised ratio is significantly different from 100, at the 95% level.

Table 4.14   Cigarette smoking status by neighbourhood social capital score and sex
Adults aged 16 and over

Cigarette smoking status	Current cigarette smoker			Ex-cigarette smoker			Never smoked			Base = 100%
	Observed %*	Expected %†	Obs/exp (%)†	Observed %*	Expected %†	Obs/exp (%)†	Observed %*	Expected %†	Obs/exp (%)†	
Neighbourhood social capital score										
Men										
Very high	24	29	85	31	31	99	45	40	111	450
High	24	29	83**	32	31	103	44	40	110**	738
Medium	28	29	97	30	29	104	42	42	100	694
Low	39	30	130**	26	28	93	35	42	83**	661
Total	29	29	100	30	30	100	41	41	100	2543
Women										
Very high	18	25	73**	21	21	97	61	54	114**	578
High	22	25	90	21	21	98	57	54	105	903
Medium	26	26	102	21	20	106	52	54	97	888
Low	33	27	124**	19	19	98	48	54	89**	868
Total	26	26	100	20	20	100	54	54	100	3237

*   The percentages refer to the proportions of the subgroups reporting each smoking status, so do not add to 100.

†   See Appendix C for a full explanation of age-standardisation.

**   Age-standardised ratio is significantly different from 100, at the 95% level.

Table 4.15   Cigarette smoking status by area deprivation category and sex
Adults aged 16 and over

Cigarette smoking status	Current cigarette smoker			Ex-cigarette smoker			Never smoked			Base = 100%
	Observed %*	Expected %†	Obs/exp (%)†	Observed %*	Expected %†	Obs/exp (%)†	Observed %*	Expected %†	Obs/exp (%)†	
Area deprivation category										
Men										
1 More affluent	19	29	66**	33	30	111	48	41	116	491
2	26	29	89	31	30	102	44	41	107	460
3	31	29	105	29	30	95	41	41	100	653
4	36	30	123**	28	29	94	36	41	87	560
5 More deprived	35	30	117	29	29	99	37	42	89	390
Total	29	29	100	30	30	100	41	41	100	2554
Women										
1 More affluent	15	24	61**	23	22	105	62	54	115**	569
2	24	26	91	21	20	106	55	54	102	636
3	25	25	100	19	21	93	56	54	103	804
4	32	26	119**	20	20	102	48	54	90**	726
5 More deprived	34	27	130**	18	19	94	47	54	88**	514
Total	26	26	100	20	20	100	54	54	100	3249

*   The percentages refer to the proportions of the subgroups reporting each smoking status, so do not add to 100.

†   See Appendix C for a full explanation of age-standardisation.

**   Age-standardised ratio is significantly different from 100, at the 95% level.

Table 4.16   Logistic regression for cigarette smoking status variables - model 1.
Adults aged 16 and over

Characteristics	Number of cases	Current cigarette smoker		Never smoked	
Baseline odds		0.414		1.125	
		Multiplying factors	95% Confidence intervals	Multiplying factors	95% Confidence intervals
Sex					
Male (R)	2356	1.00		1.00	
Female	2878	0.80*	0.69 -0.92	1.85*	1.63 -2.10
Age					
16-24 (R)	346	1.00		1.00	
25-34	1002	0.90	0.68 - 1.18	0.94	0.72 - 1.23
35-44	988	0.65*	0.49 - 0.87	1.08	0.82 - 1.43
45-54	834	0.57*	0.42 - 0.77	0.89	0.67 - 1.18
55-64	729	0.37*	0.27 - 0.51	0.80	0.59 - 1.07
65-74	722	0.18*	0.12 - 0.25	0.81	0.60 - 1.09
75 and over	613	0.09*	0.06 - 0.13	1.22	0.89 - 1.67
Marital status					
Single(R)	851	1.00		1.00	
Married/cohabiting	3091	0.86	0.71 - 1.05	0.86	0.72 - 1.03
Widowed, divorced, separated	1292	1.32*	1.04 - 1.66	0.73*	0.60 - 0.91
Social class					
I & II (R)	1699	1.00		1.00	
III (Non-manual)	1236	1.01	0.83 - 1.24	1.16	0.98 - 1.37
III (Manual)	1016	1.44*	1.17 - 1.77	0.86	0.72 - 1.03
IV & V	1283	1.37*	1.11 - 1.69	0.92	0.77 - 1.11
Gross household income					
£20000 or more (R)	2032	1.00		-	- -
£10,000 - £19,999	1371	1.24*	1.04 - 1.47	-	- -
£5,000 - £9,999	1140	1.39*	1.11 - 1.74	-	- -
Under £5,000	691	1.54*	1.17 - 2.02	-	- -
Highest qualification level					
'A'Level or above (R)	1788	1.00		1.00	
GCSE A-G or below	1960	1.29*	1.09 - 1.53	0.70*	0.61 - 0.81
No qualifications	1486	1.73*	1.39 - 2.15	0.64*	0.53 - 0.77
Housing tenure					
Owner-occupier (R)	3674	1.00		1.00	
Rents local authority	901	1.86*	1.54 - 2.25	0.51*	0.43 - 0.60
Rents privately	659	1.84*	1.51 - 2.24	0.58*	0.48 - 0.69
Number of cases in the model		5234		5234	

* Significant at the 95% level.

(R) reference category

Table 4.17 Logistic regression for cigarette smoking status variables - model 2.
Adults aged 16 and over

Characteristics	Number of cases	Current cigarette smoker		Never smoked	
Baseline odds		0.182		1.929	
		Multiplying factors	95% Confidence intervals	Multiplying factors	95% Confidence intervals
Sex					
Male (R)	2515	-	- -	1.00	
Female	3201	-	- -	1.94*	1.73 - 2.18
Age					
16-24 (R)	346	1.00		1.00	
25-34	1002	0.81	0.61 - 1.08	0.95	0.73 - 1.23
35-44	988	0.67*	0.50 - 0.90	0.98	0.75 - 1.29
45-54	834	0.55*	0.40 - 0.75	0.81	0.61 - 1.07
55-64	729	0.37*	0.26 - 0.51	0.72*	0.54 - 0.97
65-74	722	0.21*	0.15 - 0.30	0.71*	0.53 - 0.97
75 and over	613	0.10*	0.07 - 0.15	0.99	0.72 - 1.36
Marital status					
Single(R)	851	1.00		1.00	
Married/cohabiting	3091	0.91	0.70 - 1.18	0.68*	0.54 - 0.86
Widowed, divorced, separated	1292	1.30*	1.03 - 1.66	0.77*	0.62 - 0.95
Social class					
I & II (R)	1699	1.00		-	- -
III (Non-manual)	1236	1.01	0.83 - 1.23	-	- -
III (Manual)	1016	1.44*	1.18 - 1.76	-	- -
IV & V	1283	1.35*	1.10 - 1.65	-	- -
Highest qualification level					
'A'Level or above (R)	1788	1.00		1.00	
GCSE A-G or below	1960	1.21*	1.02 - 1.44	0.76*	0.67 - 0.87
No qualifications	1486	1.62*	1.31 - 2.01	0.68*	0.58 - 0.80
Housing tenure					
Owner-occupier (R)	3674	1.00		1.00	
Rents local authority	901	1.72*	1.43 - 2.06	0.59*	0.50 - 0.69
Rents privately	659	1.83*	1.52 - 2.21	0.63*	0.53 - 0.75
Household type					
One person household (R)	1512	1.00		1.00	
Living with others (no dependent children)	2516	1.03	0.79 - 1.34	1.18	0.94 - 1.49
Living with others Lone parent	297	1.42*	1.04 - 1.92	0.48*	0.36 - 0.65

continued

Table 4.17 *(Continued)* **Logistic regression for cigarette smoking status variables - model 2.**
Adults aged 16 and over

Characteristics	Number of cases	Current cigarette smoker		Never smoked	
Baseline odds		**0.414**		**1.125**	
		Multiplying factors	95% Confidence intervals	Multiplying factors	95% Confidence intervals
Personal support group					
9 or more people (R)	1255	-	-	1.00	
4-8 people	2601	-	-	1.13	0.98 - 1.30
1-3 people	1771	-	-	1.29*	1.11 - 1.51
No support	89	-	-	1.22	0.76 - 1.95
Community activity					
Some community activity (R)	1646	1.00		1.00	
No community activity	4070	1.76*	1.50 - 2.06	0.68*	0.60 - 0.77
Whether satisfied with amount of control over decisions that affect life					
Agree (R)	4423	1.00		1.00	
Neither agree nor disagree	537	1.11	0.89 - 1.38	0.89	0.74 - 1.07
Disagree	756	1.49*	1.24 - 1.79	0.67*	0.57 - 0.80
Whether can influence decisions that affect neighbourhood					
Agree (R)	1317	1.00		-	-
Neither agree nor disagree	1414	0.76*	0.63 - 0.91	-	-
Disagree	2765	0.90	0.76 - 1.06	-	-
Neighbourhood social capital score					
Very High (R)	1013	1.00		1.00	
High	1625	1.05	0.85 - 1.29	0.95	0.81 - 1.12
Medium	1570	1.12	0.92 - 1.38	0.85	0.72 - 1.01
Low	1508	1.50*	1.22 - 1.84	0.75*	0.63 - 0.89
Area deprivation category					
1 More affluent (R)	1054	1.00		1.00	
2	1085	1.45*	1.15 - 1.83	0.84*	0.70 - 1.00
3	1431	1.51*	1.21 - 1.87	0.85	0.72 - 1.01
4	1271	1.73*	1.39 - 2.16	0.71*	0.59 - 0.84
5 More deprived	875	1.56*	1.23 - 1.99	0.78*	0.64 - 0.95
Number of cases in the model		5496		5716	

* Significant at the 95% level.

(R) reference category

Table 4.18 Whether current smokers would like to give up smoking altogether by age and sex
Current cigarette smokers aged 16 and over

Age	16-24	25-34	35-44	45-54	55-64	65-74	75 and over	Total
Whether current smokers would like to give up smoking altogether	%	%	%	%	%	%	%	%
Men								
Yes	65	75	73	78	56	60	22	69
No	30	19	24	18	37	33	78	26
Don't know	6	6	3	4	7	7	-	5
Base = 100%	*97*	*164*	*137*	*122*	*102*	*67*	*33*	*722*
Women								
Yes	69	72	74	70	56	55	44	68
No	18	22	23	29	39	40	44	26
Don't know	13	6	4	1	4	4	11	6
Base = 100%	*118*	*228*	*170*	*134*	*96*	*68*	*43*	*857*
All								
Yes	67	74	73	74	56	58	34	68
No	24	20	23	23	38	37	60	26
Don't know	9	6	3	3	6	6	6	6
Base = 100%	*215*	*392*	*307*	*256*	*198*	*135*	*76*	*1579*

Table 4.19 Whether would like to give up smoking by number of cigarettes currently smoked per day and sex
Current cigarette smokers aged 16 and over

Number of cigarettes smoked per day	0 - 9	10 - 19	20 or more	All*
Whether would like to give up smoking	%	%	%	%
Men				
Yes	62	71	72	69
No	33	24	23	26
Don't know	6	5	5	5
Base = 100%	*174*	*265*	*279*	*718*
Women				
Yes	61	71	72	68
No	28	26	24	26
Don't know	11	3	4	6
Base = 100%	*265*	*339*	*252*	*856*
All				
Yes	62	71	72	68
No	30	25	23	26
Don't know	8	4	5	6
Base = 100%	*439*	*604*	*531*	*1574*

* Includes a few smokers who did not say how many cigarettes a day they smoked.

Table 4.20   When smokers intend to give up smoking by age and sex
Current cigarette smokers aged 16 and over

Age	16-24	25-34	35-44	45-54	55-64	65-74	75 and over	Total
When smokers intend to give up smoking	%	%	%	%	%	%	%	%
Men								
Within the next month	17	10	6	6	6	8	5	9
Within the next six months	19	22	14	9	9	4	-	15
Within the next year	19	18	15	18	6	8	5	16
Intends to give up but not in the next year	24	24	21	24	11	10	14	21
Unlikely to give up smoking	20	27	43	43	68	69	76	39
Base = 100%	*97*	*162*	*135*	*121*	*100*	*67*	*33*	*715*
Women								
Within the next month	16	12	5	6	9	3	8	10
Within the next six months	20	15	16	12	8	9	2	14
Within the next year	22	15	18	14	6	7	4	15
Intends to give up but not in the next year	22	24	19	17	12	10	8	19
Unlikely to give up smoking	20	34	41	51	65	70	79	43
Base = 100%	*117*	*226*	*165*	*133*	*95*	*67*	*42*	*845*
All								
Within the next month	17	10	6	6	7	6	5	9
Within the next six months	20	19	15	10	8	6	1	15
Within the next year	20	17	17	16	6	8	4	15
Intends to give up but not in the next year	23	24	20	21	12	10	10	20
Unlikely to give up smoking	20	30	42	47	67	70	79	41
Base = 100%	*214*	*388*	*300*	*254*	*195*	*134*	*75*	*1560*

Table 4.21 When smokers intend to give up smoking by number of cigarettes currently smoked per day and sex

Current cigarette smokers aged 16 and over

Number of cigarettes smoked per day	0 - 9	10 - 19	20 or more	All*
When smokers intend to give up smoking	%	%	%	%
Men				
Within the next month	15	7	7	9
Within the next six months	20	16	10	15
Within the next year	15	19	12	16
Intends to give up but not in the next year	18	24	21	21
Unlikely to give up smoking	32	33	50	39
Base = 100%	*173*	*262*	*276*	*711*
Women				
Within the next month	15	7	6	9
Within the next six months	17	16	8	14
Within the next year	16	16	11	15
Intends to give up but not in the next year	18	20	17	19
Unlikely to give up smoking	33	41	58	43
Base = 100%	*262*	*336*	*246*	*844*
All				
Within the next month	15	7	7	9
Within the next six months	19	16	9	15
Within the next year	16	18	12	15
Intends to give up but not in the next year	18	22	19	20
Unlikely to give up smoking	33	37	53	41
Base = 100%	*435*	*598*	*522*	*1555*

* Includes a few smokers who did not say how many cigarettes a day they
  smoked.

Table 4.22 When smokers intend to give up smoking by whether they want to give up smoking

Current cigarette smokers aged 16 and over

Whether to give up smoking	Wants to give up smoking	Does not want to give up smoking	Don't know	Total
When smokers intend to give up smoking	%	%	%	%
Within the next month	13	1	7	9
Within the next six months	20	2	10	14
Within the next year	20	3	11	15
Intends to give up but not in the next year	21	16	28	20
Unlikely to give up smoking	27	77	44	41
Base = 100%	*1056*	*427*	*77*	*1560*

5 Drinking

Summary of main findings

■ Mean weekly alcohol consumption was higher for men (18.4 units) than for women (7.7 units per week).

■ The age-groups with the highest mean alcohol consumption were those aged 16–34 among men (just over 22 units per week) and those aged 16–24 among women (just over 13 units). (Section 5.3)

■ Among men, mean weekly alcohol consumption was highest for those in Social Classes IV/V and among women, for those in Social Classes I/II. (Section 5.4)

■ Having taken account of age, drinking behaviour varied in relation to a number of demographic and socio-economic factors. The likelihood of drinking over 21 units per week for men and over 14 units for women was relatively greater among those with a gross household income of £20,000 or more. The proportions drinking these amounts were also greater for women in Social Classes I/II, women who were single and women with 'A' levels or higher qualifications. (Sections 5.4 and 5.5)

■ Conversely, having taken account of age, the likelihood of being a non-or occasional drinker was relatively greater among those who were in Social Classes IV/V, those with a gross household income below £10,000, the economically inactive, those who had no qualifications and women who lived alone. (Sections 5.4 and 5.5)

■ These specific measures of alcohol consumption were associated with only a few of the factors describing people's social environment. After taking account of age, the likelihood of drinking over 21 units per week for men and over 14 units for women was relatively greater for the small numbers of men with no personal support, men who lived alone, women who lived with other adults but no children, and men who were not active in their local community. The likelihood of being a non-or occasional drinker was relatively greater for those with a personal support group of 1–3 people and for men who were active in the community.

■ Logistic regression analysis was used to look at the relative importance of the different characteristics. It showed that characteristics of the respondent's social environment, such as whether they were happy with the amount of control they had over their own life, and whether their area was classified as deprived, were much less strongly related to drinking behaviour than were social class, income and tenure. (Section 5.5)

■ Significant factors in predicting the odds of drinking more than 21 units per week for men and 14 units for women were: sex, age, income, community activity, size of personal support group and household type. (Section 5.6)

continued

■ Those most likely to agree that 'drinking was an important part of having a good social life' and that 'it's OK to get drunk from time to time' were men, younger people, and those who drank more than 21 units per week (men) and 14 units per week (women). (Section 5.7)

■ Those most likely to agree that they felt 'comfortable drinking soft drinks when their friends were drinking alcohol' were women, older people, and those who were non- or occasional drinkers. (Section 5.7)

5.1 Alcohol consumption and health

Sustained excessive drinking can affect both physical and mental health. It causes several diseases such as cirrhosis of the liver and (especially when combined with the use of tobacco and/or 'paan') cancer of the mouth, throat, and gullet. Excessive alcohol consumption can increase the risk of high blood pressure, strokes and possibly heart disease. It is also a contributory factor in some accidents and can cause psychological problems such as depression, suicide and amnesia[1,2].

There is also evidence that modest alcohol consumption can be beneficial in protecting against coronary heart disease (CHD) for men over 40 and women past the menopause.

Building upon the earlier Green Paper *Our Healthier Nation*, the White Paper *Saving Lives: Our Healthier Nation* outlined four main priority areas for improvement in health - cancer, CHD and strokes, accidents, and mental illness[3,4]. The White Paper also confirmed the Government's intention to develop a new strategy to tackle alcohol misuse. It sets out the three main aims for the strategy as:

- to encourage people who drink to do so sensibly in line with our [Department of Health] guidance, so as to avoid alcohol-related problems
- to protect individuals and communities from anti-social and criminal behaviour related to alcohol misuse
- to provide services of proven effectiveness that enable people to overcome their alcohol misuse problems.

Previous HEMS reports have briefly described the associations between alcohol consumption and demographic and socio-economic characteristics such as marital status, employment status, social class, and qualification level. This chapter focuses on results from the 1998 HEMS and looks at alcohol consumption in relation to these personal characteristics and to respondents' social environment. It also looks at attitudes towards drinking.

5.2 Measurement of alcohol consumption

In order to measure alcohol consumption, HEMS uses a similar methodology to that developed for use by the General Household Survey (GHS) and the Health Survey for England (HSE). As in previous years, respondents were asked about six types of alcoholic drink, how often they consumed each type, and how much they usually consumed on any one day. From this information, an estimate of the average number of units usually consumed per week can be made[5]. This information on estimated units consumed per week is then grouped into bands of alcohol consumption (AC) levels.

It is known that surveys which collect data on reported drinking behaviour underestimate the amount of alcohol consumed when compared to estimates based on alcohol sales. Respondents may unintentionally underestimate the amount they drink in two main ways. Firstly, they may undercount the amount they drink at home. Secondly, respondents may have problems in recalling the amount they have drunk in any one day or on any one occasion, either due to general memory effects or due to the amount of alcohol that they consumed[6].

The HEMS surveys were set up in the wake of the 1992 White Paper *Health of the Nation*[7]. This report set recommendations for alcohol consumption based upon weekly levels. The levels were a maximum of 21 units per week for men and 14 units per week for women. In 1995, another report, *Sensible drinking*[1], introduced daily benchmarks[8] in order to avoid the previous recommendations being interpreted as allowing 'binge' drinking. The Department of Health's advice on sensible drinking is now based on these daily benchmarks. Following the publication of *Saving Lives: Our Healthier Nation*, the Government is developing a new strategy to tackle alcohol misuse in all its forms.

This chapter will refer to usual mean weekly units consumed (including a nil consumption for non-drinkers as well as consumption for drinkers). The chapter also refers to alcohol consumption (AC) levels (in terms of units per week). The 1998 HEMS did not collect data on daily alcohol consumption. However, the use of weekly AC levels not only allows some comparability with previous HEMS reports but also identifies broad groups with different drinking patterns. The AC levels shown in the tables for this chapter relate to the following number of units usually consumed per week:

Less than one unit usually consumed per week/ non-drinker
1–21 units for men and 1–14 units for women
22–35 units for men and 15–25 units for women
36–50 units for men and 26–35 units for women
51 or more units for men and 36 or more units for women

In order to simplify findings this chapter will also refer to the pre-1995 recommended levels (i.e. over 21 units per week for men and over 14 units per week for women), but this is not shown explicitly in the tables.

It should be noted that the data include a few cases with very high estimates of weekly alcohol consumption. In all, 34 cases (26 men and 8 women), had alcohol consumption ranging from 101 to 268 units per week. Although the cases were spread across all age-groups, half of the respondents were aged under 35. The pattern of answers given was consistent and believable so there was no justification for excluding them from the data. The means shown here will be affected by the inclusion of these cases.

5.3 Alcohol consumption in relation to sex and age

Sex

Mean weekly alcohol consumption was higher for men (18.4 units per week) than for women (7.7 units). Women were more likely than men to be non- or occasional drinkers (28% of women compared with only 13% of men). Almost a third of men (30%) reported drinking more than 21 units per week, compared with just under a fifth (17%) of women who reported drinking more than 14 units per week. **(Table 5.1)**

Age

For both men and women, alcohol consumption was higher among those aged under 35 than it was among those aged 35–64, and was lowest among those aged 65 and over. Mean weekly consumption for men aged 16–34 was just over 22 units, compared with just under 11 units per week among men aged 75 and over. Women aged 16–24 had a consumption of 13.4 units per week, compared with 3.7 units for women aged 75 and over.

Figure 5.1 Alcohol consumption (mean usual weekly units) by age and sex: adults aged 16 and over

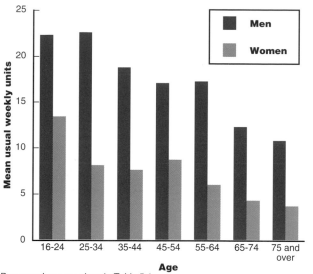

Base numbers are given in Table 5.1.

Men and women aged 75 and over were most likely to be non- or occasional drinkers. Just over a quarter of men (28%) and half of women (54%) aged 75 and over were, compared with only a tenth (8%) of men aged 25-34 and a sixth (17%) of women aged 16-24.

For both sexes, the proportions drinking more than 21/14 units per week were generally lower among the older age-groups. For example, almost two-fifths (38%) of men aged 25–34 drank over 21 units per week compared with just under a fifth (17%) of men aged 75 or over. Similarly, 34% of women aged 16–24 drank over 14 units per week compared with only 8% of women aged 75 and over. **(Figure 5.1 and Table 5.1)**

Trends by sex and age

In 1998, the HEMS included for the first time people aged 75 and over. Provided that respondents in this age-group are excluded from the 1998 data, we can compare alcohol consumption for three years of the survey (1995, 1996 and 1998). Table 5.2 shows that the pattern of mean weekly consumption and the number of units consumed per week, for men, is broadly the same across all three years. For women, mean weekly consumption rose from 7.0 units in 1995 to 7.7 units in 1996 and 8.1 units per week in 1998. The most recent GHS report showed that there had been a gradual increase in mean consumption for women since 1992[9]. The HEMS figures appear to fit into this pattern. **(Table 5.2)**

5.2 Alcohol consumption in relation to other demographic and socio-economic characteristics of individuals

Age-standardisation

The previous section showed that alcohol consumption varied with age. In this next section, alcohol consumption will be looked at in relation to a number of other characteristics of individuals, including for example, the respondents' marital status, employment status, social class, income, and qualification level. However, each of these variables is also related to the respondent's age (for example, higher proportions of younger respondents would be single, and of older respondents married or widowed). Therefore, it is helpful to take account of this by age-standardising the data.

Tables 5.5 to 5.17 present age-standardised data and show the actual, or 'observed', percentages as well as the percentage that would be expected, given the age composition of the subgroup. The ratio of these two percentages indicates whether the observed percentage is higher (if it is greater than 100) or lower (if it is less than 100) than would be expected on the basis of age alone. The tables also indicate if the ratio of observed to expected values is significantly different from 100. If it does differ significantly this suggests that the observed variation is not explained by age alone. For further details on age-standardisation see Appendix C in this report.

In addition, Tables 5.3 and 5.4 show the data in terms of the mean weekly units of alcohol consumed for each analysis variable. These mean amounts are not age-standardised.

Marital status

Among the different marital status groups, single people had the highest mean consumption (24.3 units per week for men and 12.6 units for women). Among men, married men had the lowest consumption of 16.4 mean weekly units. However, among women, the widowed, divorced or separated had the lowest mean consumption of 5.1 units per week. **(Table 5.3)**

After controlling for age, married or cohabiting men were less likely than expected to drink over 21 units per week and single women were more likely than expected to drink over 14 units per week. For example, 31% of single women drank over 14 units per week compared with only 11% of widowed, divorced or separated women. **(Table 5.5)**

Social class

For men, mean weekly alcohol consumption was higher for the manual social classes, with men in Social Classes IV/ V having the highest consumption (19.8 units per week). Conversely, for women, those in the professional classes had the highest level of consumption (8.7 units per week for women in Social Classes I / II and 8.2 units for women in Social Class III non-manual). **(Table 5.3)**

Women in Social Classes I / II were more likely than expected on the basis of age alone to drink over 14 units per week: 22% did so, compared with only 13% of women in Social Classes IV/ V. After taking age into account, both men and women in Social Classes IV/ V had a greater than expected likelihood of being non- or occasional drinkers. **(Table 5.6)**

Gross household income

The pattern of mean weekly consumption was U-shaped, with people in households with an annual income of £20,000 or more having the highest weekly consumption (20.2 units per week for men and 9.6 units for women). The pattern of mean consumption then fell as income decreased and rose again for those with a household income of under £5,000. This group had the second highest levels of consumption (16.9 units per week for men and 7.0 units for women). **(Table 5.3)**

Given their ages, people in households with an income of £20,000 or more were most likely to drink over 21/14 units per week. Around a third of men (35%) and a quarter of women (23%) drank at this level, compared with a fifth of men and a tenth of women with a household income of £5,000–£9,999. **(Table 5.7)**

Economic activity

Taking into account that the economically inactive are more likely to be older, it was not surprising that this group had the lowest mean weekly consumption (14.9 units for men and 5.2 for women). Although mean weekly consumption was highest for employed respondents, the difference compared with other economic status groups was only significant for women. **(Table 5.3)**

After allowing for age, there was little difference amongst men who were drinkers by economic activity. Among women, the employed were more likely than expected, given their ages, to drink over 14 units. For both men and women, being economically inactive meant a greater likelihood of being a non- or occasional drinker, even after taking into account the age structure of the groups. **(Table 5.8)**

Highest qualification level

For men there was very little significant difference in mean alcohol consumption by qualification level. However, among women, mean consumption was lowest amongst those without qualifications (4.8 units per week) and was around half that of women with 'A' levels or higher (9.4 units). **(Table 5.3)**

Among men, after taking account of their ages, there were few differences for drinkers by qualification level. However, among women, those with 'A' levels or higher qualifications were the most likely, and women with no qualifications the least likely, to drink over 14 units of alcohol per week.

Even allowing for qualifications being more common amongst younger age-groups, those who did not have any qualifications were more likely and those with 'A' levels or higher qualifications were less likely to be non- or occasional drinkers, than would be predicted by age alone. **(Table 5.9)**

Tenure

Mean weekly consumption was very different amongst those who lived in different types of rented accommodation. Those in local authority housing had the lowest mean weekly consumption (16.1 units per week for men and 5.7 units for women). Among women, mean consumption was significantly higher for those in privately rented housing (9.3 units per week) than for other tenure groups. **(Table 5.3)**

For both sexes, those who lived in local authority accommodation were less likely to drink over 21/14 units per week and more likely to be non- or occasional drinkers, than would be expected on the basis of age alone. Women who lived in owner-occupied housing were also more likely than expected to drink over 14 units per week. **(Table 5.10)**

5.5 Alcohol consumption in relation to household type and social environment

Previous HEMS reports have mainly concentrated on the demographic and socio-economic variables outlined in Section 5.4 above. However, with the 1998 HEMS, additional information was collected on the social environment of respondents, and in addition a new analysis variable was created - household type. In this section, alcohol consumption is

investigated in relation to these new variables. The new variables, which are described in detail in Chapter 2, were as follows:

- Household type.
- Personal support group – that is, the number of people the respondent could call on at a time of serious personal crisis.
- Community activity – that is, participation in the last two weeks in adult education, voluntary or community groups or religious activities.
- Satisfaction with amount of control over decisions affecting own life.
- Perceived ability to influence decisions affecting the neighbourhood.
- Neighbourhood social capital score – derived from level of respondents' agreement with statements about their neighbourhood (see Appendix C).
- Area deprivation category – based on the HEMS area deprivation score for postcode sectors, which takes into account the 1991 Census rates of unemployment, car ownership, overcrowding and social class (see Appendix C).

On the whole, these factors were much less strongly related to drinking behaviour than were those discussed earlier, such as marital status, social class, household income and tenure. The main associations were with household type, personal support group and community activity. There was very little difference in alcohol consumption by any of the other variables, including the HEMS area deprivation category. **(Tables 5.4, 5.11–5.17)**

Household type

Among men, those who lived with at least one other adult and dependent children had the lowest mean weekly consumption (16.5 units per week). Conversely, among women, those who lived alone had the lowest mean consumption (6.0 units). Women with the highest consumption were lone mothers (8.5 units per week) and women who lived with other adults but without children (8.1 units). **(Table 5.4)**

After taking account of the age structure of the groups, men who lived alone were more likely than other men to drink over 21 units per week and women who lived with other adults but no children were more likely than other women to drink over 14 units per week. Given their ages, those who lived with other adults and dependent children were least likely to drink over 21/ 14 units per week. **(Table 5.11)**

Personal support group

The pattern of mean weekly consumption by size of personal support group was U-shaped for both men and women. The highest mean consumption was for those with no personal social support (though, the sample of respondents was too small to draw any firm conclusions, as the differences were not statistically significant).

Respondents with a support group of nine or more people had the next highest mean consumption (21.0 units per week for men and 8.9 for women). Those with a support group of one to three people had the lowest mean consumption (16.2 units for men and 6.0 units for women). **(Table 5.4)**

Men with no social support were most likely to drink over 21 units per week (this was significant even though the sample size was small). Almost half (48%) of men did so, and this remained significant even after taking into account the age structure of the group. After controlling for age, those with a support group of one to three people were less likely than expected to drink over 21/14 units per week and more likely than expected to be non- or occasional drinkers. (**Table 5.12**)

Community activity

For both men and women, those who were active in their communities had lower mean alcohol consumption than those who were not active locally. Mean weekly consumption for men who took part in community activities was 15.8 units and for women 6.7 units. Conversely, those who were not active in their local community had mean consumption of 19.2 units per week for men and 8.1 units for women. (**Table 5.4**)

Among women drinkers, after taking account of their ages, there were few differences by level of community activity. However, among men, those who did not participate in any form of community activity were more likely than those who did participate to drink over 21 units per week (32% compared with 25%, respectively). Conversely, men who were active in the community were more likely than those who were not active in their communities to be non- or occasional drinkers. Both of these patterns held even after taking the age structure of the group into account. These findings for men and the mean consumption pattern for both sexes are consistent with other research which has shown that membership of a voluntary organisation is associated with decreased levels of current drinking[10]. (**Table 5.13**)

5.6 Assessing the relative importance of different characteristics associated with drinking behaviour

The previous sections have shown that a number of variables are associated with alcohol consumption but, of course, many of these factors will be inter-related. This section uses logistic regressions to look at the relative importance of the different factors associated with alcohol consumption. The following levels of usual weekly alcohol consumption have been used as the dependent variables for the logistic regression models[11]:

> 1–21 units for men and 1–14 units for women
> Over 21 units for men and 14 units for women
> Over 35 units for men and 25 units for women

Odds ratios and logistic regression

Logistic regression is a multivariate technique which can be used to predict the odds of a behaviour occurring for people with different combinations of the characteristics. Odds are the ratio of the probability that an event will occur (for example, having a certain alcohol consumption level) to the probability that an event will not occur. This technique indicates whether each analysis variable makes a significant contribution to explaining the variation in the outcome variable (the health behaviour in question), having held all of the other analysis variables under consideration constant.

Two sets of logistic regressions were carried out, the first included the variables discussed in Section 5.4, and the second

included the new variables discussed in Section 5.5. Once Model 2 had been run to identify significant variables it was re-run to obtain relative odds for only those variables which had been significant (that is, those which had an independent association with drinking behaviour).

The results of the logistic regression analysis are shown in Tables 5.18 and 5.19. The columns headed 'multiplying factors' can be thought of as 'weights'; they represent the factor by which the odds of someone drinking above a certain level of consumption increase with the attribute shown compared with a reference category. For each variable, the reference category (shown with a value of 1.00) was taken to be the first category for each attribute. The baseline odds shown at the top of each table represent the average odds for the respondents with all of the reference categories shown[12]. For each category of the variable, a 95% confidence interval is also shown. If the interval contains the value 1.00, then that odds ratio is not significantly different from the reference category. Undue weight should not be given to the significance or otherwise of particular categories, as this depends to some extent on which was chosen as the reference category. A more detailed explanation of logistic regression is given in Appendix C.

Logistic regression model including the demographic and socio-economic variables - Model 1

Table 5.18 shows the first logistic regression model for the three levels of alcohol consumption. Figure 5.2 shows the variables which had independent effects in Model 1.

Two of the variables, age and marital status, were significant for all three levels of consumption. For the higher levels, sex also had an independent effect. Qualification level and tenure were related to the likelihood of drinking 1–21 units (men) and 1–14 units (women). Household income was related to the likelihood of drinking more than this level per week. Social class was not retained as significant in any of the models; this may have been due to the different drinking patterns of men and women by social class as shown in Section 5.4.

The pattern of odds in the logistic regression model for those who drank over 21/14 units was similar to that for those who drank 35/25 units. Men had higher odds than women; single people had higher odds than those in other marital status groups; and the odds decreased as age increased. In addition, for the model for drinking over 21/14 units, the odds decreased as income level decreased.

The pattern of odds of drinking 1–21/1–14 units (the ratio of the probabilities of drinking at this level to not drinking at this level) was different from the other two models. For this model, those aged 25–34 had the highest odds (1.17) and those aged 75 or over had the lowest odds (0.76). Married or cohabiting people had higher odds than those in other marital status groups; those with 'A' level or higher qualifications had higher odds than those with lower qualifications; and those in owner-occupied housing had the highest odds (for this variable) of drinking at this level. (**Table 5.18**)

Logistic regression model including all the analysis variables - Model 2

Model 2 included all of the variables from Model 1 plus the new variables discussed in Section 5.5. The variables with significant independent effects are marked with an asterisk in Figure 5.3.

The pattern of odds for the demographic and socio-economic variables was similar to Model 1, except that marital status was not retained by the models for the two higher levels of consumption, probably reflecting the inclusion in these models of household type.

Of the new variables added in Model 2, household type and personal support group were included for all three consumption levels. Among the different household types, lone parents had the highest odds for drinking 1–21 /1–14 units (1.63). At the higher

consumption levels, one person households had odds which were higher than the odds for other household types.

Those with no personal support had lower odds of drinking 1–21/1–14 units than other personal support groups. Conversely, those with no personal support had the highest odds for the two other models. In addition, whether the respondent agreed that 'I can influence decisions that affect my neighbourhood' was included for drinking 1–21/1–14 units, and community activity was included in the models for the higher levels of consumption. **(Table 5.19)**

Figure 5.2 Logistic regression Model 1 for alcohol consumption - variables with independent effects

Usual number of units consumed per week

	1–21 for men/ 1–14 for women	Over 21 for men/ Over 14 for women	Over 35 for men/ Over 25 for women
Sex	-	*	*
Age	*	*	*
Marital status	*	*	*
Social class	-	-	-
Gross household income	-	*	-
Economic activity	-	-	-
Highest qualification level	*	-	-
Housing tenure	*	-	-

* Has an independent effect

- Has no independent effect

Figure 5.3 Logistic regression Model 2 for alcohol consumption - variables with independent effects

Usual number of units consumed per week

	1–21 for men/ 1–14 for women	Over 21 for men/ Over 14 for women	Over 35 for men/ Over 25 for women
Demographic and socio-economic variables:			
Sex	-	*	*
Age	*	*	*
Marital status	*	-	-
Social class	-	-	-
Gross household income	-	*	-
Economic activity	-	-	-
Highest qualification level	*	-	-
Housing tenure	*	-	-
Household type	*	*	*
Social environment variables:			
Personal support group	*	*	*
Community activity	-	*	*
Satisfaction with control over own life decisions	-	-	-
Influence over decisions affecting neighbourhood	*	-	-
Neighbourhood social capital score	-	-	-
Area deprivation category	-	-	-

* Has a independent effect

- Has no independent effect

5.7 Attitudes towards drinking

Respondents were asked whether they agreed or disagreed with the following statements:

- Drinking alcohol is an important part of having a good social life.
- I feel comfortable drinking soft drinks when my friends are drinking alcohol.
- It's OK to get drunk from time to time.

This section explores these attitudes towards drinking by sex, age and alcohol consumption level. However, this brief exploration does not touch upon the wider analysis variables used elsewhere in this chapter. It is recommended that further analysis should be conducted to investigate the relationship between attitudes towards drinking by a wider range of factors.

Sex

Men were more likely than women to agree with the first and last statements and women were more likely than men to agree with the middle one. For example:

- A third of men agreed that drinking alcohol was an important part of having a good social life compared with just under one fifth of women. Over two-thirds (68%) of women and only half (48%) of men disagreed with this statement.

- Four fifths of women but only two-thirds of men agreed with the statement 'I feel comfortable drinking soft drinks when my friends are drinking alcohol'.

- 56% of men compared with 43% of women agreed with the statement 'it's OK to get drunk from time to time'.

Age

Among women, those aged 16–24 were least likely to agree (76%) and most likely to disagree (17%) with the statement about soft drinks, compared with 83% and 12% respectively of all women.

Respondents aged 75 and over were least likely to agree that 'it's OK to get drunk from time to time'. Only 18% of men and 6% of women in this age-group agreed with the statement compared with 80% of men aged 25–34 and 74% of women aged 16–24. **(Table 5.20)**

Attitudes towards drinking and alcohol consumption

The above analysis suggests that, those groups most likely to drink alcohol or to have high levels of consumption were most likely to agree with the first and last statements and disagree with the middle one. However, Table 5.21 shows that there was a relatively high proportion of drinkers who did not hold positive views about drinking. For example, although almost two-thirds of men who drank 51 units or more a week and almost a half of women who drank 36 units or more agreed that 'drinking is an important part of having a good social life', a fifth of men and a third of women in this group disagreed with this statement. **(Table 5.21)**

Notes and References

1   Department of Health. *Sensible drinking: The report of an inter-departmental working group.* (1995).

2   Health Education Authority. *Health update: Alcohol.* Health Education Authority (London: 1997).

3   Department of Health. *Our Healthier Nation.* TSO (London: 1998).

4   Department of Health. *Saving Lives: Our healthier nation.* TSO (London: 1999).

5   The method used to calculate the alcohol consumption rating is to multiply the number of units of each type of drink consumed on a usual occasion by the frequency with which it was drunk, using the factors shown below, and totalling across all drinks.

    Multiplying factors for converting drinking frequency and number of units consumed on a usual occasion into number of units consumed per week.

Drinking frequency	Multiplying factor
Almost every day	7.0
or 6 days a week	5.5
or 4 days a week	3.5
Once or twice a week	1.5
Once or twice a month	0.375
Once every couple of months	0.115
Once or twice a year	0.029

    The number of units of each type of drink consumed on a 'usual' occasion is multiplied by the factor corresponding to the frequency with which the drink was consumed. In all except the first category, the factors are averages of the range of frequencies shown in the category, for example where a drink was consumed '3-4 days a week', the amount drunk was multiplied by 3.5.

6   Goddard E. Detailed recall of drinking behaviour over seven days. *Survey Methodology Bulletin* (1992), 31.

7   Department of Health. *Health of the Nation: a strategy for health in England.* HMSO (London: 1992).

8   The report sets benchmarks for sensible drinking, stating that regular consumption of between three and four units of alcohol a day for men and two to three units for women will not accrue significant health risk. However, consistently drinking this number of units a day is not recommended because of the progressive health risk this carries.

9   Thomas M, Walker A, Wilmot A and Bennett, N. *Living in Britain: results from the 1996 General Household Survey.* TSO (London: 1998).

10 Broman C L. Social Relationships and Health-Related Behaviour. *Journal of Behavioural Medicine* (1993), 16, 4.

11 There were two aims in choosing these levels of consumption: to explore the associations with the highest levels of consumption as defined by the survey (35/25 units per week) and to explore the associations with consumption below 22/15

units. A preliminary analysis of consumption below 22/15 units which included non- or occasional drinkers, had results which were simply the converse of the model for drinking over 21/14 units and since non-drinkers are a very different group to drinkers it was decided to only explore consumption between 1–21 and 1–14 units.

12 For example in Model 1, the odds of drinking 1–21 units for men and 1–14 units for women for people with different characteristics can be calculated by multiplying the baseline odds shown at the top of the table by the appropriate factors. So, for example, a single male aged 25-34, who holds 'A' level or higher qualifications and is privately renting would have odds calculated as shown below:

$$1.274 \times 1.00 \times 1.17 \times 1.00 \times 0.84 = 1.25$$

This would give odds of 1.25 to one that a man with these characteristics would drink 1-21 units per week.

Table 5.1 Alcohol consumption level (AC rating) and mean weekly number of units by age and sex
Adults aged 16 and over

Age	16-24	25-34	35-44	45-54	55-64	65-74	75 and over	Total
Alcohol consumption in units per week	%	%	%	%	%	%	%	%
Men								
Non-drinker	9	3	5	5	7	8	13	6
Under one	3	6	5	8	9	8	15	7
1-10	31	30	32	33	36	44	33	33
11-21	20	24	26	25	22	20	21	23
22-35	14	17	18	15	11	11	11	15
36-50	9	11	9	8	8	4	3	8
51 and over	14	10	6	6	7	5	3	7
Mean weekly units	*22.3*	*22.6*	*18.8*	*17.0*	*17.3*	*12.3*	*10.8*	*18.4*
Standard error of the mean	*1.0*	*0.8*	*0.7*	*0.6*	*0.9*	*0.7*	*0.8*	*0.3*
Median	*12.7*	*15.4*	*13.1*	*12.0*	*9.3*	*7.2*	*6.0*	*11.7*
Base=100%	*233*	*432*	*468*	*433*	*390*	*350*	*252*	*2558*
Women								
Non-drinker	8	7	8	10	13	18	24	12
Under one	9	11	12	12	26	24	30	16
1-7	30	44	43	38	34	36	28	37
8-14	19	20	22	19	13	14	9	17
15-25	19	13	9	12	10	6	7	11
26-35	7	3	3	6	1	2	1	3
36 and over	8	3	2	4	3	1	1	3
Mean weekly units	*13.4*	*8.1*	*7.6*	*8.6*	*6.0*	*4.3*	*3.7*	*7.7*
Standard error of the mean	*0.7*	*0.4*	*0.4*	*0.4*	*0.4*	*0.3*	*0.4*	*0.2*
Median	*8.3*	*4.5*	*4.1*	*4.7*	*1.6*	*1.1*	*0.4*	*3.4*
Base=100%	*272*	*630*	*571*	*463*	*406*	*445*	*457*	*3244*

**Table 5.2 Alcohol consumption level (AC rating) and
mean weekly number of units by year and sex**
Adults aged 16-74

Year	1995	1996	1998
Alcohol consumption in units per week	%	%	%
Men			
Non-drinker	6	7	6
Under one	6	7	6
1-10	34	31	33
11-21	23	24	23
22-35	16	17	15
36-50	8	7	8
51 and over	6	7	8
Mean weekly units	*18.2*	*18*	*18.9*
Standard error			
of the mean	*0.4*	*0.3*	*0.3*
Median	*11.5*	*12.2*	*12.1*
Base=100%	*2119*	*2007*	*2306*
Women			
Non-drinker	9	10	10
Under one	17	17	15
1-7	42	39	38
8-14	17	17	18
15-25	10	11	12
26-35	3	3	4
36 and over	2	3	3
Mean weekly units	*7.0*	*7.7*	*8.1*
Standard error of			
the mean	*0.2*	*0.2*	*0.2*
Median	*3.1*	*3.1*	*3.8*
Base=100%	*2548*	*2560*	*2787*

Table 5.3 Mean weekly alcohol consumption by demographic and socio-economic variables and sex
Adults aged 16 and over

	Mean weekly units		Bases = 100%*	
	Men	Women	Men	Women
Demographic and socio-economic variables				
Marital status				
Single	24.3	12.6	502	551
Married/cohabiting	16.4	7.0	1634	1668
Widowed, divorced, separated	19.6	5.1	417	1023
Social class (based on own current or last job)				
I & II	18.2	8.7	947	827
III (Non-manual)	17.2	8.2	273	1062
III (Manual)	18.9	6.8	789	292
IV & V	19.8	6.6	463	925
Gross household income (annual)				
£20,000 or more	20.2	9.6	1090	982
£10,000 - £19,999	17.7	6.7	680	723
£5,000 - £9,999	14.1	4.9	440	737
Under £5,000	16.9	7.0	196	542
Economic activity				
Employed	19.9	9.2	1566	1785
Unemployed	18.4	7.0	91	79
Economically inactive	14.9	5.2	886	1375
Highest qualification level				
'A' Level or above	19.4	9.4	1005	895
GCSE A-G or below	18.1	8.5	904	1276
No qualifications	17.2	4.8	636	1062
Housing tenure				
Owner-occupier	18.6	7.8	1888	2163
Rents from local authority	16.1	5.7	364	619
Rents privately	20.5	9.3	297	455
Total	18.4	7.7	2553	3242

*   Base for total is taken from marital status, bases may vary slightly for other items.

Table 5.4 Mean weekly alcohol consumption by household type and social environment variables and sex
Adults aged 16 and over

Household type and social environment variables	Mean weekly units		Bases = 100%*	
	Men	Women	Men	Women
Household type				
One person household	21.3	6.0	593	958
Living with others (no dependent children)	19.0	8.1	1304	1243
Living with others (with dependent children)	16.5	7.7	635	763
Lone adult (with dependent children)	[6.5]†	8.5	21	278
Personal support group				
9 or more people	21.0	8.9	577	689
4-8 people	18.2	8.1	1101	1515
1-3 people	16.2	6.0	804	993
No support	[30.1]†	[9.1]†	55	35
Community activity				
Some community activity	15.8	6.7	577	1087
No community activity	19.2	8.1	1976	2155
Whether agrees that 'I am satisfied with the amount of control I have over decisions that affect my life'				
Agree	18.5	7.4	1887	2558
Neither agree nor disagree	17.0	9.7	251	293
Disagree	19.2	8.4	397	368
Whether agrees that 'I can influence decisions that affect my neighbourhood'				
Agree	16.6	7.8	582	772
Neither agree nor disagree	19.1	8.1	652	814
Disagree	19.0	7.4	1291	1616
Neighbourhood social capital score				
Very High	19.2	6.7	449	572
High	17.3	7.6	735	902
Medium	18.3	7.3	692	889
Low	19.5	8.7	662	865
Area deprivation category				
1 More affluent	19.8	8.3	491	567
2	17.2	7.9	460	634
3	17.4	6.4	651	807
4	19.4	9.1	563	722
5 More deprived	18.5	6.6	388	512
Total	18.4	7.7	2525	3202

* Base for total is taken from whether agrees that 'I can influence decisions that affect my neighbourhood', bases may vary slightly for other items.

† The small bases for these categories imply that these means should be treated with caution.

Table 5.5 Alcohol consumption by marital status and sex
Adults aged 16 and over

Alcohol consumption / Marital status	Does not drink or drinks less than one unit per week			Drinks 1 - 21 units (men) / 1 - 14 units (women)			Drinks 22 - 35 units (men) / 15 - 25 units (women)			Drinks 36 - 50 units (men) / 26 - 35 units (women)			Drinks 51 units or more (men)/ 36 units or more (women)			Base = 100%
	Observed %*	Expected %†	Obs/exp (%)†	Observed %*	Expected %†	Obs/exp (%)†	Observed %*	Expected %†	Obs/exp (%)†	Observed %	Expected %*	Obs/exp (%)†	Observed %	Expected* %	Obs/exp (%)†	
Men																
Single	14	12	116	49	57	87**	13	15	88	10	9	108	14	11	132**	502
Married/cohabiting	12	13	94	60	57	106**	15	15	103	8	8	95	5	7	76**	1634
Widowed/divorced/separated	18	17	108	50	57	88	14	13	109	8	6	122	10	6	177**	417
Total	13	13	100	57	57	100	15	15	100	8	8	100	7	7	100	2553
Women																
Single	20	20	99	49	53	92**	18	16	114**	5	5	100	7	5	137**	551
Married/cohabiting	26	27	97	58	57	103**	10	11	97	3	3	103	2	3	75**	1668
Widowed/divorced/separated	42	39	107	47	49	97	7	8	86	2	2	84	2	2	115	1023
Total	28	28	100	54	54	100	11	11	100	3	3	100	3	3	100	3242

* The percentages refer to the proportion of the subgroups reporting each level of alcohol consumption, so do not add to 100.

† See Appendix C for a full explanation of age-standardisation.

** Age-standardised ratio is significantly different from 100, at the 95% level.

Table 5.6 Alcohol consumption by social class based on own current or last job and sex
Adults aged 16 and over

Alcohol consumption	Does not drink or drinks less than one unit per week			Drinks 1 - 21 units (men) / 1 - 14 units (women)			Drinks 22 - 35 units (men) / 15 - 25 units (women)			Drinks 36 - 50 units (men) / 26 - 35 units (women)			Drinks 51 units or more (men) / 36 units or more (women)			Base = 100%††
	Observed %*	Expected %†	Obs/exp (%)†	Observed %*	Expected %†	Obs/exp (%)†	Observed %*	Expected %†	Obs/exp (%)†	Observed %	Expected %*	Obs/exp (%)†	Observed %	Expected* %	Obs/exp (%)†	
Social class																
Men																
I & II	9	12	77**	59	58	102	18	15	116**	8	8	96	6	7	96	947
III (Non-manual)	10	11	91	62	57	109	12	15	81	10	9	122	5	8	60**	273
III (Manual)	14	12	110	56	57	97	15	15	99	8	8	100	8	7	109	789
IV & V	16	12	135**	54	57	96	12	15	80	8	8	94	10	8	120	463
Total	12	12	100	57	57	100	15	15	100	8	8	100	7	7	100	2472
Women																
I & II	18	26	71**	60	57	105	16	11	142**	4	3	112	2	3	88	827
III (Non-manual)	23	26	88**	58	55	106**	11	12	97	3	4	83	4	3	129	1062
III (Manual)	32	29	110	50	53	92	12	11	109	4	3	137	2	3	58	292
IV & V	39	29	134**	48	54	90**	7	11	62**	3	3	102	2	3	84	925
Total	27	27	100	55	55	100	11	11	100	4	4	100	3	3	100	3106

* The percentages refer to the proportion of the subgroups reporting each level of alcohol consumption, so do not add to 100.

† See Appendix C for a full explanation of age-standardisation.

** Age-standardised ratio is significantly different from 100, at the 95% level.

†† Members of the Armed Forces, persons in inadequately described occupations and persons who have never worked are excluded from this analysis and from the bases shown.

Table 5.7 Alcohol consumption by gross household income and sex
Adults aged 16 and over

Alcohol consumption	Does not drink or drinks less than one unit per week			Drinks 1 - 21 units (men) 1 - 14 units (women)			Drinks 22 - 35 units (men) / 15 - 25 units (women)			Drinks 36 - 50 units (men) / 26 - 35 units (women)			Drinks 51 units or more (men)/ 36 units or more (women)			Base = 100%
	Observed %*	Expected %†	Obs/exp (%)†	Observed %*	Expected %†	Obs/exp (%)†	Observed %*	Expected %†	Obs/exp (%)†	Observed %	Expected %*	Obs/exp (%)†	Observed %	Expected* %	Obs/exp (%)†	
Gross household income																
Men																
£20,000 or more	7	10	69**	58	57	102	19	16	117**	9	9	98	8	8	97	1092
£10,000-£19,999	12	13	94	60	58	104	12	15	85	9	8	107	7	7	104	682
£5,000-£9,999	27	16	169**	53	59	90**	8	13	65**	6	6	98	6	6	93	440
Under £5,000	21	15	139	53	58	92	11	14	79	7	7	89	8	6	138	197
Total	12	12	100	57	57	100	15	15	100	8	8	100	7	7	100	2411
Women																
£20,000 or more	14	22	65**	62	58	107**	16	12	124**	4	4	121	3	3	99	982
£10,000-£19,999	27	27	100	58	56	105	10	12	89	2	3	83	2	3	77	723
£5,000-£9,999	45	35	128**	44	51	86**	7	9	78	2	2	88	2	2	83	738
Under £5,000	44	35	127**	43	50	86**	6	10	62**	2	3	66	4	2	190	543
Total	28	28	100	55	55	100	11	11	100	3	3	100	3	3	100	2986

* The percentages refer to the proportion of the subgroups reporting each level of alcohol consumption, so do not add to 100.

† See Appendix C for a full explanation of age-standardisation.

** Age-standardised ratio is significantly different from 100, at the 95% level.

Table 5.8 Alcohol consumption by economic activity and sex
Adults aged 16 and over

Alcohol consumption	Does not drink or drinks less than one unit per week			Drinks 1 - 21 units (men) / 1 - 14 units (women)			Drinks 22 - 35 units (men) / 15 - 25 units (women)			Drinks 36 - 50 units (men) / 26 - 35 units (women)			Drinks 51 units or more (men) / 36 units or more (women)			Base = 100%
	Observed %*	Expected %†	Obs/exp (%)†	Observed %*	Expected %†	Obs/exp (%)†	Observed %*	Expected %†	Obs/exp (%)†	Observed %	Expected %*	Obs/exp (%)†	Observed %	Expected* %	Obs/exp (%)†	
Economic activity status																
Men																
Employed	8	11	76**	58	56	104**	16	16	104	10	9	104	7	8	94	1566
Unemployed	20	11	178	50	55	90	12	16	79	11	9	123	8	9	79	91
Economically inactive	23	18	131**	54	58	92**	11	12	90	5	6	81	8	6	124	886
Total	13	13	100	57	57	100	15	15	100	8	8	100	7	7	100	2543
Women																
Employed	20	23	88**	59	58	102	13	12	107**	4	4	113**	4	4	102	1785
Unemployed	24	20	117	59	58	101	14	14	106	1	4	16**	3	4	72	79
Economically inactive	42	38	111**	47	49	95**	8	9	84**	2	2	77	2	2	99	1375
Total	28	28	100	54	54	100	11	11	100	3	3	100	3	3	100	3239

* The percentages refer to the proportion of the subgroups reporting each level of alcohol consumption, so do not add to 100.

† See Appendix C for a full explanation of age-standardisation.

** Age-standardised ratio is significantly different from 100, at the 95% level.

Health in England 1998: investigating the links between social inequalities and health

Table 5.9 Alcohol consumption by highest qualification level and sex
Adults aged 16 and over

Highest qualification level	Does not drink or drinks less than one unit per week			Drinks 1 - 14 units (men) / 1 - 21 units (women)			Drinks 22 - 35 units (men) / 15 - 25 units (women)			Drinks 36 - 50 units (men) / 26 - 35 units (women)			Drinks 51 units or more (men) / 36 units or more (women)			Base = 100%
	Observed %*	Expected %†	Obs/exp (%)†	Observed %*	Expected %†	Obs/exp (%)†	Observed %*	Expected %†	Obs/exp (%)†	Observed %	Expected %*	Obs/exp (%)†	Observed %	Expected* %	Obs/exp (%)†	
Men																
'A' Level or above	8	12	66**	60	57	106**	16	16	104	9	9	108	7	8	93	1005
GCSE A-G or below	13	13	104	56	56	100	16	15	106	8	8	92	7	8	93	904
No qualifications	22	16	144**	52	58	89**	11	13	80	7	7	99	8	6	131	636
Total	13	13	100	57	57	100	15	15	100	8	8	100	7	7	100	2545
Women																
'A' Level or above	14	24	57**	62	57	108**	17	12	145**	4	4	112	3	3	94	895
GCSE A-G or below	24	25	95	58	56	103	11	12	90	4	4	116	4	3	105	1276
No qualifications	47	36	133**	43	50	86**	6	9	64**	1	3	50**	2	2	97	1062
Total	28	28	100	55	55	100	11	11	100	3	3	100	3	3	100	3233

* The percentages refer to the proportion of the subgroups reporting each level of alcohol consumption, so do not add to 100.

† See Appendix C for a full explanation of age-standardisation.

** Age-standardised ratio is significantly different from 100, at the 95% level.

Table 5.10 Alcohol consumption by housing tenure and sex
Adults aged 16 and over

Alcohol consumption	Does not drink or drinks less than one unit per week			Drinks 1 - 21 units (men) / 1 - 14 units (women)			Drinks 22 - 35 units (men) / 15 - 25 units (women)			Drinks 36 - 50 units (men) / 26 - 35 units (women)			Drinks 51 units or more (men) / 36 units or more (women)			Base = 100%
Housing tenure	Observed %*	Expected %†	Obs/exp (%)†	Observed %*	Expected %†	Obs/exp (%)§†	Observed %*	Expected %†	Obs/exp (%)†	Observed %	Expected %*	Obs/exp (%)†	Observed %	Expected* %	Obs/exp (%)†	
Men																
Owner-occupier	10	13	82**	59	57	103**	15	15	103	8	8	104	7	7	96	1888
Rents from local authority	25	14	177**	51	57	91	10	14	71**	7	8	89	7	7	95	364
Rents privately	16	12	129	49	55	88**	17	15	112	7	9	82	11	9	130	297
Total	13	13	100	57	57	100	15	15	100	8	8	100	7	7	100	2549
Women																
Owner-occupier	24	28	86**	58	55	105**	12	11	113**	3	3	106	2	3	83**	2163
Rents from local authority	46	30	152**	42	53	78**	7	11	62**	3	3	102	3	3	97	619
Rents privately	29	27	108	53	54	97	9	12	78	2	4	68	6	3	190**	455
Total	28	28	100	54	54	100	11	11	100	3	3	100	3	3	100	3237

* The percentages refer to the proportion of the subgroups reporting each level of alcohol consumption, so do not add to 100.

† See Appendix C for a full explanation of age-standardisation.

** Age-standardised ratio is significantly different from 100, at the 95% level.

Table 5.11 Alcohol consumption by household type and sex
Adults aged 16 and over

Alcohol consumption / Household type	Does not drink or drinks less than one unit per week			Drinks 1 - 21 units (men) / 1 - 14 units (women)			Drinks 22 - 35 units (men) / 15 - 25 units (women)			Drinks 36 - 50 units (men) / 26 - 35 units (women)			Drinks 51 units or more (men) / 36 units or more (women)			Base = 100%
	Observed %*	Expected %†	Obs/exp (%)†	Observed %*	Expected %†	Obs/exp (%)†	Observed %*	Expected %†	Obs/exp (%)†	Observed %	Expected %	Obs/exp (%)†	Observed %	Expected %*	Obs/exp (%)†	
Men																
One person household	16	15	108	50	57	87**	14	14	101	10	7	129	10	6	159**	593
Living with others (no dependent children)	13	14	92	57	57	100	14	14	101	8	8	102	8	7	113**	1304
Living with others (with dependent children)	12	10	115	59	56	105	16	17	99	8	9	90	4	8	59**	635
Lone adult (with dependent children)	[5]	-	-	[14]	-	-	[2]	-	-	[0]	-	-	[0]	-	-	21
Total	13	13	100	57	57	100	15	15	100	8	8	100	7	7	100	2553
Women																
One person household	42	47	91**	44	61	72**	8	11	75**	3	3	102	3	2	110	958
Living with others (no dependent children)	27	30	92**	53	53	102	13	11	113**	3	3	90	4	3	112	1243
Living with others (with dependent children)	22	20	113**	61	61	101	10	12	83**	4	4	110	2	3	59**	763
Lone adult (with dependent children)	22	19	111	60	61	99	11	13	86	2	4	71	5	3	151	278
Total	28	28	100	54	54	100	11	11	100	3	3	100	3	3	100	3242

* The percentages refer to the proportion of the subgroups reporting each level of alcohol consumption, so do not add to 100.

† See Appendix C for a full explanation of age-standardisation.

** Age-standardised ratio is significantly different from 100, at the 95% level.

Table 5.12 Alcohol consumption by size of personal support group and sex
Adults aged 16 and over

Alcohol consumption / Personal support group	Does not drink or drinks less than one unit per week			Drinks 1 - 21 units (men) / 1 - 14 units (women)			Drinks 22 - 35 units (men) / 15 - 25 units (women)			Drinks 36 - 50 units (men) / 26 - 35 units (women)			Drinks 51 units or more (men) / 36 units or more (women)			Base = 100%
	Observed %*	Expected %†	Obs/exp (%)†	Observed %*	Expected %†	Obs/exp (%)†	Observed %*	Expected %†	Obs/exp (%)†	Observed %	Expected* %	Obs/exp (%)†	Observed %	Expected* %	Obs/exp (%)†	
Men																
9 or more people	13	13	101	53	57	94	16	15	105	8	8	96	11	8	138**	579
4 - 8 people	11	13	83**	58	57	103	15	15	103	8	8	102	7	7	95	1102
1 - 3 people	15	13	119**	59	57	103	14	15	92	7	8	89	5	7	71**	804
No support	24	13	177	28	57	49**	12	15	87	23	8	275**	14	7	196	55
Total	13	13	100	57	57	100	15	15	100	8	8	100	8	7	100	2540
Women																
9 or more people	26	28	92	55	55	101	12	11	108	4	3	115	4	3	119	689
4 - 8 people	23	27	85**	57	55	105**	13	11	112**	3	3	92	4	3	116	1515
1 - 3 people	37	29	127**	50	54	93**	8	11	74**	3	3	104	2	3	57**	993
No support	38	29	133	44	55	81	12	10	113	2	3	63	4	3	137	35
Total	28	28	100	55	55	100	11	11	100	3	3	100	3	3	100	3232

* The percentages refer to the proportion of the subgroups reporting each level of alcohol consumption, so do not add to 100.

† See Appendix C for a full explanation of age-standardisation.

** Age-standardised ratio is significantly different from 100, at the 95% level.

Table 5.13 Alcohol consumption by community activity and sex
Adults aged 16 and over

Alcohol consumption	Does not drink or drinks less than one unit per week			Drinks 1 - 21 units (men) / 1 - 14 units (women)			Drinks 22 - 35 units (men) / 15 - 25 units (women)			Drinks 36 - 50 units (men) / 26 - 35 units (women)			Drinks 51 units or more (men) / 36 units or more (women)			Base = 100%
	Observed %*	Expected %†	Obs/exp (%)†	Observed %*	Expected %†	Obs/exp (%)†	Observed %*	Expected %†	Obs/exp (%)†	Observed %	Expected %*	Obs/exp (%)†	Observed %	Expected* %	Obs/exp (%)†	
Community activity																
Men																
Some community activity	17	13	125**	58	57	102	14	15	98	5	8	61**	6	7	89	577
No community activity	12	13	93	56	57	99	15	15	101	9	8	111**	8	7	103	1976
Total	13	13	100	57	57	100	15	15	100	8	8	100	7	7	100	2553
Women																
Some community activity	26	29	91**	58	55	105	12	11	109	3	3	93	2	3	60**	1087
No community activity	29	28	104	53	54	97**	11	11	96	4	3	103	4	3	118**	2155
Total	28	28	100	54	54	100	11	11	100	3	3	100	3	3	100	3242

* The percentages refer to the proportion of the subgroups reporting each level of alcohol consumption, so do not add to 100.

† See Appendix C for a full explanation of age-standardisation.

** Age-standardised ratio is significantly different from 100, at the 95% level.

Table 5.14 Alcohol consumption by whether agrees with the statement 'I am satisfied with the amount of control I have over decisions that affect my life' and sex

Adults aged 16 and over

Alcohol consumption	Does not drink or drinks less than one unit per week			Drinks 1 - 21 units (men) 1 - 14 units (women)			Drinks 22 - 35 units (men) / 15 - 25 units (women)			Drinks 26 - 35 units (women) Drinks 36 - 50 units (men) /			Drinks 51 units or more (men)/ 36 units or more (women)			Base = 100%
Whether agrees is satisfied with the amount of control over decisions that affect own life	Observed %*	Expected %†	Obs/exp (%)†	Observed %*	Expected %†	Obs/exp (%)†	Observed %*	Expected %†	Obs/exp (%)†	Observed %	Expected %*	Obs/exp (%)†	Observed %	Expected* %	Obs/exp (%)†	
Men																
Agree	12	13	97	57	57	100	15	15	99	8	8	102	8	8	102	1887
Neither agree nor disagree	12	12	94	57	57	100	19	15	126	7	8	83	5	7	72	251
Disagree	15	12	119	56	57	98	13	15	88	8	8	100	8	7	108	397
Total	13	13	100	57	57	100	15	15	100	8	8	100	7	7	100	2535
Women																
Agree	29	28	103	54	54	99	11	11	102	3	3	90	3	3	92	2558
Neither agree nor disagree	25	27	92	55	55	99	10	11	93	3	3	97	6	3	215**	293
Disagree	21	26	82**	60	56	108	10	11	92	6	3	168	2	3	69	368
Total	28	28	100	55	55	100	11	11	100	3	3	100	3	3	100	3219

* The percentages refer to the proportion of the subgroups reporting each level of alcohol consumption, so do not add to 100.

† See Appendix C for a full explanation of age-standardisation.

** Age-standardised ratio is significantly different from 100, at the 95% level.

Table 5.15 Alcohol consumption by whether agrees with the statement 'I can influence decisions that affect my neighbourhood' and sex
Adults aged 16 and over

Alcohol consumption	Does not drink or drinks less than one unit per week			Drinks 1 - 21 units (men) / 1 - 14 units (women)			Drinks 22 - 35 units (men) / 15 - 25 units (women)			Drinks 36 - 50 units (men) / 26 - 35 units (women)			Drinks 51 units or more (men) / 36 units or more (women)			Base = 100%
	Observed %*	Expected %†	Obs/exp (%)†	Observed %*	Expected %†	Obs/exp (%)†	Observed %*	Expected %†	Obs/exp (%)†	Observed %	Expected %*	Obs/exp (%)†	Observed %	Expected %	Obs/exp (%)†	
Whether can influence decisions that affect own neighbourhood																
Men																
Agree	14	13	104	59	57	103	15	15	104	7	8	83	5	7	79	582
Neither agree nor disagree	9	12	76**	60	56	106	14	15	92	10	9	112	7	8	94	652
Disagree	14	13	110	54	57	95**	15	15	103	8	8	100	8	8	112	1291
Total	13	13	100	57	57	100	15	15	100	8	8	100	8	7	100	2525
Women																
Agree	26	28	91	58	55	105	11	11	98	3	3	94	3	3	108	772
Neither agree nor disagree	23	26	87**	58	55	105	12	12	104	4	4	106	3	3	95	814
Disagree	32	29	111**	51	54	95**	11	11	98	3	3	100	3	3	99	1616
Total	28	28	100	54	54	100	11	11	100	3	3	100	3	3	100	3202

* The percentages refer to the proportion of the subgroups reporting each level of alcohol consumption, so do not add to 100.

† See Appendix C for a full explanation of age-standardisation.

** Age-standardised ratio is significantly different from 100, at the 95% level.

Table 5.16 Alcohol consumption by neighbourhood social capital score and sex
Adults aged 16 and over

Neighbourhood social capital score	Does not drink or drinks less than one unit per week			Drinks 1 - 21 units (men) / 1 - 14 units (women)			Drinks 22 - 35 units (men) / 15 - 25 units (women)			Drinks 36 - 50 units (men) / 26 - 35 units (women)			Drinks 51 units or more (men) / 36 units or more (women)			Base = 100%
	Observed %*	Expected %†	Obs/exp (%)†	Observed %*	Expected %†	Obs/exp (%)†	Observed %*	Expected %†	Obs/exp (%)†	Observed %	Expected %*	Obs/exp (%)†	Observed %	Expected %*	Obs/exp (%)†	
Men																
Very high	11	13	88	61	57	108	10	15	68**	9	8	114	8	7	112	449
High	12	13	91	56	57	99	18	15	122**	9	8	106	5	7	73**	735
Medium	13	13	100	56	57	99	15	15	101	8	8	99	8	7	105	692
Low	15	13	118	55	56	97	14	15	97	7	8	86	9	8	114	662
Total	13	13	100	57	57	100	15	15	100	8	8	100	7	7	100	2538
Women																
Very high	27	29	94	58	55	105	10	10	94	3	3	95	2	3	87	572
High	27	29	95	55	55	100	12	11	110	3	3	105	3	3	98	902
Medium	26	28	94	56	54	103	12	11	103	4	3	109	2	3	68	889
Low	31	27	115**	50	54	93**	11	12	91	3	4	90	5	3	139**	865
Total	28	28	100	54	54	100	11	11	100	3	3	100	3	3	100	3228

* The percentages refer to the proportion of the subgroups reporting each level of alcohol consumption, so do not add to 100.

† See Appendix C for a full explanation of age-standardisation.

** Age-standardised ratio is significantly different from 100, at the 95% level.

Table 5.17 Alcohol consumption by area deprivation category and sex
Adults aged 16 and over

Alcohol consumption	Does not drink or drinks less than one unit per week			Drinks 1 - 21 units (men) / 1 - 14 units (women)			Drinks 22 - 35 units (men) / 15 - 25 units (women)			Drinks 36 - 50 units (men) / 26 - 35 units (women)			Drinks 51 units or more (men) / 36 units or more (women)			Base = 100%
	Observed %*	Expected %†	Obs/exp (%)†	Observed %*	Expected %†	Obs/exp (%)†	Observed %*	Expected %†	Obs/exp (%)†	Observed %	Expected %*	Obs/exp (%)†	Observed %	Expected %	Obs/exp (%)†	
Area deprivation category																
Men																
1 More Affluent	8	14	63**	57	56	101	17	14	118	9	8	111	8	8	110	491
2	13	13	106	60	57	105	12	15	83	8	8	95	7	7	89	460
3	12	13	90	59	57	104	15	15	102	8	8	99	6	7	82	651
4	17	13	133**	52	57	92**	15	15	99	8	8	95	8	8	109	563
5 More Deprived	15	13	117	54	56	95	14	15	94	8	8	99	9	8	118	388
Total	13	13	100	57	57	100	15	15	100	8	8	100	7	7	100	2553
Women																
1 More Affluent	22	30	73**	58	54	107	13	11	128**	4	3	117	4	3	122	567
2	22	27	81**	60	55	108**	12	11	108	4	3	110	2	3	83	634
3	30	29	106	56	54	103	10	11	88	3	3	101	1	3	36**	807
4	31	28	114**	49	54	90**	12	12	103	4	3	109	4	3	140	722
5 More Deprived	36	27	133**	50	55	90**	8	11	71**	1	3	49**	4	3	144	512
Total	28	28	100	54	54	100	11	11	100	3	3	100	3	3	100	3242

* The percentages refer to the proportion of the subgroups reporting each level of alcohol consumption, so do not add to 100.

† See Appendix C for a full explanation of age-standardisation.

** Age-standardised ratio is significantly different from 100, at the 95% level.

Table 5.18 Logistic regression for alcohol consumption - model 1
Adults aged 16 and over

Characteristics	No. of cases	Drinking 1 - 21 units (men)/ 1 - 14 units (women)		Drinking over 21 units (men)/ 14 units (women)		Drinking over 35 units (men)/ 25 units (women)	
Baseline odds		**1.274**		**1.343**		**0.432**	
		Multiplying factors	95% confidence intervals	Multiplying factors	95% confidence intervals	Multiplying factors	95% confidence intervals
Sex							
Male (R)	2348	-	- -	1.00		1.00	
Female	2870	-	- -	0.46*	0.40 - 0.53	0.31*	0.25 - 0.38
Age							
16-24 (R)	342	1.00		1.00		1.00	
25-34	999	1.17	0.90 - 1.51	0.71*	0.54 - 0.94	0.83	0.58 - 1.20
35-44	987	1.15	0.88 - 1.51	0.61*	0.45 - 0.82	0.69	0.47 - 1.02
45-54	832	1.04	0.79 - 1.38	0.69*	0.51 - 0.93	0.78	0.52 - 1.15
55-64	727	0.92	0.69 - 1.23	0.54*	0.39 - 0.75	0.57*	0.37 - 0.87
65-74	720	1.13	0.84 - 1.51	0.39*	0.28 - 0.55	0.35*	0.22 - 0.55
75 and over	611	0.76	0.56 - 1.03	0.34*	0.23 - 0.49	0.22*	0.12 - 0.38
Marital status							
Single(R)	845	1.00		1.00		1.00	
Married/cohabiting	3086	1.39*	1.17 - 1.65	0.59*	0.48 - 0.72	0.54*	0.42 - 0.69
Widowed, divorced, separated	1287	1.11	0.91 - 1.36	0.83	0.65 - 1.06	0.80	0.58 - 1.11
Gross household income							
£20000 or more (R)	2029	-	- -	1.00		-	- -
£10,000 - £19,999	1365	-	- -	0.74*	0.63 - 0.88	-	- -
£5,000 - £9,999	1136	-	- -	0.53*	0.42 - 0.66	-	- -
Under £5,000	688	-	- -	0.51*	0.39 - 0.67	-	- -
Highest qualification level							
'A'Level or above (R)	1785	1.00		-	- -	-	- -
GCSE A-G or below	1953	0.89	0.78 - 1.01	-	- -	-	- -
No qualifications	1480	0.61*	0.52 - 0.71	-	- -	-	- -
Housing tenure							
Owner-occupier (R)	3667	1.00		-	- -	-	- -
Rents local authority	896	0.77*	0.66 - 0.91	-	- -	-	- -
Rents privately	655	0.84*	0.70 - 1.00	-	- -	-	- -
Number of cases in the model		5218		5225		5218	

* Significant at the 95% level.

(R) reference category

Table 5.19 Logistic regression for alcohol consumption - model 2
Adults aged 16 and over

Characteristics	No. of cases	Drinking 1 - 21 units (men)/ 1 - 14 units (women)		Drinking over 21 units (men)/ 14 units (women)		Drinking over 35 units (men)/ 25 units (women)	
Baseline odds		1.274		1.343		0.432	
		Multiplying factors	95% confidence intervals	Multiplying factors	95% confidence intervals	Multiplying factors	95% confidence intervals
Sex							
Male (R)	2400	-	- -	1.00		1.00	
Female	2981	-	- -	0.48*	0.42 - 0.55	0.36*	0.30 - 0.44
Age							
16-24 (R)	494	1.00		1.00		1.00	
25-34	1050	1.08	0.84 - 1.39	0.69*	0.53 - 0.89	0.73*	0.53 - 0.99
35-44	1023	1.10	0.85 - 1.44	0.59*	0.45 - 0.76	0.63*	0.45 - 0.87
45-54	883	1.02	0.77 - 1.34	0.57*	0.44 - 0.74	0.56*	0.41 - 0.78
55-64	777	0.94	0.70 - 1.25	0.41*	0.31 - 0.55	0.40*	0.28 - 0.57
65-74	787	1.16	0.87 - 1.57	0.29*	0.21 - 0.40	0.22*	0.15 - 0.33
75 and over	679	0.78	0.58 - 1.07	0.25*	0.18 - 0.36	0.15*	0.09 - 0.25
Marital status							
Single(R)	1031	1.00		-	- -	-	- -
Married/cohabiting	3260	1.42*	1.13 - 1.78	-	- -	-	- -
Widowed, divorced, separated	1402	1.06	0.87 - 1.30	-	- -	-	- -
Gross household income							
£20,000 or more (R)	2066	-	- -	1.00		-	- -
£10,000 - £19,999	1404	-	- -	0.75*	0.63 - 0.88	-	- -
£5,000 - £9,999	1175	-	- -	0.55*	0.44 - 0.69	-	- -
Under £5,000	736	-	- -	0.50*	0.38 - 0.66	-	- -
Highest qualification level							
'A'Level or above (R)	1883	1.00		-	- -	-	- -
GCSE A-G or below	2156	0.89	0.78 - 1.01	-	- -	-	- -
No qualifications	1654	0.63*	0.54 - 0.74	-	- -	-	- -
Housing tenure							
Owner-occupier (R)	4007	1.00		-	-	-	
Rents local authority	947	0.75*	0.64 - 0.87	-	-	-	
Rents privately	739	0.84	0.71 - 1.00	-	- -	-	- -
Household type							
One person household (R)	1507	1.00		1.00		1.00	
Living with others (no dependent children)	2508	1.01	0.81 - 1.27	0.68*	0.56 - 0.82	0.66*	0.53 - 0.82
Living with others (with dependent children)	1382	1.04	0.79 - 1.36	0.47*	0.38 - 0.58	0.43*	0.32 - 0.56
Lone parent	296	1.63*	1.23 - 2.16	0.65*	0.45 - 0.93	0.48*	0.29 - 0.80
Personal support group							
9 or more people (R)	1247	1.00		1.00		1.00	
4-8 people	2592	1.14	0.99 - 1.31	0.88	0.74 - 1.04	0.82	0.66 - 1.03
1-3 people	1766	1.00	0.86 - 1.16	0.70*	0.58 - 0.84	0.68*	0.53 - 0.88
No support	88	0.47*	0.29 - 0.75	1.35	0.81 - 2.25	1.51	0.85 - 2.68
Community activity							
Some community activity (R)	1543	-	- -	1.00		1.00	
No community activity	3838	-	- -	1.31*	1.12 - 1.53	1.58*	1.26 - 1.99
Whether agrees that 'I can influence decisions that affect my neighbourhood'							
Agree (R)	1352	1.00		-	- -	-	- -
Neither agree nor disagree	2886	1.04	0.89 - 1.21	-	- -	-	- -
Disagree	1455	0.89	0.78 - 1.02	-	- -	-	- -
Number of cases in the model		5218		5381		5769	

*   Significant at the 95% level.

(R) reference category

Health in England 1998: investigating the links between social inequalities and health   93

Table 5.20 Attitudes towards drinking by age and sex
Adults aged 16 and over

Age	16-24	25-34	35-44	45-54	55-64	65-74	75 and over	Total
Attitudes towards drinking	%	%	%	%	%	%	%	%
Men								
Drinking alcohol is an important part of having a good social life								
Agree	37	32	30	29	37	34	41	33
Neither agree nor disagree	20	21	22	20	15	13	13	19
Disagree	43	47	48	51	48	53	47	48
I feel comfortable drinking soft drinks when my friends are drinking alcohol								
Agree	62	60	64	67	65	66	66	64
Neither agree nor disagree	15	10	8	10	10	10	13	11
Disagree	23	30	28	22	26	24	21	26
It is OK to get drunk from time to time								
Agree	74	80	66	47	36	24	18	56
Neither agree nor disagree	15	11	14	17	11	8	12	13
Disagree	11	9	20	36	53	68	70	31
*Base=100%**	*233*	*431*	*464*	*431*	*389*	*349*	*252*	*2549*
Women								
Drinking alcohol is an important part of having a good social life								
Agree	19	17	14	14	17	17	22	17
Neither agree nor disagree	18	18	17	15	10	13	12	15
Disagree	63	64	69	71	73	70	65	68
I feel comfortable drinking soft drinks when my friends are drinking alcohol								
Agree	76	80	85	83	87	88	85	83
Neither agree nor disagree	6	6	4	4	5	6	6	5
Disagree	17	14	12	12	8	6	8	12
It is OK to get drunk from time to time								
Agree	74	73	51	35	25	10	6	43
Neither agree nor disagree	14	12	17	16	10	8	7	13
Disagree	12	15	31	49	65	82	87	44
*Base=100%**	*272*	*630*	*572*	*463*	*406*	*445*	*453*	*3241*
All								
Drinking alcohol is an important part of having a good social life								
Agree	28	25	22	22	27	25	29	25
Neither agree nor disagree	19	20	19	18	12	13	13	17
Disagree	53	56	58	61	61	62	59	58
I feel comfortable drinking soft drinks when my friends are drinking alcohol								
Agree	69	69	74	75	76	78	78	74
Neither agree nor disagree	11	8	6	8	7	8	9	8
Disagree	20	22	20	17	17	14	13	18
It is OK to get drunk from time to time								
Agree	74	76	59	41	30	17	10	49
Neither agree nor disagree	15	12	16	17	10	8	9	13
Disagree	11	12	26	42	59	76	81	38
*Base=100%**	*505*	*1061*	*1036*	*894*	*795*	*794*	*705*	*5790*

*   Bases are shown from 'It's Ok to get drunk from time to time' - bases may vary slightly for other items.

Table 5.21 Attitudes towards drinking by alcohol consumption level and sex
Adults aged 16 and over

Alcohol consumption level	Does not drink or occasional drinker	Drinks 1-21 (men)/1-14 units (women)	Drinks 22-35 (men)/15-25 units (women)	Drinks 36-50 (men)/26-35 units (women)	Drinks 51 units or more (men)/36 units or more (women)	Total
Attitudes towards drinking	%	%	%	%	%	%
Men						
Drinking alcohol is an important part of having a good social life						
Agree	9	29	45	52	63	33
Neither agree nor disagree	9	20	25	17	15	19
Disagree	82	51	29	32	22	48
I feel comfortable drinking soft drinks when my friends are drinking alcohol						
Agree	83	69	51	44	36	64
Neither agree nor disagree	7	10	13	13	11	11
Disagree	10	20	36	44	52	26
It is OK to get drunk from time to time						
Agree	23	54	68	77	82	56
Neither agree nor disagree	19	14	12	6	7	13
Disagree	58	33	20	17	11	31
Base=100%*	*344*	*1442*	*373*	*202*	*180*	*2541*
Women						
Drinking alcohol is an important part of having a good social life						
Agree	8	15	33	37	46	17
Neither agree nor disagree	9	16	23	17	20	15
Disagree	83	68	45	45	34	68
I feel comfortable drinking soft drinks when my friends are drinking alcohol						
Agree	92	84	67	67	55	83
Neither agree nor disagree	4	5	10	6	10	5
Disagree	4	11	23	27	34	12
It is OK to get drunk from time to time						
Agree	23	46	63	60	73	43
Neither agree nor disagree	12	14	10	11	11	13
Disagree	64	40	27	29	16	44
Base=100%*	*967*	*1748*	*335*	*95*	*86*	*3231*
All						
Drinking alcohol is an important part of having a good social life						
Agree	8	22	40	47	58	25
Neither agree nor disagree	9	18	24	17	17	17
Disagree	83	60	36	36	26	58
I feel comfortable drinking soft drinks when my friends are drinking alcohol						
Agree	90	77	58	51	42	74
Neither agree nor disagree	5	8	12	11	11	8
Disagree	6	16	30	39	47	18
It is OK to get drunk from time to time						
Agree	23	50	66	72	79	49
Neither agree nor disagree	14	14	11	8	8	13
Disagree	62	36	23	20	13	38
Base=100%*	*1311*	*3190*	*708*	*297*	*266*	*5772*

*   Bases are shown from 'It's Ok to get drunk from time to time' - bases may vary slightly for other items.

Physical activity

Summary of main findings

- In 1998, 27% of men and 35% of women aged 16 and over were classified as sedentary - they participated less than once a week in 30 minutes or more of at least moderate-intensity activity. (Section 6.3)

- Overall, a similar proportion took part in at least moderate-intensity activity on five or more days a week, but the proportions of men and women doing so were almost reversed - 36% of men and 24% of women had done so. (Section 6.3)

- Only 17% of men and 6% of women took part in vigorous physical activity lasting 20 minutes or more at least three times a week. (Section 6.3)

- The characteristic most closely associated with the likelihood of being physically active was the respondent's age, and in all age-groups, women were less likely to be physically active than were men. Thus, for example, 64% of men and 72% of women aged 75 and over were classed as sedentary, compared with 15% of men and 34% of women aged 16-24. (Section 6.3)

- Having taken account of age, the likelihood of participating in physical activity to one of the recommended levels was relatively greater among those with higher household incomes, those with educational qualifications, and with indicators of relative affluence, such as being in employment, and not living in local authority housing. (Section 6.4)

- An exception to this pattern was that, the likelihood of participating in physical activity to one of the recommended levels was not higher among those in non-manual social classes: on the whole, the reverse was true, probably because physical activity at work is taken into account. Thus, for example, 44% of men in Social Classes IV / V had participated in at least moderate-intensity activity lasting at least 30 minutes on at least five days a week, compared with only 27% of men in Social Classes I / II. (Section 6.4)

- In addition, after taking age into account, the likelihood of being classified as sedentary was relatively low for men with personal support groups of 9 or more people, and for lone mothers. It was relatively greater, on the other hand, for those not involved in community activities, for men with low neighbourhood social capital, and men living in more deprived areas. (Section 6.5)

continued

■ Logistic regression analysis was used to look at the relative importance of the different characteristics. It showed that levels of physical activity were much more strongly related to the demographic and socio-economic variables, than to people's social environment as measured by the survey. Only involvement in community activities was independently related to participation in moderate-intensity physical activity. (Section 6.6)

■ The variables with significant independent effects on the likelihood of being sedentary were age (by far the strongest effect), social class, household income, qualification level, economic activity, household type and involvement in community activities. Two additional variables - sex and marital status - were also associated with the measures of participation to the recommended levels. (Section 6.6)

■ Respondents were asked whether they thought that they were getting enough exercise to keep fit, and whether they would like to take more exercise. On the whole, older people and those who were more physically active were more likely than others to think that they were getting enough exercise. However, as many as two fifths of those classified as sedentary thought that they were getting enough exercise. (Section 6.7)

■ Just over two thirds of both men and women said that they would like to take more exercise. The proportions saying this were highest among men and women under age 55. (Section 6.7)

■ Overall, 28% of respondents said that they intended to start taking more exercise in the next month, and a further 21% that they intended to do so within six months. (Section 6.7)

6.1 Introduction and background

Physical activity and health

The role of increased physical activity in the promotion of good health and the prevention and control of chronic diseases is well documented. Physical activity and exercise have been most clearly associated with the control and prevention of coronary heart disease[1], stroke, hypertension, non insulin-dependent diabetes mellitus, cancer of the colon, obesity and improved mental health[2,3]. There is also evidence that physical activity may reduce the risk of developing osteoporosis and that muscle strengthening activity reduces the risk of falling and fractures among older people[2]. Since it helps to maintain functional ability and to prevent disability, immobility and isolation, physical activity improves quality of life, especially among older people[4].

Recommendations for physical activity

The Health of the Nation Physical Activity Task Force consultation paper[5] set out proposals for developing a comprehensive physical activity strategy for England. As part of this strategy the Health Education Authority developed a national promotional programme aimed at encouraging people to be more physically active. Physical activity at the following levels was recommended as providing a benefit to health:

- five or more occasions a week of at least moderate intensity activity lasting at least 30 minutes per occasion; or

- three or more occasions per week of vigorous intensity activity lasting at least 20 minutes per occasion.

These recommendations were based on current US guidelines and agreed by an international panel of experts at an HEA symposium which examined the scientific evidence associated with physical activity and health[6]. The symposium agreed three national objectives:

- to reduce the proportion of the population who are sedentary (that is, who exercise at moderate intensity less than once a week),

- to increase the proportion of the population achieving the recommended level of at least moderate intensity activity; and

- to increase the proportion of the population achieving the recommended level of vigorous activity.

Population based studies have shown that there appears to be a gradient of benefits as activity increases both in quantity and intensity and that although, in general, those at the upper end of the activity scale gain the greatest benefits, in population terms the greatest relative gains are to be obtained from encouraging those who are sedentary

to become moderately active[7]. Furthermore, moderate intensity activity represents a more realistic target at an individual level, particularly for the least active.

6.2 Measurement of physical activity

Levels of physical activity have been measured by HEMS since 1995. In 1995 and 1996, the survey covered adults aged 16–74, but in 1998, coverage was extended to adults aged 75 and over. The topic was also included on the Health Survey for England from 1991 to 1994[8] and again in 1997 for adults aged 16–24[9] (and in 1998, although, at the time of writing, published results are not yet available for the 1998 survey).

Appendix C gives full details of the derivation of the measures of physical activity used on the survey, but the key points are given here. Physical activity includes:

- activity at work;
- activity at home (including heavy gardening, DIY and heavy housework);
- walks lasting 30 minutes or more;
- sports and exercise activities (including cycling).

Moderate intensity activity includes brisk or fast walking for at least 30 minutes; heavy housework, heavy gardening or DIY; sports and exercise (if they did not make the respondent out of breath or sweaty); and some specified occupations. The duration criteria of 30 minutes or more used for the summary of at least moderate intensity activity applies only to sports and exercise activities and walking.

Vigorous intensity activity includes running; sports and exercise (if they made the respondent out of breath or sweaty); and some specified occupations.

The reference period for both was the four weeks prior to interview, and data are presented as average weekly frequencies.

The three measures of physical activity used in this analysis are the proportions who took part in:

- at least moderate-intensity activity lasting at least 30 minutes, on less than one day a week, so classified as 'sedentary',

- at least moderate-intensity activity lasting at least 30 minutes, on five or more days a week,

- vigorous activity lasting at least 20 minutes, on at least three days a week.

6.3 Physical activity in relation to sex and age

Sex

In 1998, 27% of men and 35% of women aged 16 and over were classified as sedentary - they participated less than once a week in 30 minutes or more of moderate-intensity activity. Overall, a similar proportion took part in at least moderate-intensity activity on five or more days a week, but the proportions of men and women doing so were almost reversed - 36% of men and 24% of women had done so.

Only 17% of men and 6% of women took part in vigorous physical activity lasting 20 minutes or more at least three times a week. (Table 6.1)

Sex and age

In all age-groups, men were more likely than women to be physically active, and among both men and women, the proportion who were sedentary (i.e. were moderately active for at least 30 minutes less than once a week) increased sharply with age: 64% of men and 72% of women aged 75 and over were classed as sedentary, compared with 15% of men and 34% of women aged 16–24. The association between vigorous activity and age was even more striking: 38% of men and 24% of women aged 16–24 participated in vigorous activity lasting at least 20 minutes at least three times a week, compared with fewer than 0.5% of men and women aged 75 and over. (Figure 6.1 and Table 6.1)

Trends by sex and age

Provided that those aged 75 and over are excluded from the 1998 data, the results can be compared with those for 1995 and 1996. Table 6.2 shows that the 1998 data for those aged 16-74 are very similar to those presented in the earlier reports. (Table 6.2)

It is not apparent from the table shown, but, compared with earlier years, a much higher proportion of young women aged 16–24, 34%, were classified as sedentary than previously: the equivalent figure for 1995 was 23% and for 1996, 20%. The apparent drop in 1996 is probably explained by a change in the survey measure for 'walking' at a moderate level of activity. (The measure was changed from a distance-based measure of 2 or more miles in 1995, to a shorter distance, 1–2 miles, in 1996, and to a time-based measure of 30 minutes or more – equivalent to 1.5 miles or more, in 1998.)

The increase in the proportion of women aged 16–24 who were 'sedentary' in 1998, over 1995, is mainly due to a fall in the proportion of this group who took part in sport or exercise at this 'moderate' level, rather than a fall in the proportions taking part in physical activities in the home or at work. The findings of the Health Survey for England (HSE) suggest that the increase may be real, rather due to sampling fluctuations. The HSE found a similar, though smaller, increase between the 1994 and 1997 surveys, with the proportion 'sedentary' increasing from 27% to 31%[9]. Even so, data for further years would be required to confirm any trend.

Physical activity in relation to other demographic and socio-economic variables

Age-standardisation

As in previous years, level of physical activity was also considered in relation to other characteristics of respondents – in particular, their marital status, employment status, social class (derived from their current or most recent occupation) income, and educational attainment. Since these are also related to the respondent's age (for example, older respondents tend to have lower educational qualifications) it is helpful to take account of this by age-standardising the data.

As well as the measured percentage for a particular subgroup, Tables 6.3 to 6.15 also show the percentage that would be expected, given the age composition of the subgroup. The ratio of these two percentages indicates whether the observed percentage is higher (if it is greater than 100) or lower (if it is less than 100) than would be expected on the basis of age alone. The tables also indicate if the ratio of observed to expected values is significantly different from 100. If it does differ significantly, this suggests that the observed variation is not explained by age alone. The technique is discussed further in Appendix C.

Figure 6.1 Level of physical activity by age and sex: adults aged 16 and over

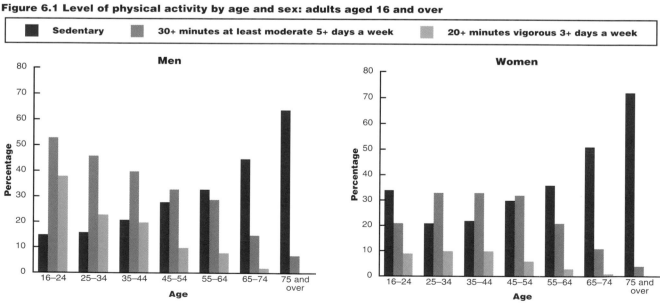

Base numbers are given in Table 6.1.

Marital status

On the whole, having taken into account the fact that, for example, single people are younger on average than married people, there was little difference according to marital status in the likelihood of being classified as sedentary or of participating in at least moderate-intensity activity at the recommended level. However, among both men and women, those who were widowed, divorced or separated were more likely to participate in vigorous activity than would be expected on the basis of their ages alone. (**Table 6.3**)

Social class

On the whole, men in manual social classes were more likely to be physically active than were men whose social class was non-manual. This might not perhaps at first be expected – surveys generally show that those in non-manual classes are more likely than others to follow advice about maintaining a healthy lifestyle. However, it is largely attributable to the fact that physical activity at work is taken into account, and manual occupations are more likely than non-manual ones to be physically demanding. Thus 44% of men in Social Classes IV/V had participated in at least moderate-intensity activity lasting at least 30 minutes on at least five days a week, compared with only 27% of men in Social Classes I/II. Even allowing for differences in the age composition of the social classes (for example, those in Social Classes I/II tend to be older, on average), there were wide differences between the social classes. However, there was no significant association for men between social class and participation in vigorous activity, nor between social class and the likelihood of being sedentary.

The picture for women in relation to social class was somewhat different. Women in Social Classes I/II were less likely to be sedentary, and more likely to participate in vigorous activity than would be expected on the basis of their ages alone, but they were no more likely to participate in at least moderate intensity activity. Women in Social Classes IV/V, in contrast, were more likely to have taken part in moderate-intensity activity (possibly because of the type of work they were doing), but less likely to have participated in vigorous activity, than would be expected from their ages. (**Table 6.4**)

Gross household income

Men in low income households (those with less than £5,000 gross income a year) were more than twice as likely as were men in high income households (those with £20,000 or more a year) to be sedentary, and about half as likely to have participated in at least moderate physical activity. The difference in relation to vigorous activity was even more marked - 22% of men in the high income households, compared with only 6% of men in the low income households had participated in vigorous activity lasting at least 20 minutes on at least three days a week. Some of these differences were due to the fact that those in low income households tended to be older, on average, but a similar, though less marked, pattern was evident when this was taken into account. Differences among women before controlling for age were similar, but even less marked when age differences were allowed for. (**Table 6.5**)

Economic activity

Working people were more likely to be physically active, and less likely to be sedentary than were the unemployed and the economically inactive. For example, among working men, 18%

were sedentary and 21% had participated in vigorous activity to the recommended level, compared with 49% and 8% respectively of the economically inactive. The pattern was similar among women, but a little less marked. Economically inactive people are much older, on average, than those working (most of them are retired), but even when this was taken into account, working people were more likely to be active, and the economically inactive were more likely to be sedentary, than would be expected on the basis of their ages. Because of the relatively small number of unemployed people in the sample (fewer than 200 in total) significant differences are more difficult to detect. Nonetheless, both men and women who were unemployed were less likely to participate in moderate or vigorous activity than would be expected from their ages alone. (**Table 6.6**)

Highest qualification level

Men and women with any qualifications at all were much more likely than those with none to be physically active, and correspondingly less likely to be sedentary. On the whole, these differences remained when the ages of those with and those without qualifications were taken into account. There was little difference in levels of physical activity between those with 'A' level or higher qualifications, and those with other types of qualification. (**Table 6.7**)

Housing tenure

Those renting from a local authority were more likely to be classified as sedentary, and less likely to participate in either moderate or vigorous intensity activity at the specified level, and this association remained even when age was taken into account. (Table 6.8)

6.5 Physical activity in relation to household type and social environment

Analysis in previous HEMS reports has focused on the demographic and socio-economic characteristics of respondents described in the section above. However, for the 1998 survey, information was also collected about the social environment of respondents, and in addition, a new analysis variable was created - household type. In this next section, diet is investigated in relation to these new variables. The variables, which are described in detail in Chapter 2, are as follows:

- Household type
- Personal support group – that is, the number of people the respondent could call on at a time of serious personal crisis
- Community activity – that is, participation in the last two weeks in adult education, voluntary or community groups or religious activities
- Satisfaction with amount of control over decisions affecting own life
- Perceived ability to influence decisions affecting the neighbourhood
- Neighbourhood social capital score – derived from level of respondents' agreement with statements about their neighbourhood (see Appendix C).
- Area deprivation category – based on the HEMS area deprivation score for postcode sectors, which takes into account the 1991 Census rates of unemployment, car ownership, overcrowding and social class (see Appendix C).

On the whole, these factors were much less strongly related to the likelihood of a respondent being physically active than were those discussed earlier, such as social class, employment status, and income.

Furthermore, where there were associations, they were predominantly with the likelihood of being sedentary, rather than with the likelihood of participating in moderate-intensity or vigorous activity at the specified levels. For example, both men and women were less likely to be sedentary than would be expected on the basis of their age alone if they also participated in community activities such as voluntary work or adult education classes, but although they were slightly more likely to have done vigorous physical activity of the type specified in the last four weeks, the difference was not large enough to be statistically significant. There was a similarly weak association between being sedentary and living in an area classified as 'more deprived'.

In addition, after taking age into account, the proportions classified as sedentary were relatively lower among lone mothers, and among men with personal support groups of nine or more, but relatively higher among men with low neighbourhood social capital scores. **(Tables 6.9 – 6.15)**

Assessing the relative importance of different characteristics in determining whether people are likely to be sedentary or physically active

The analysis presented so far shows that the single characteristic most strongly associated with the likelihood of participation in physical activity is the respondent's age. Clearly it is not realistic to expect most men and women aged 70 to be as physically active as people 50 years younger, but there is no a *prior* reason why being in a particular social class, income group or employment status category should predispose an individual to be more or less physically active. For that reason, the preceding analyses took account of the different age composition of categories of the various characteristics under consideration.

However, in the same way that these other characteristics are related to age, they are also in some cases related to each other. Thus it would be expected, for example, that those in Social Classes I/II would on average have a higher household income than those in Social Classes IV/V. The analysis presented so far throws little light on the relative importance of each of the factors in predicting the likelihood of an individual being physically active, nor the extent to which each has an effect which is independent of the others (except for age, which has been taken account of by age standardisation). This section uses logistic regression to look at the relative importance of the different factors.

Odds ratios and logistic regression

Logistic regression is a multivariate technique which can be used to predict the odds of a behaviour occurring for people with different combinations of the characteristics. Odds are the ratio of the probability that an event will occur (for example, being 'sedentary') to the probability that an event will not occur. This technique is valuable because it indicates whether each analysis variable makes a significant contribution to explaining the variation in the outcome variable (the health behaviour in question), having held all of the other analysis variables under consideration constant.

Two sets of logistic regressions relating to the physical activity measures were carried out. The first included only the demographic and socio-economic variables discussed in Section 6.4, and the second included the new variables discussed in Section 6.5. Once Model 2 had been run to identify significant variables it was re-run to obtain relative odds for only those variables which had been significant (that is, those which had an independent association with the aspect of physical activity).

The results of the logistic regression analysis are shown in Tables 6.16 and 6.17. The columns headed 'multiplying factors' can be thought of as 'weights'. For example, they represent the factor by which the odds of someone having a 'less healthy diet' increase with the characteristic shown compared with a reference category. For each variable, the reference category (shown with a value of 1.00) was taken to be the first category. The baseline

Figure 6.2 Logistic Regression Model 1 for physical activity - variables with significant independent effects

	'Sedentary' (moderate activity lasting at least 30 minutes, less than one day a week)	At least moderate activity lasting at least 30 minutes, on at least 5 days a week	Vigorous activity lasting at least 20 minutes, on at least 3 days a week
Demographic and socio-economic variables:			
Sex	-	*	*
Age	*	*	*
Marital status	*	*	*
Social class	*	*	*
Gross household income	-	-	*
Economic activity	*	*	-
Highest qualification level	*	*	-
Housing tenure	*	*	-

* Had an independent affect

- Had no independent effect

Figure 6.3 Logistic Regression Model 2 for physical activity - variables with significant independent effects

	'Sedentary' (moderate activity lasting at least 30 minutes, less than one day a week)	At least moderate activity lasting at least 30 minutes, on at least 5 days a week	Vigorous activity lasting at least 20 minutes, on at least 3 days a week
Demographic and socio-economic variables:			
Sex	-	*	*
Age	*	*	*
Marital status	-	*	*
Social class	*	*	-
Gross household income	*	-	*
Economic activity	*	*	-
Highest qualification level	*	*	-
Housing tenure	-	-	-
Household type	*	-	-
Social environment variables:			
Personal support group	-	-	-
Community activity	*	*	-
Satisfaction with control over own life decisions	-	-	-
Influence over decisions affecting neighbourhood	-	-	-
Neighbourhood social capital score	-	-	-
Area deprivation category	-	-	-

* Had an independent affect

- Had no independent effect

odds shown at the top of each table represent the average odds for the respondents with all of the reference categories shown. For each category of the variable, a 95% confidence interval is also shown. If the interval contains the value 1.00, then that odds ratio is not significantly different from the reference category. Undue weight should not be given to the significance or otherwise of particular categories, as this depends to some extent on which was chosen as the reference category. A more detailed explanation of logistic regression is given in Appendix C.

Logistic regression model including the demographic and socio-economic variables – Model 1

Table 6.16 gives the details of the first logistic regression model, for the three measures relating to respondents' physical activity. Figure 6.2 gives a summary, indicating which of the variables had significant independent effects in this model.

The first thing to note is that with one exception, all the variables that were significant in explaining the proportion of respondents classified as sedentary were also significant in explaining the proportion who participated in at least moderate-intensity activity lasting 30 minutes or more on at least 5 days a week. This might be expected because these two indicators are categories of the same variable. The exception is the sex of the respondent, which was not significantly associated with being sedentary, but was associated with participating in moderate intensity activity. Thus, age, marital status, employment status, social class, educational attainment and tenure were all independently associated with the likelihood of being sedentary, and in reverse,

with participating in moderate intensity activity at the specified level. Apart from age, the characteristic showing the most variation in participation was employment status (after all other characteristics had been controlled for).

It is interesting that, apart from age, the only characteristics significantly associated with vigorous activity were sex, marital status and household income. The association with income was particularly strong, even though it was not associated with either of the other two measures. Having controlled for all the other variables, the odds of those in the highest income group participating in vigorous activity were 3.6 times the odds of those in the lowest group doing so. Variation according to sex and marital status was less marked. However, taking all the variables into account, for a given age and income group, the relative odds of a widowed, divorced or separated man participating in vigorous activity, compared with a married woman, were about 5.5. (**Table 6.16**)

Logistic regression model including all the analysis variables - Model 2

Model 2 included the additional variables discussed in Section 6.5. Full details of the logistic regression analysis are shown in Table 6.17. The variables which had significant independent effects are shown in Figure 6.3.

Only two of the new variables - household type and whether the respondent had participated in community activities - had an independent association with any of the three physical activity indicators. Housing tenure was no longer significant when the new variables were included, suggesting that it was related to other environment variables which had a slightly stronger association with participation in physical activity.

The new variables - household type, and community activity - were less strongly related to participation in physical activity than were characteristics such as social class and employment status (this is consistent with the pattern of results in the age-standardised cross-tabulations presented earlier), and neither was significant in relation to participation in vigorous activity. Being a lone parent reduced the likelihood of being classified as sedentary, but was not significantly associated with increased odds of participating in the recommended levels of at least moderate-intensity activity. Taking part in community activities such as adult education classes or voluntary work reduced the odds of being sedentary, and correspondingly increased the odds of participating in the recommended levels of at least moderate-intensity activity.

It is interesting that these two new variables were both ones which related more closely to the individuals themselves than to the characteristics of their neighbourhood or their feelings about it. For example, it is perhaps not surprising that those who have sufficient motivation to take part in community activities such as voluntary work, can also motivate themselves to take exercise. **(Table 6.17)**

6.7 Attitudes towards physical activity

Assessment of own level of physical activity

Respondents were asked whether they thought they were getting enough exercise to keep fit. Just over one half of all men, and just under one half of all women said that they thought they were getting enough exercise. On the whole, the older people were, the more likely they were to think they were getting enough exercise, but the proportion was also high, at 56%, among young men aged 16–24. **(Tables 6.18 and 6.19)**

People were somewhat more likely to think they were getting enough exercise if they were physically active: 70% of men who participated in at least five occasions of moderate intensity activity lasting 30 minutes or more thought they were getting enough exercise, compared with 38% of men who were classified as sedentary. However, it is perhaps surprising that the difference according to level of activity was not more marked - that even among men who were meeting the recommended level of activity (five or more occasions of at least moderate-intensity activity) 30% did not think they were getting enough exercise. Of more concern, perhaps, is that, as many as two fifths of those classified as sedentary thought they were getting enough exercise.

Whether would like to take more exercise, and when intends to do so

Just over two thirds of both men and women said that they would like to take more exercise. The proportions saying this were highest among men and women under age 55, and then among those aged 55 and over the proportion declined quite sharply the older they were.

Overall, 28% of respondents said that they intended to start taking more exercise in the next month, and a further 21% that they intended to do so within six months. Differences between men and women were slight, and not statistically significant, but younger respondents of both sexes were much more likely than older people to say they intended to take more exercise: for example, 42% of those aged 16–24 intended to take more exercise within the next month, compared with only 9% of those aged 75 and over.

Perhaps surprisingly, there was little association between current level of physical activity and either the wish to take more exercise, or the intention to do so. **(Tables 6.20 and 6.21)**

Notes and references

1. Powell KE *et al*. Physical activity and the incidence of coronary heart disease. *Annual Review of Public Health*, (1987), 8, 253–87

2. U.S. Department of Health and Human Services. *Physical Activity and Health: A Report of the Surgeon General*. US department of Health and Human Services and Centers for Disease Control and Prevention, (Atlanta, GA. 1996).

3. Health Education Authority. Health Update 5: Physical Activity. Health Education Authority (London: 1995).

4. Young A. Exercise. In Ebrahim S and Kalache A (eds). *Epidemiology in old age*. BMJ Publishing Group (London: 1996).

5. Department of Health. *More people, more active, more often; Physical activity in England - A consultation paper*. Department of Health (London: 1995).

6. Killoran A *et al* (eds). *Moving on: international perspectives on promoting physical activity*. Health Education Authority (London: 1994).

7. Blair S and Connelly J. How much physical activity should we do? The case for moderate amounts and intensities of physical activity. In Killoran A *et al* (eds). *Moving on: international perspectives on promoting physical activity*. Health Education Authority (London: 1994).

8. Colhoun H et al. *Health Survey for England 1994*. HMSO (London: 1996).

9. Prescott-Clarke P and Primatesta P (eds) *Health Survey for England - The health of young people '95-'97*. TSO (London: 1998).

Table 6.1   Physical activity by age and sex
Adults aged 16 and over

Age	16-24	25-34	35-44	45-54	55-64	65-74	75 and over	Total
Frequency of at least moderate intensity activity for 30 minutes or more	%	%	%	%	%	%	%	%
Men								
Less than one day a week (sedentary)	15	16	21	28	33	45	64	27
1-2 days a week	20	24	23	26	28	29	22	24
3-4 days a week	13	14	16	12	10	10	7	12
5 or more days a week	53	46	40	33	29	15	7	36
Base = 100%	*233*	*432*	*464*	*432*	*390*	*350*	*254*	*2555*
Women								
Less than one day a week (sedentary)	34	21	22	30	36	51	72	35
1-2 days a week	33	30	31	27	31	30	20	29
3-4 days a week	12	16	14	12	13	8	4	12
5 or more days a week	21	33	33	32	21	11	4	24
Base = 100%	*272*	*631*	*572*	*463*	*406*	*447*	*456*	*3247*
All								
Less than one day a week (sedentary)	24	18	22	29	35	48	69	31
1-2 days a week	26	27	27	26	29	30	21	27
3-4 days a week	13	15	15	12	11	9	5	12
5 or more days a week	37	40	37	32	25	13	5	30
Base = 100%	*505*	*1063*	*1036*	*895*	*796*	*797*	*710*	*5802*
Vigorous activity for 20 minutes or more, at least 3 times a week								
Men	38	23	20	10	8	2	0	17
Base = 100%	*233*	*432*	*464*	*432*	*390*	*350*	*254*	*2555*
Women	9	10	10	6	3	1	-	6
Base = 100%	*272*	*631*	*572*	*463*	*406*	*447*	*456*	*3247*
All	24	17	15	8	6	2	0	12
Base = 100%	*505*	*1063*	*1036*	*895*	*796*	*797*	*710*	*5802*

Table 6.2 Physical activity by year and sex
Adults aged 16-74

Year	Men 1995	Men 1996	Men 1998	Women 1995	Women 1996	Women 1998	All 1995	All 1996	All 1998
Frequency of at least moderate intensity activity for 30 minutes or more	%	%	%	%	%	%	%	%	%
Less than one day a week (sedentary)	25	24	25	29	26	30	27	25	28
1-2 days a week	25	23	25	31	30	30	28	27	27
3-4 days a week	13	12	13	13	14	13	13	13	13
5 or more days a week	38	41	38	27	31	26	32	36	32
Base = 100%	2119	2043	2301	2547	2599	2791	4666	4642	5092
Percentage participating in vigorous activity for 20 minutes or more, at least 3 times a week	18	18	18	7	8	7	12	13	13
Base = 100%	2119	2043	2301	2547	2599	2791	4666	4642	5092

Table 6.3 Physical activity by marital status and sex
Adults aged 16 and over

Level of physical activity	Participation in at least moderate activity — Sedentary (moderate activity lasting at least 30 minutes less than one day a week) Observed %*	Expected %†	Obs/exp (%)†	At least moderate activity lasting at least 30 minutes on at least 5 days a week Observed %*	Expected %†	Obs/exp (%)†	Participation in vigorous activity — Vigorous activity lasting at least 20 minutes on at least 3 days a week Observed %*	Expected %†	Obs/exp (%)†	Base = 100%
Marital status										
Men										
Single	19	18	108	45	47	95	32	30	105	584
Married/cohabiting	28	29	97	34	34	102	13	14	94	1295
Widowed/divorced/ separated	42	38	109	28	25	110	11	9	130	652
Total	27	27	100	36	36	100	17	17	100	2531
Women										
Single	30	32	96	24	24	102	10	9	111	775
Married/cohabiting	33	31	104	26	27	97	6	7	88**	1617
Widowed/divorced/ separated	45	48	94	18	16	113	5	3	147	818
Total	35	35	100	24	24	100	6	6	100	3210

* The percentages refer to the proportions of the subgroups reporting each level of physical activity, so do not add to 100.

† See Appendix C, for a full explanation of age-standardisation.

** Age-standardised ratio is significantly different from 100, at the 95% level.

Table 6.4 Physical activity by social class based on own current or last job and sex
Adults aged 16 and over

Level of physical activity	Participation in at least moderate activity						Participation in vigorous activity			Base = 100% ††
	Sedentary (moderate activity lasting at least 30 minutes less than one day a week)			At least moderate activity lasting at least 30 minutes on at least 5 days a week			Vigorous activity lasting at least 20 minutes on at least 3 days a week			
	Observed %*	Expected %†	Obs/exp (%)†	Observed %*	Expected %†	Obs/exp (%)†	Observed %*	Expected %†	Obs/exp (%)†	
Social class										
Men										
I & II	27	28	96	27	35	78**	14	15	98	948
III (Non-manual)	24	24	101	33	40	84**	22	20	112	274
III (Manual)	28	28	101	43	35	123**	16	16	106	792
IV & V	28	26	105	44	38	116**	16	19	88	467
Total	27	27	100	36	36	100	16	16	100	2495
Women										
I & II	25	31	80**	27	27	101	10	7	135**	830
III (Non-manual)	36	34	107	20	25	79**	6	7	95	1063
III (Manual)	36	37	96	30	23	130**	5	6	87	292
IV & V	40	36	109**	27	23	117**	4	6	73**	930
Total	34	34	100	25	25	100	6	6	100	3117

* The percentages refer to the proportions of the subgroups reporting each level of physical activity, so do not add to 100.

† See Appendix C, for a full explanation of age-standardisation.

** Age-standardised ratio is significantly different from 100, at the 95% level.

†† Members of the Armed Forces, persons in inadequately described occupations and persons who have never worked are not shown as separate categories but are included in the bases for all persons.

Table 6.5 Physical activity by gross household income and sex
Adults aged 16 and over

Level of physical activity	Participation in at least moderate activity						Participation in vigorous activity			Base = 100%
	Sedentary (moderate activity lasting at least 30 minutes less than one day a week)			At least moderate activity lasting at least 30 minutes on at least 5 days a week			Vigorous activity lasting at least 20 minutes on at least 3 days a week			
	Observed %*	Expected %†	Obs/exp (%)†	Observed %*	Expected %†	Obs/exp (%)†	Observed %*	Expected %†	Obs/exp (%)†	
Gross household income										
Men										
£20,000 or more	19	23	85**	40	40	102	22	20	112	1093
£10,000-£19,999	28	28	100	37	34	110	14	16	86	683
£5,000-£9,999	45	37	120**	20	26	79**	8	11	74**	441
Under £5,000	48	34	138**	18	29	62**	6	12	52**	197
Total	27	27	100	36	36	100	17	17	100	2414
Women										
£20,000 or more	24	27	87**	29	29	100	11	8	128**	982
£10,000-£19,999	33	32	103	25	25	101	6	7	86	726
£5,000-£9,999	49	43	115**	18	19	94	2	4	54**	740
Under £5,000	42	44	97	19	18	108	3	5	56**	544
Total	34	34	100	24	24	100	7	7	100	2992

*   The percentages refer to the proportions of the subgroups reporting each level of physical activity, so do not add to 100.

†   See Appendix C, for a full explanation of age-standardisation.

**   Age-standardised ratio is significantly different from 100, at the 95% level.

Table 6.6 Physical activity by economic activity and sex
Adults aged 16 and over

Level of physical activity	Participation in at least moderate activity						Participation in vigorous activity			Base = 100%
	Sedentary (moderate activity lasting at least 30 minutes less than one day a week)			At least moderate activity lasting at least 30 minutes on at least 5 days a week			Vigorous activity lasting at least 20 minutes on at least 3 days a week			
	Observed %*	Expected %†	Obs/exp (%)†	Observed %*	Expected %†	Obs/exp (%)†	Observed %*	Expected %†	Obs/exp (%)†	
Economic activity status										
Men										
Employed	**18**	22	83**	**44**	40	110**	**21**	20	106**	*1571*
Unemployed	**27**	20	136	**29**	43	68**	**14**	24	60**	*91*
Economically inactive	**49**	40	122**	**15**	24	64**	**8**	10	82	*890*
Total	**27**	27	100	**36**	36	100	**17**	17	100	*2552*
Women										
Employed	**26**	27	94**	**32**	29	109**	**9**	8	112**	*1786*
Unemployed	**25**	27	92	**25**	29	86	**4**	9	32**	*81*
Economically inactive	**50**	48	106**	**12**	16	74**	**2**	3	65**	*1378*
Total	**35**	35	100	**24**	24	100	**6**	6	100	*3245*

*   The percentages refer to the proportions of the subgroups reporting each level of physical activity, so do not add to 100.

†   See Appendix C, for a full explanation of age-standardisation.

**   Age-standardised ratio is significantly different from 100, at the 95% level.

Table 6.7 Physical activity by highest qualification level and sex
Adults aged 16 and over

Level of physical activity	Participation in at least moderate activity						Participation in vigorous activity			Base = 100%
	Sedentary (moderate activity lasting at least 30 minutes less than one day a week)			At least moderate activity lasting at least 30 minutes on at least 5 days a week			Vigorous activity lasting at least 20 minutes on at least 3 days a week			
	Observed %*	Expected %†	Obs/exp (%)†	Observed %*	Expected %†	Obs/exp (%)†	Observed %*	Expected %†	Obs/exp (%)†	
Highest qualification level										
Men										
'A' Level or above	22	24	90**	36	38	93**	20	18	106	1007
GCSE A-G or below	23	26	90**	43	38	113**	19	19	100	908
No qualifications	44	35	126**	25	28	88	9	12	81	639
Total	27	27	100	36	36	100	17	17	100	2554
Women										
'A' Level or above	26	30	89**	28	27	101	10	8	132**	897
GCSE A-G or below	30	32	95	26	26	101	7	7	95	1279
No qualifications	49	44	112**	18	18	97	2	4	51**	1067
Total	35	35	100	24	24	100	6	6	100	3243

* The percentages refer to the proportions of the subgroups reporting each level of physical activity, so do not add to 100.
† See Appendix C, for a full explanation of age-standardisation.
** Age-standardised ratio is significantly different from 100, at the 95% level.

Table 6.8 Physical activity by housing tenure and sex
Adults aged 16 and over

Level of physical activity	Participation in at least moderate activity						Participation in vigorous activity			Base = 100%
	Sedentary (moderate activity lasting at least 30 minutes less than one day a week)			At least moderate activity lasting at least 30 minutes on at least 5 days a week			Vigorous activity lasting at least 20 minutes on at least 3 days a week			
	Observed %*	Expected %†	Obs/exp (%)†	Observed %*	Expected %†	Obs/exp (%)†	Observed %*	Expected %†	Obs/exp (%)†	
Housing tenure										
Men										
Owner-occupier	25	27	93**	36	36	102	18	17	107**	1890
Rents from local authority	37	29	128**	30	34	88	11	17	67**	365
Rents privately	27	24	112	39	40	99	19	21	91	295
Total	27	27	100	36	36	100	17	17	100	2550
Women										
Owner-occupier	33	34	97	25	25	101	7	6	105	2166
Rents from local authority	44	38	117**	19	22	87	4	6	62**	620
Rents privately	33	35	95	26	24	112	8	7	114	457
Total	35	35	100	24	24	100	6	6	100	3243

* The percentages refer to the proportions of the subgroups reporting each level of physical activity, so do not add to 100.
† See Appendix C, for a full explanation of age-standardisation.
** Age-standardised ratio is significantly different from 100, at the 95% level.

Table 6.9 Physical activity by household type and sex
Adults aged 16 and over

Level of physical activity	Participation in at least moderate activity						Participation in vigorous activity			Base = 100%
	Sedentary (moderate activity lasting at least 30 minutes less than one day a week)			At least moderate activity lasting at least 30 minutes on at least 5 days a week			Vigorous activity lasting at least 20 minutes on at least 3 days a week			
	Observed %*	Expected %†	Obs/exp (%)†	Observed %*	Expected %†	Obs/exp (%)†	Observed %*	Expected %†	Obs/exp (%)†	
Household type										
Men										
One person household	34	33	104	30	30	99	15	12	120	592
Living with others (no dependent children)	30	30	102	33	34	97	16	16	101	1308
Living with others (with dependent children)	19	21	92	44	42	105	20	21	95	634
Lone adult (with dependent children)	[3]	-	-	[11]	-	-	[2]	-	-	21
Total	27	27	100	36	36	100	17	17	100	2555
Women										
One person household	48	50	95	16	14	111	5	3	190**	962
Living with others (no dependent children)	37	36	101	23	23	99	6	5	107	1241
Living with others (with dependent children)	27	25	109	30	31	97	8	10	84	764
Lone adult (with dependent children)	17	24	71**	33	31	107	7	10	72	280
Total	35	35	100	24	24	100	6	6	100	3247

* The percentages refer to the proportions of the subgroups reporting each level of physical activity, so do not add to 100.

† See Appendix C, for a full explanation of age-standardisation.

** Age-standardised ratio is significantly different from 100, at the 95% level.

Table 6.10 Physical activity by size of personal support group and sex
Adults aged 16 and over

Level of physical activity	Participation in at least moderate activity						Participation in vigorous activity			Base = 100%
	Sedentary (moderate activity lasting at least 30 minutes less than one day a week)			At least moderate activity lasting at least 30 minutes on at least 5 days a week			Vigorous activity lasting at least 20 minutes on at least 3 days a week			
	Observed %*	Expected %†	Obs/exp (%)†	Observed %*	Expected %†	Obs/exp (%)†	Observed %*	Expected %†	Obs/exp (%)†	
Personal support group										
Men										
9 or more people	23	26	86**	42	37	113**	20	18	110	579
4 - 8 people	26	27	96	34	36	94	17	17	100	1104
1 - 3 people	32	28	115**	34	35	97	16	16	94	805
No support	34	28	117	37	35	106	9	16	55	55
Total	27	27	100	36	36	100	17	17	100	2543
Women										
9 or more people	31	34	92	27	25	109	6	6	96	691
4 - 8 people	35	34	101	23	24	95	7	6	104	1518
1 - 3 people	38	36	104	24	23	103	6	6	100	995
No support	31	34	96	18	25	69	0	6	0	35
Total	35	35	100	24	24	100	6	6	100	3239

*   The percentages refer to the proportions of the subgroups reporting each level of physical activity, so do not add to 100.
†   See Appendix C, for a full explanation of age-standardisation.
**   Age-standardised ratio is significantly different from 100, at the 95% level.

Table 6.11 Physical activity by community activity and sex
Adults aged 16 and over

Level of physical activity	Participation in at least moderate activity						Participation in vigorous activity			Base = 100%
	Sedentary (moderate activity lasting at least 30 minutes less than one day a week)			At least moderate activity lasting at least 30 minutes on at least 5 days a week			Vigorous activity lasting at least 20 minutes on at least 3 days a week			
	Observed %*	Expected %†	Obs/exp (%)†	Observed %*	Expected %†	Obs/exp (%)†	Observed %*	Expected %†	Obs/exp (%)†	
Community activity										
Men										
Some community activity	24	28	85**	35	35	100	20	17	118	576
No community activity	28	27	104**	36	36	100	16	17	95	1979
Total	27	27	100	36	36	100	17	17	100	2555
Women										
Some community activity	30	35	86**	25	24	106	7	6	107	1088
No community activity	37	35	107**	23	24	97	6	6	97	2159
Total	35	35	100	24	24	100	6	6	100	3247

*   The percentages refer to the proportions of the subgroups reporting each level of physical activity, so do not add to 100.
†   See Appendix C, for a full explanation of age-standardisation.
**   Age-standardised ratio is significantly different from 100, at the 95% level.

Table 6.12 Physical activity by whether agrees with the statement 'I am satisfied with the amount of control I have over decisions that affect my life' and sex

Adults aged 16 and over

| Level of physical activity | Participation in at least moderate activity | | | | | | Participation in vigorous activity | | | Base = 100% |
| | Sedentary (moderate activity lasting at least 30 minutes less than one day a week) | | | At least moderate activity lasting at least 30 minutes on at least 5 days a week | | | Vigorous activity lasting at least 20 minutes on at least 3 days a week | | | |
	Observed %*	Expected %†	Obs/exp (%)†	Observed %*	Expected %†	Obs/exp (%)†	Observed %*	Expected %†	Obs/exp (%)†	
Whether satisfied with amount of control overdecisions that affect life										
Men										
Agrees	27	27	100	36	36	101	18	17	103	*1894*
Neither agrees nor disagrees	28	27	103	35	36	97	15	16	92	*252*
Disagrees	26	26	100	35	36	98	15	16	91	*397*
Total	27	27	100	36	36	100	17	17	100	*2543*
Women										
Agrees	35	35	100	24	24	99	6	6	99	*2566*
Neither agrees nor disagrees	33	34	98	24	25	97	7	7	109	*294*
Disagrees	33	32	104	28	26	107	7	7	102	*368*
Total	35	35	100	24	24	100	6	6	100	*3228*

*   The percentages refer to the proportions of the subgroups reporting each level of physical activity, so do not add to 100.

†   See Appendix C, for a full explanation of age-standardisation.

** Age-standardised ratio is significantly different from 100, at the 95% level.

Table 6.13 Physical activity by whether agrees with the statement 'I can influence decisions that affect my neighbourhood' and sex

Adults aged 16 and over

Level of physical activity	Participation in at least moderate activity						Participation in vigorous activity			Base = 100%
	Sedentary (moderate activity lasting at least 30 minutes less than one day a week)			At least moderate activity lasting at least 30 minutes on at least 5 days a week			Vigorous activity lasting at least 20 minutes on at least 3 days a week			
	Observed %*	Expected %†	Obs/exp (%)†	Observed %*	Expected %†	Obs/exp (%)†	Observed %*	Expected %†	Obs/exp (%)†	
Whether can influence decisions that affect neighbourhood										
Men										
Agrees	26	29	91	35	34	104	14	15	92	584
Neither agrees nor disagrees	24	25	95	39	38	102	20	19	102	652
Disagrees	29	27	107	35	36	97	17	17	102	1295
Total	27	27	100	36	36	100	17	17	100	2531
Women										
Agrees	31	34	90**	25	25	102	7	6	110	775
Neither agrees nor disagrees	33	33	101	26	25	103	7	7	98	818
Disagrees	37	36	104	23	23	97	6	6	96	1617
Total	35	35	100	24	24	100	6	6	100	3210

*   The percentages refer to the proportions of the subgroups reporting each level of physical activity, so do not add to 100.

†   See Appendix C, for a full explanation of age-standardisation.

** Age-standardised ratio is significantly different from 100, at the 95% level.

Table 6.14 Physical activity by neighbourhood social capital score and sex
Adults aged 16 and over

| Level of physical activity | Participation in at least moderate activity | | | | | | Participation in vigorous activity | | | Base = 100% |
| | Sedentary (moderate activity lasting at least 30 minutes less than one day a week) | | | At least moderate activity lasting at least 30 minutes on at least 5 days a week | | | Vigorous activity lasting at least 20 minutes on at least 3 days a week | | | |
	Observed %*	Expected %†	Obs/exp (%)†	Observed %*	Expected %†	Obs/exp (%)†	Observed %*	Expected %†	Obs/exp (%)†	
Neighbourhood social capital score										
Men										
Very high	24	28	86	38	35	108	16	16	100	*450*
High	28	28	99	34	35	98	17	16	103	*738*
Medium	26	27	97	38	36	104	20	18	110	*694*
Low	30	26	115**	35	37	93	16	18	87	*662*
Total	27	27	100	36	36	100	17	17	100	*2544*
Women										
Very high	31	35	90	27	24	113	8	6	123	*577*
High	35	35	101	21	24	88**	6	6	87	*902*
Medium	36	35	104	23	24	97	7	6	105	*888*
Low	35	34	101	26	24	107	6	7	93	*868*
Total	35	35	100	24	24	100	6	6	100	*3235*

*   The percentages refer to the proportions of the subgroups reporting each level of physical activity, so do not add to 100.

†   See Appendix C, for a full explanation of age-standardisation.

**   Age-standardised ratio is significantly different from 100, at the 95% level.

Table 6.15 Physical activity by area deprivation category and sex
Adults aged 16 and over

Level of physical activity	Participation in at least moderate activity						Participation in vigorous activity			Base = 100%
	Sedentary (moderate activity lasting at least 30 minutes less than one day a week)			At least moderate activity lasting at least 30 minutes on at least 5 days a week			Vigorous activity lasting at least 20 minutes on at least 3 days a week			
	Observed %*	Expected %†	Obs/exp (%)†	Observed %*	Expected %†	Obs/exp (%)†	Observed %*	Expected %†	Obs/exp (%)†	
Area deprivation category										
Men										
1 More affluent	**22**	28	81**	**35**	36	99	**18**	17	107	*491*
2	**25**	27	93	**35**	36	97	**17**	17	102	*460*
3	**27**	27	99	**36**	36	101	**15**	17	88	*653*
4	**28**	27	105	**39**	36	107	**18**	17	105	*561*
5 More deprived	**35**	26	131**	**34**	37	92	**18**	18	100	*390*
Total	**27**	27	100	**36**	36	100	**17**	17	100	*2555*
Women										
1 More affluent	**34**	36	92	**20**	23	87	**7**	6	127	*569*
2	**30**	34	90	**29**	25	117**	**8**	7	117	*636*
3	**37**	36	103	**25**	24	104	**6**	6	106	*803*
4	**36**	35	104	**25**	24	103	**6**	7	88	*725*
5 More deprived	**38**	33	113	**20**	25	82**	**4**	7	58**	*514*
Total	**35**	35	100	**24**	24	100	**6**	6	100	*3247*

* The percentages refer to the proportions of the subgroups reporting each level of physical activity, so do not add to 100.

† See Appendix C, for a full explanation of age-standardisation.

** Age-standardised ratio is significantly different from 100, at the 95% level.

Table 6.16 Logistic regression for physical activity - model 1
Adults aged 16 and over

Characteristics	No. of cases	Sedentary Multiplying factors	Sedentary 95% confidence intervals	Moderate activity Multiplying factors	Moderate activity 95% confidence intervals	Vigorous activity Multiplying factors	Vigorous activity 95% confidence intervals
Baseline odds		0.167		0.630		0.647	
Sex							
Male (R)	2356	-	- -	1.00		1.00	
Female	2878	-	- -	0.78 *	0.68 - 0.90	0.45 *	0.37 - 0.55
Age							
16 - 24 (R)	346	1.00		1.00		1.00	
25 - 34	1002	0.84	0.61 - 1.17	1.04	0.79 - 1.36	0.79	0.56 - 1.10
35 - 44	988	1.08	0.77 - 1.50	0.87	0.65 - 1.16	0.63 *	0.44 - 0.91
45 - 54	834	1.47 *	1.05 - 2.06	0.73 *	0.54 - 0.99	0.35 *	0.23 - 0.52
55 - 64	729	1.64 *	1.16 - 2.31	0.57 *	0.42 - 0.79	0.26 *	0.17 - 0.41
65 - 74	722	1.76 *	1.21 - 2.57	0.46 *	0.31 - 0.67	0.11 *	0.06 - 0.20
75 and over	613	3.96 *	2.67 - 5.85	0.17 *	0.10 - 0.28	0.01 *	0.00 - 0.06
Marital status							
Single(R)	851	1.00		1.00		1.00	
Married/cohabiting	3091	1.18	0.96 - 1.45	1.02	0.84 - 1.23	0.62 *	0.48 - 0.81
Widowed, divorced, separated	1292	0.95	0.75 - 1.20	1.35 *	1.06 - 1.72	1.55 *	1.09 - 2.18
Social class							
I & II (R)	1699	1.00		1.00		-	- -
III (Non - manual)	1236	1.32 *	1.09 - 1.58	0.92	0.76 - 1.13	-	- -
III (Manual)	1016	0.93	0.76 - 1.14	2.13 *	1.74 - 2.59	-	- -
IV & V	1283	1.09	0.89 - 1.33	1.86 *	1.52 - 2.28	-	- -
Gross household income							
£20,000 or more (R)	2032	-	- -	-	- -	1.00	
£10,000 - £19,999	1371	-	- -	-	- -	0.67 *	0.53 - 0.84
£5,000 - £9,999	1140	-	- -	-	- -	0.37 *	0.26 - 0.53
Under £5,000	691	-	- -	-	- -	0.28 *	0.18 - 0.44
Economic activity							
Employed (R)	3163	1.00		1.00		-	- -
Unemployed	148	0.98	0.65 - 1.46	0.65 *	0.45 - 0.95	-	- -
Economically inactive	1923	1.97 *	1.63 - 2.38	0.44 *	0.35 - 0.54	-	- -
Highest qualification level							
'A'Level or above (R)	1788	1.00		1.00		-	- -
GCSE A - G or below	1960	1.03	0.87 - 1.22	1.02	0.87 - 1.20	-	- -
No qualifications	1486	1.54 *	1.26 - 1.87	0.77 *	0.62 - 0.96	-	- -
Housing tenure							
Owner - occupier (R)	3674	1.00		1.00		-	- -
Rents local authority	901	1.36 *	1.13 - 1.62	0.75 *	0.61 - 0.92	-	- -
Rents privately	659	1.16	0.95 - 1.42	0.97	0.79 - 1.19	-	- -
Number of cases in the model		5234		5234		5234	

* Significant at the 95% level.

(R) reference category

Table 6.17 Logistic regression for physical activity - model 2
Adults aged 16 and over

Characteristics	No. of cases	Sedentary — Multiplying factors	Sedentary — 95% confidence intervals	Moderate activity — Multiplying factors	Moderate activity — 95% confidence intervals	Vigorous activity — Multiplying factors	Vigorous activity — 95% confidence intervals
Baseline odds		0.141		0.685		0.643	
Sex							
Male (R)	2345	-	- -	1.00		1.00	
Female	2872	-	- -	0.76 *	0.66 - 0.88	0.45 *	0.37 - 0.55
Age							
16-24 (R)	346	1.00		1.00		1.00	
25-34	999	0.93	0.68 - 1.28	1.03	0.78 - 1.35	0.78	0.56 - 1.10
35-44	985	1.16	0.85 - 1.59	0.86	0.65 - 1.15	0.63 *	0.44 - 0.90
45-54	833	1.48 *	1.08 - 2.02	0.74 *	0.55 - 0.99	0.35 *	0.23 - 0.52
55-64	724	1.57 *	1.13 - 2.17	0.58 *	0.42 - 0.80	0.26 *	0.17 - 0.41
65 - 74	718	1.58 *	1.10 - 2.27	0.46 *	0.31 - 0.67	0.11 *	0.06 - 0.20
75 and over	612	3.42 *	2.34 - 4.99	0.17 *	0.10 - 0.28	0.01 *	0.00 - 0.06
Marital status							
Single (R)	847	-	- -	1.00			
Married/cohabiting	3080	-	- -	1.04	0.86 - 1.27	0.63 *	0.48 - 0.82
Widowed, divorced, separated	1290	-	- -	1.34 *	1.05 - 1.70	1.55 *	1.10 - 2.19
Social class							
I & II (R)	1694	1.00		1.00		-	- -
III (Non - manual)	1231	1.29 *	1.07 - 1.56	0.92	0.75 - 1.11	-	- -
III (Manual)	1011	0.89	0.73 - 1.09	2.12 *	1.73 - 2.58	-	- -
IV & V	1281	1.06	0.87 - 1.30	1.79 *	1.47 - 2.19	-	- -
Gross household income							
£20,000 or more (R)	2024	1.00		-	- -	1.00	
£10,000 - £19,999	1369	1.15	0.97 - 1.37	-	- -	0.67 *	0.54 - 0.85
£5,000 - £9,999	1137	1.49 *	1.20 - 1.85	-	- -	0.37 *	0.26 - 0.53
Under £5,000	687	1.42 *	1.08 - 1.87	-	- -	0.28 *	0.18 - 0.45
Economic activity							
Employed (R)	3157	1.00		1.00		-	- -
Unemployed	148	0.91	0.60 - 1.38	0.62 *	0.43 - 0.89	-	- -
Economically inactive	1912	1.98 *	1.62 - 2.41	0.42 *	0.34 - 0.52	-	- -
Highest qualification level							
'A'Level or above (R)	1781	1.00		1.00		-	- -
GCSE A - G or below	1957	0.99	0.83 - 1.17	1.03	0.87 - 1.21	-	- -
No qualifications	1479	1.41 *	1.15 - 1.74	0.77 *	0.62 - 0.95	-	- -
Household type							
One person household (R)	1412	1.00		-	- -	-	- -
Living with others (no dependent children)	2239	1.17	0.98 - 1.38	-	- -	-	- -
Living with others (with dependent children)	1284	1.13	0.90 - 1.42	-	- -	-	- -
Lone parent	282	0.59 *	0.41 - 0.86	-	- -	-	- -
Community activity							
Some community activity (R)	1488	1.00		1.00		-	- -
No community activity	3729	1.23 *	1.07 - 1.43	0.86 *	0.74 - 0.99	-	- -
Number of cases in the model		5217		5217		5217	

* Significant at the 95% level.

(R) reference category

Table 6.18 Whether thinks is getting enough exercise to keep fit by age and sex
Adults aged 16 and over

Age	16-24	25-34	35-44	45-54	55-64	65-74	75 and over	Total
Whether thinks is getting enough exercise to keep fit	%	%	%	%	%	%	%	%
Men								
Yes	56	46	45	47	58	66	70	53
No	44	54	54	50	37	26	15	44
Can't take exercise	-	1	1	3	5	9	14	3
Base = 100%	*232*	*430*	*464*	*432*	*386*	*349*	*253*	*2546*
Women								
Yes	41	41	40	47	52	65	60	48
No	59	58	58	50	44	27	19	48
Can't take exercise	-	1	2	3	4	8	21	4
Base = 100%	*272*	*630*	*570*	*463*	*406*	*444*	*455*	*3240*
All								
Yes	49	44	43	47	55	66	64	50
No	51	56	56	50	40	26	18	46
Can't take exercise	-	1	1	3	5	8	18	4
Base = 100%	*504*	*1060*	*1034*	*895*	*792*	*793*	*708*	*5786*

Table 6.19 Whether thinks is getting enough exercise to keep fit, by frequency of participation in at least moderate-intensity activity for 30 minutes or more and sex

Adults aged 16 and over

Frequency of activity	Less than one day a week (sedentary)	1-2 days a week	3-4 days a week	5 or more days a week	Total
Whether getting enough exercise to keep fit	%	%	%	%	%
Men					
Yes	38	43	52	70	53
No	51	56	47	30	44
Can't take exercise	11	1	1	0	3
Base = 100%	*773*	*638*	*304*	*831*	*2546*
Women					
Yes	38	43	54	64	48
No	50	56	45	35	48
Can't take exercise	11	1	1	0	4
Base = 100%	*1160*	*936*	*384*	*760*	*3240*

Table 6.20 Percentage who would like to take more exercise, and when intends to do so, by age and sex
Adults aged 16 and over

Age	16-24	25-34	35-44	45-54	55-64	65-74	75 and over	Total
	%	%	%	%	%	%	%	%
Men								
Percentage who would like to take more exercise:	69	81	76	70	53	45	38	67
Base = 100%	232	426	458	420	364	320	217	2437
When intends to take more exercise*								
Within the next month	38	37	34	28	17	18	8	29
Within the next six months	24	25	23	19	15	9	5	20
Within the next year	10	9	8	9	7	5	4	8
Intends to take more exercise but not in the next year	2	3	4	3	4	4	1	3
Unlikely to take more exercise	26	26	31	40	56	64	81	40
Base = 100%	231	425	457	418	361	319	217	2428
Women								
Percentage who would like to take more exercise:	82	79	76	71	62	47	38	68
Base = 100%	271	627	560	445	384	410	363	3060
When intends to take more exercise*								
Within the next month	46	30	31	20	30	14	9	27
Within the next six months	30	30	24	26	14	14	8	23
Within the next year	6	11	10	10	7	5	1	8
Intends to take more exercise but not in the next year	2	4	5	4	5	4	2	4
Unlikely to take more exercise	15	26	29	40	43	64	80	38
Base = 100%	271	625	558	442	383	410	361	3050
All								
Percentage who would like to take more exercise:	75	80	76	70	58	46	38	68
Base = 100%	503	1053	1018	865	748	730	580	5497
When intends to take more exercise*								
Within the next month	42	33	33	24	24	16	9	28
Within the next six months	27	27	24	22	15	12	7	21
Within the next year	8	10	9	10	7	5	2	8
Intends to take more exercise but not in the next year	2	4	4	4	5	4	2	4
Unlikely to take more exercise	20	26	30	40	49	64	80	39
Base = 100%	502	1050	1015	860	744	729	578	5478

* Excludes respondents who did not know whether they wanted to take more exercise.

Table 6.21 Percentage who would like to take more exercise, and when intends to do so, by frequency of participation in at least moderate-intensity activity for 30 minutes or more and sex

Adults aged 16 and over

Frequency of activity	Less than one day a week (sedentary)	1-2 days a week	3-4 days a week	5 or more days a week	Total
	%	%	%	%	%
Men					
Percentage who would like to take more exercise:	68	73	72	61	67
Base = 100%	672	633	302	830	2437
When intends to take more exercise*					
Within the next month	25	27	34	32	29
Within the next six months	16	25	19	19	20
Within the next year	9	8	9	7	8
Intends to take more exercise but not in the next year	4	4	2	3	3
Unlikely to take more exercise	46	36	35	40	40
Base = 100%	667	631	301	829	2428
Women					
Percentage who would like to take more exercise:	67	72	74	64	68
Base = 100%	1003	919	380	758	3060
When intends to take more exercise*					
Within the next month	24	29	28	29	27
Within the next six months	20	24	29	20	23
Within the next year	8	8	8	8	8
Intends to take more exercise but not in the next year	4	5	3	3	4
Unlikely to take more exercise	44	33	31	40	38
Base = 100%	998	916	378	758	3050

* Excludes respondents who did not know whether they wanted to take more exercise.

Diet

Summary of main findings

- In 1998, 18% of adults had a 'less healthy diet', and 15% had a 'more healthy diet', based on the survey diet score. Overall, 15% mentioned at least three of the four main components of a healthy diet. (Section 7.2)

- Among men, 21% reported a 'less healthy diet', compared with 16% of women. Similarly, only 12% of men had a 'more healthy diet', compared with 17% of women. In every sub-group investigated, men were more likely than women to have a 'less healthy diet'. (Section 7.3)

- Lower proportions of men than women usually ate high-fibre breads (36%, compared with 48%), and fruit or vegetables daily (59% compared with 74%). (Section 7.3)

- The levels of knowledge about diet differed between the sexes for only one aspect. Men were less likely than women to mention the need to 'eat lots of fruit, vegetables or salad', (62%, compared with 74%). Hence, 14% of men mentioned at least three out of four components of a healthy diet, compared with 16% of women. (Section 7.3)

- Age was the characteristic most closely associated with diet quality. Those in the younger and older age-groups were more likely than those in the middle age-groups to have a 'less healthy diet'. For example, among those aged 16-24, nearly a third of the men, and nearly a quarter of the women, had a 'less healthy diet'. Diet quality improved with increasing age until the 55–64 age-group, but declined in the two oldest age-groups. (Section 7.3)

- People's knowledge about diet also varied with age, with the oldest age-group having the lowest levels. (Section 7.3)

- Having taken age into account, diet quality varied in relation to a wide range of other demographic and socio-economic variables. It decreased with decreasing levels of household income, qualifications, and social class. In addition, it was relatively lower among the widowed divorced and separated, the unemployed, and those in local authority housing. It was also relatively lower among men in privately rented accommodation, among lone mothers and, to a lesser extent, among women who were economically inactive and women living alone. (Section 7.4)

- Differences in levels of knowledge about diet followed a broadly similar pattern, with a few exceptions. For example, they were not any lower among lone mothers than among women in other household types. (Section 7.4)

continued

- Diet quality and knowledge varied only slightly with aspects of people's social environment. They were relatively lower among those with small personal support groups, those not involved in community activities, those who lacked influence over neighbourhood decisions, those with low neighbourhood social capital and those in more deprived areas. (Section 7.5)

- Logistic regression analysis was used to look at the relative importance of the different factors. Four of the variables – sex, age, income and qualification level - had independent effects on all three of the diet measures. Age had the strongest effects. Most other factors had effects on just one of the diet measures. Two additional variables – tenure and neighbourhood social capital – were independently associated with having a 'less healthy diet', while community involvement and control over decisions affecting life were associated with having a 'more healthy diet'. (Section 7.6)

- The social environment variables were slightly more likely to have significant independent effects on knowledge about diet than on diet quality. Three of them – personal support group, community activity and area deprivation category – had independent effects on this measure. (Section 7.6)

7.1 Introduction and background

Diet and health

Diet and nutrition affect to varying extents all of the four priority areas targeted in the Government's White Paper *Saving Lives – Our Healthier Nation*[1]. For some cancers, and for coronary heart disease and stroke, diet and nutrition are major risk factors. It is estimated that diet accounts for about a quarter of cancer deaths, while a number of the risk factors for coronary heart disease and stroke are diet-related, for example, high serum cholesterol, high blood pressure and obesity. In addition, diet and nutrition can affect indirectly other aspects of health identified in the White Paper. For example, obesity and anorexia can be associated with impaired mental health, and nutrition can affect the risk of osteoporosis, which is a risk factor for injury due to falls. There are also links between obesity and other health problems, such as osteoarthritis, gallstones and non-insulin dependent diabetes.

Improving people's diet is seen as one way to help reduce health risks. One of the Government's aims is to encourage people to eat a balanced diet. They also aim to improve people's access to foods to make up a balanced diet[2].

Recommendations for a healthy diet

Following the publication of the White Paper *The Health of the Nation* in 1992, guidelines for a balanced diet were drawn up[3]. Foods were classified into five main groups, those being:

- Bread, other cereals and potatoes
- Fruit and vegetables
- Milk and dairy foods
- Meat, fish and alternatives
- Foods containing fat, and foods containing sugar.

It is recommended that in order to have a healthy diet, people should eat a variety of foods every day from the first four groups listed, while cutting back on those in the fifth group. Advice also states, for example, that the starchy foods in the first group, (particularly those high in fibre), should make up the main part of all meals. At least five portions of fruit and vegetables should be eaten daily. Lower fat versions of milk and dairy products and fish, and lean and lower fat meat products, should be chosen. Of the fats in foods, saturated fats should be kept to a minimum. In addition, a reduction in salt intake is required in most people's diets.

HEMS diet questions

The HEMS surveys since 1995 have asked a series of questions about diet. The range of questions has varied in the different years, but in each year, some key questions about people's eating habits and their knowledge of what constitutes a healthy diet have been included. Previous reports have analysed these data in some detail[4].

For this present analysis, people's answers about diet in the 1998 survey have been summarised to obtain just three dietary indicators so that these can be investigated in relation to a number of analysis variables. Thus the quality of people's diet, based on their reported eating habits, and their knowledge about what constitutes a healthy diet are looked at in relation to their personal characteristics and aspects of their social environment.

The three dietary indicators investigated are the proportions of adults who:

- had a 'less healthy diet' (based on the summary diet score), or
- a 'more healthy diet' (based on the summary diet score),
- mentioned at least three components of a healthy diet, (that is, three out of the four main components selected for this analysis).

The derivation of these dietary measures is described in detail below.

7.2 Measurement of diet quality and of knowledge about diet

Measurement of diet quality – the HEMS diet score

For this analysis, a diet score has been derived as a summary measure of diet quality. The score is similar to that created by Dowler and Calvert in 1995[5], and subsequently developed by Cooper et al for their analysis of the 1993 and 1994 Health Surveys for England[6]. The derivation of the score has been adapted to reflect the particular questions about diet that are included in the HEMS.

The HEMS diet score was derived for each respondent based on their answers to nine of the survey questions: four about the types of foods that they said they usually ate, and five about how often they ate certain foods. (See Appendix C for details of the derivation of the score.) Although respondents' answers may not accurately reflect their actual food consumption, it can be expected to give a broad indication of the likely quality of their diet[7].

The diet scores derived in this way potentially range from -8 to +11. In practice, they ranged from -5 to +11. On the basis of these scores, respondents have been allocated to one of four categories, as shown in Figure 7.1. The analysis in this report concentrates on those in the two extreme groups – those with a 'less healthy diet' (scoring -5 to 0), and those with a 'more healthy diet' (scoring +5 to +11). These groups account for 18% and 15% of the sample of adults respectively. **(Figure 7.1)**

Figure 7.1 Diet quality – diet score groups
Adults aged 16 and over

Diet score group		%
(–5 to 0):	A – 'Less healthy diet'	18
(+1 to +2):	B	36
(+3 to +4):	C	31
(+5 to +11):	D – 'More healthy diet'	15
Base = 100%		*5762*

Figure 7.2 gives details about the diets of respondents in these two groups. It shows the percentages giving selected answers to the nine questions which make up the diet score. As might be expected, it shows, for example, that the group with a 'less healthy diet' were more likely than those with a 'more healthy diet' to have a diet low in fruit and vegetables and high in fat.

Figure 7.2 Positive and negative aspects of respondents' usual diets by diet quality
Adults aged 16 and over

Diet quality*	'Less healthy diet'	'More healthy diet'	Total
Aspects of usual diet	Percentage consuming each food		
Aspects with a positive diet score			
Eats brown, granary, wholemeal, wheatmeal or S.Asian breads	13	79	42
Has skimmed or semi-skimmed milk	40	92	71
Eats bread or rolls daily†	64	93	83
Eats potatoes, rice or pasta daily†	26	77	54
Eats fruit or vegetables or salads daily†	27	97	67
Aspects with a negative diet score			
Spreads butter or hard margarine on bread	51	4	25
Has fried foods fried in solid fat	28	1	10
Eats chips and other fried food daily†	7	0	2
Eats biscuits, cakes or confectionery daily†	56	20	38
Base	*1065*	*866*	*5762*

*   These groups are derived from the survey diet score grouped into four groups (see Section 7.4).

†   Frequency of eating foods 'daily' means at least once every day.

They were also less likely to choose high–fibre breads, and more likely to eat 'biscuits, cakes and confectionery' at least once a day. **(Figure 7.2)**

(In Part B of this report, Table B.7.1 shows the information in Figure 7.2 separately for men and women.)

Measurement of knowledge about what constitutes a healthy diet

The survey measure of people's knowledge about what constitutes a healthy diet is derived from answers to the question:

- 'In a few words, how would you describe a healthy diet?'

In the interview, this question was asked after the detailed questions about the respondent's actual diet. Interviewers were briefed not to prompt respondents in any way, but to record the answers to this question verbatim. If people gave only a general answer, such as 'eat a balanced diet' or 'eat everything in moderation', the interviewers were instructed to ask what they meant by this, and to probe fully. The interviewers then coded the answers using a coding list. Answers which were not covered by the coding list were coded later, at the analysis stage[8].

Figure 7.3 shows the percentages of respondents who gave each answer. It also shows the summary measure adopted for the present analysis, that is, whether respondents:
'mentioned at least three of the four main components of a healthy diet', coded as:

- Eat lots of fruit, vegetables or salad,
- Cut down on fatty or fried foods, eat grilled food,
- Eat lots of fibre, cereals, wholemeal food,
- Eat lots of starch, carbohydrates, potatoes, pasta or rice.

The proportions who mentioned each of these components varied, from 68% for 'eat more fruit and vegetables' to only 20% for 'eat

Figure 7.3   Knowledge about diet
Adults aged 16 and over

Percentage giving each answer	All adults aged 16 and over
Components of a healthy diet mentioned*	
Eat lots of fruit, vegetables or salad	68
Cut down on fatty or fried foods, eat grilled food	39
Eat lots of fibre, cereals, wholemeal food	26
Eat lots of starch, carbohydrates, potatoes, pasta or rice	21
Mentioned at least three of the four main components above	**15**
Eat a balanced diet	25
Eat everything in moderation	13
Avoid red meat, eat white meat, fish	18
Cut down on sugar, cakes and confectionery	9
Eat lots of meat, eggs, cheese, drink lots of milk	8
Drink lots of water, fruit juice, liquid	6
Cut down on salt	2
Other	23
Including:	
Food which is full of vitamins and minerals	3
Eat regularly, 3 meals a day, not between meals	2
Eat fresh food, avoid convenience foods and takeaways	1
Eat whatever you like	1
Alcohol (changing types of drink or cutting down)	1
No meat, meat free diet	1
Don't know	1
Base†	*5750*

*   Respondents answers were recorded verbatim, then coded into the eleven precodes or as 'other'. Other' answers mentioned by at least 1% of respondents are listed here.

†   Percentages total to more than 100% because more than one answer could be given.

Figure 7.4 Diet quality by knowledge about diet and sex
Adults aged 16 and over

Number of components of a healthy diet mentioned	None	One	Two	Three or more	Total
Diet quality based on diet score	%	%	%	%	%
Men					
A - 'less healthy diet'	33	22	17	13	21
B -	38	40	37	36	38
C -	23	28	30	33	29
D - 'more healthy diet'	6	10	15	18	12
Base = 100%	475	807	887	341	2510
Women					
A - 'less healthy diet'	25	18	13	9	16
B -	31	38	32	28	33
C -	32	31	36	37	34
D - 'more healthy diet'	12	13	18	27	17
Base = 100%	*389*	*1077*	*1242*	*493*	*3201*
All					
A - 'less healthy diet'	30	20	15	11	18
B -	35	39	34	31	36
C -	27	30	34	35	32
D - 'more healthy diet'	8	12	17	23	15
Base = 100%	*864*	*1884*	*2129*	*834*	*5711*

more starch'. Only a minority of respondents, 15%, mentioned as many as three of the four components. **(Figure 7.3)**

It should be noted that, while this survey measure provides a useful indicator of people's probable knowledge about diet, there may be a number of reasons why some respondents do not mention all these components of a healthy diet. While some may not have known all the components, others may have known them all but not thought to mention them. Certainly the results of the 1995 HEMS suggest that if respondents had been asked about specific types of food, the vast majority would have been able to say whether or not it was best to eat plenty of them or to cut down on them[9].

The relationship between diet quality and knowledge about diet

The aim of health education programmes, is to help people make informed choices about what to eat, and to improve their diets. It is recognised, of course, that knowledge is not the only factor which influences diet quality. For example, having access to affordable food is also a factor. The survey results suggest, however, that the people with greater knowledge tended to have the 'more healthy diets': among those who mentioned at least three of the four main components of a healthy diet, 23% had a 'more healthy diet', and 11% had a 'less healthy diet'. In contrast, among adults who mentioned none of the four main components, only 8% had a 'more healthy diet', and as many as 30% had a 'less healthy diet'. **(Figure 7.4)**

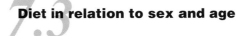

Diet in relation to sex and age

Sex

The quality of men's diets, as measured by the survey diet score, tended to be lower than the quality of women's diets: 21% of men reported a 'less healthy diet', compared with 16% of women. Similarly, only 12% of men had a 'more healthy diet', compared with 17% of women. **(Table 7.1)**

Closer examination of the different aspects of their diets suggests that men's diets vary in a number of ways from those of women. For example, a lower proportion of men usually ate high-fibre breads (36% of men, compared with 48% of women). Similarly, a lower proportion of men than of women ate fruit or vegetables daily (59% compared with 74%). The proportion who said that they ate fruit or vegetables more than once every day was also lower, (only 21% of men, compared with 34% of women, - figures not shown in tables). **(Table 7.2)**

The levels of knowledge about the four main components of a healthy diet differed between the sexes in only one respect. Men were less likely than women to mention the need to 'eat lots of fruit, vegetables or salad', (62% of men mentioned this, compared with 74% of women). This was the main reason for the proportion of men reaching the summary measure of 'mentioning at least three of the four main components' being slightly lower than among women (14% compared with 16%). **(Table 7.3)**

Sex and age

The quality of diets varied with age. The pattern was similar for men and women, though in each age-group the quality of men's diets was consistently slightly lower than the quality of women's.

Those in the younger and older age-groups were more likely than those in the middle age-groups to have a 'less healthy diet'. Nearly a third of the men in this youngest group, and nearly a quarter of the women, had a 'less healthy diet'. Conversely, only 6% of the men in this youngest group, and 11% of women, had a 'more healthy diet'. Diet quality improved with increasing age until the 55–64 age-group. It began to decline again in the two oldest age–groups, so that among those aged 75 or over, 25% of men and 19% of women had a 'less healthy diet'. The proportions in this oldest group with a 'more healthy diet' were only 9% and 12% respectively. **(Figure 7.5a and Table 7.1)**

These findings are broadly in line with those from the analysis mentioned earlier of the Health Survey for England (HSE) 1993 and 1994, but with one main exception. Cooper at al suggest that, in the youngest age-group (ages 16–24), unlike in other age-groups, the quality of women's diets was lower than the quality of men's diets[10]. The HEMS 1998 suggests, however that the converse is true, and that the quality of women's diets was higher than the men's in all age-groups.

People's knowledge about what constitutes a healthy diet also varied with age, though the pattern was somewhat different than for quality of diet. It was those in the oldest age-group who were the least likely to mention at least three of the four main components of a healthy diet. Thus the proportion mentioning at least three of the four rose from 11% among those aged 16–24, to 18% among those aged 35–54, but it began to fall again and was only 5% among those aged 75 or over. **(Figure 7.5b and Table 7.3)**

There may be a number of reasons for diet quality being relatively low among the older age-group. The lower levels of

knowledge shown by the survey may play some part. For example, older people may be less likely than younger groups to hear or read recent health education information, and they may be less likely to take note of such information. They may also be less likely to recall it and mention it in a survey interview. However, some older people may also consider that they have already lived to a 'good age', and that the changes in diet suggested in health information may not be too important for them. It is also possible that some of the older people will have been advised not to follow this general guidance about diet. For example, to counter weight loss in older age, they may have been advised by doctors to eat more, rather than less, fatty foods.

Trends by sex and age

In 1998, the HEMS included for the first time people aged 75 and over. Provided that this age-group is excluded from the 1998 data, the results can be compared with those from the 1995 and 1996 surveys.

It is not possible to calculate a comparable diet score for previous years' surveys, because of changes made to a few of the questions about eating habits. However, Table 7.4 shows the data which are available about some of the aspects of people's usual diets. Although the changes are small, the results suggest some improvements in people's diets. They show an increase in the proportions who usually drink reduced-fat milks, particularly among men. There also seems to have been an increase in the proportions who reported eating 'potatoes, pasta or rice' daily, and 'fruit, vegetables or salads' daily, again particularly among men. In addition, there may have been a decline in the proportions who usually have foods fried in solid fat. **(Table 7.4)**

Because of the change in the method of measuring knowledge about diet after the 1995 survey[11], comparisons are limited to the results from the 1996 and 1998 surveys. While the figures in Table 7.5 suggest some change, it is not possible to be sure of any clear trends on the basis of two years' data. **(Table 7.5)**

Figure 7.5a Diet quality – percentage with a less healthy by age and sex: adults aged 16 and over

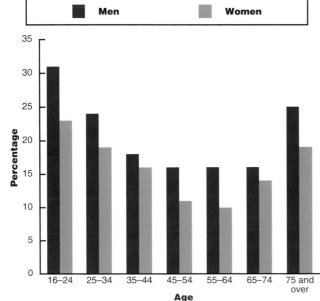

Base numbers are given in Table 7.1.

Figure 7.5b Knowledge about diet – percentage who mentioned at least three components of a healthy diet by age and sex: adults aged 16 and over

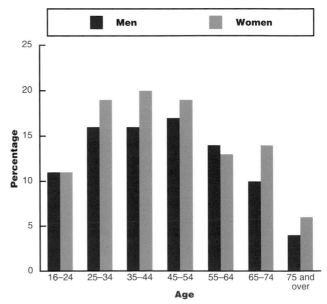

Base numbers are given in Table 7.3.

7.4 Diet in relation to other demographic and socio-economic characteristics of individuals

Age-standardisation

The previous section showed that both diet quality and knowledge about diet varied with age. In this next section, these aspects of diet will be investigated in relation to a number of other characteristics of individuals, including for example, the respondents' marital status, social class and educational attainment. Since these analysis variables are also related to the respondent's age (for example, older respondents tend to have lower levels of educational qualifications), it is helpful to take account of age by age-standardisation.

Tables 7.6 to 7.18 present age-standardised data. They show the actual, or 'observed', percentages as well as the percentage that would be 'expected', given the age composition of each subgroup. The ratio of these two percentages indicates whether the observed percentage is higher (if it is greater than 100) or lower (if it is less than 100) than would be expected on the basis of age alone. The tables also indicate if the ratio of observed to expected values is significantly different from 100. If it does differ significantly, this suggests that the observed variation is not explained by age alone. For further details on age-standardisation, see Appendix C of this report.

The data in these tables are shown separately for men and women. Interestingly, in every sub-group investigated, men were slightly more likely than women to have a 'less healthy diet'.

Marital status

Diet quality was higher among married and cohabiting people of both sexes than among the single and the widowed, divorced and separated. While diet quality was lowest among single people, this was largely related to their ages, in that single people tend to be younger than the other groups and, as shown earlier, diet quality was lowest in the youngest age-group. However the relatively low quality of diets among the widowed, divorced and separated was not explained by their ages: 28% of the men in this group had a 'less healthy diet', and 19% of the women. The corresponding figures for married and cohabiting men and women were lower, 18% and 13% respectively. (**Table 7.6**)

Differences between the marital status groups in their levels of knowledge about diet were less marked than the differences in the quality of their diets, and were largely explained by the ages of the groups. (**Table 7.6**)

Social class

Diet quality for both men and women tended to increase with increasing social class. For example, among men, as many as 28% of those in Social Classes IV/V had a 'less healthy diet', compared with 16% of those in Social Classes I /II . The corresponding figures for women were 21% and 11% respectively. These differences between the social class groups remained even when differences in age were taken into account. (**Table 7.7**)

Among men, knowledge about diet also increased with increasing social class, even after taking age into account. This pattern was not as marked among women: only among those in Social Classes IV/V was the knowledge level lower than for the other groups of women. (**Table 7.7**)

Household income

The pattern of results for the different household income groups was similar to that for the different social classes. Diet quality for both men and women increased with increasing gross household income, and the differences were not related to age alone. Thus for example, among men in the lowest income group (with less than £5,000 gross annual household income), 37% had a 'less healthy diet', nearly twice as many as would be expected on the basis of their ages alone. Similarly, only 4% of this group of men had a 'more healthy diet'. At the other extreme, among men with household incomes of £20,000 or more, 17% had a 'less healthy diet', and 15% had a 'more healthy diet'. (**Table 7.8**)

Among men, knowledge about diet also increased with increasing income, even after taking age into account. This pattern was not as marked among women: only among those in the highest income group was the knowledge level significantly higher than for the other groups of women. (**Table 7.8**)

Economic activity

Men and women who were unemployed tended to have less healthy diets than did those who were working or were economically inactive. As many as 40% of unemployed men had a 'less healthy diet', and only 5% had a 'more healthy diet'. Among unemployed women, the proportions were less extreme, 30% and 9% respectively. This pattern was not explained by the relative ages of the unemployed.

Among women, there is also some evidence that the proportion with a 'less healthy diet' was slightly higher among the economically inactive, and slightly lower among those working, than would be expected on the basis of their ages alone. (**Table 7.9**)

Levels of knowledge about diet did not vary greatly with economic activity, except that the level was relatively low among unemployed men: only 7% mentioned three of the four components of a healthy diet, half as many as would be expected on the basis of their ages alone. (**Table 7.9**)

Qualification level

The pattern of results for people with different levels of educational qualifications was similar to those for the different social class and income groups. Diet quality increased with increasing qualification levels. Those with no qualifications were more likely than others to have low quality diets: 28% of the men in this group, and 21% of the women, had a 'less healthy diet'. The corresponding proportions among men and women with 'A' levels or higher qualifications were 16% and 11%. (**Table 7.10**)

Among both men and women, levels of knowledge about diet increased with qualification level, and differences were greater than would be expected on the basis of age alone. (**Table 7.10**)

Housing tenure

Men and women in owner-occupied accommodation tended to have more healthy diets than did those in rented accommodation. Those in local authority housing had the lowest quality diets:

33% of the men in this group and 26% of the women had a 'less healthy diet'. These differences were not accounted for by age alone. (**Table 7. 11**)

Levels of knowledge about diet were also higher among men and women in owner-occupied accommodation, and lower among those in LA-rented accommodation, than would be expected on the basis of age alone. (**Table 7. 11**)

7.5 Diet in relation to household type and social environment

Analysis in previous HEMS reports has focused on the demographic and socio-economic characteristics of respondents described in the section above. However, for the 1998 survey, information was also collected about the social environment of respondents, and in addition, a new analysis variable was created – household type. In this next section, diet is investigated in relation to these new variables. The variables, which are described in detail in Chapter 2, are as follows:

- Household type.
- Personal support group – that is, the number of people the respondent could call on at a time of serious personal crisis.
- Community activity – that is, participation in the last two weeks in adult education, voluntary or community groups or religious activities.
- Satisfaction with amount of control over decisions affecting own life.
- Perceived ability to influence decisions affecting the neighbourhood.
- Neighbourhood social capital score – derived from level of respondents' agreement with statements about their neighbourhood (see Appendix C).
- Area deprivation category - based on the HEMS area deprivation score for postcode sectors, which takes into account the 1991 Census rates of unemployment, car ownership, overcrowding and social class (see Appendix C).

Household type

Diet quality and knowledge about diet were not strongly associated with household type, though associations were more marked for women than for men. Lone mothers were more likely than women in other household types to have low quality diets: 28% of lone mothers had a 'less healthy diet', compared with 16% of all women, and only 9% had a 'more healthy diet', compared with 17% of all women. These differences were greater than would be expected on the basis of age alone.

There is also some indication that, after taking age into account, women living on their own (with no dependent children) were less likely to have a 'more healthy diet' than would be expected on the basis of their ages alone. These women also had slightly lower levels of knowledge about diet than did women in the other household types. (**Table 7.12**)

Personal support group

The pattern of association between diet quality and size of personal support group is not strong. There is, however, some suggestion that diet quality was lowest among those with a small support group, particularly among the few respondents who said that they had no-one that they could turn to for help or comfort if they had a serious personal crisis. (**Table 7.13**)

Levels of knowledge about diet were very low among men in this latter group, with no support. This might be expected as this group may have relatively few social contacts with whom they share information about topics such as diet. (**Table 7. 13**)

Community activity

Diet quality was slightly higher among people who took part in community activities than among those who did not. The association was perhaps strongest among women. (Women were also more likely than men to participate in such activities.) Among women, 22% of those involved in community activities had a 'more healthy diet', compared with 14% of those not involved in such activities. These differences were not explained by the ages of the women. (**Table 7.14**)

Levels of knowledge about diet were also slightly higher among those involved in community activities, again particularly among women. (**Table 7. 14**)

Control over decisions that affect own life

Respondents were asked whether they agreed or disagreed with the following statement:

- I am satisfied with the amount of control I have over decisions that affect my life.

The associations between this attitude statement and diet quality and knowledge about diet were not marked. The data suggest slightly lower diet quality among the men and women who felt that they lacked control over their own life than among those who did not feel this. However, given the sample sizes, the differences were not statistically significant. (**Table 7.15**)

Influence over decisions that affect neighbourhood

Respondents were also asked whether they agreed or disagreed with the following statement:

- I can influence decisions that affect my neighbourhood.

Associations were a little more marked in relation to this second statement. Men and women who felt that they could not influence decisions affecting their neighbourhood tended to have the lower quality diets. For example, 18% of the women in this group had a 'less healthy diet', compared with 13% of women who felt they could influence such decisions. These differences were not explained by the ages of the women. (Table 7.16)

Neighbourhood social capital score

Diet quality was not strongly related to neighbourhood social capital as measured by the survey, though the data suggests a stronger association for women than for men. Among women, 20% of those with a low neighbourhood social capital score had a 'less healthy diet', compared with only 12% of those with either high or very high scores, a difference not explained by age alone. (**Table 7.17**)

Levels of knowledge about diet tended to rise, though not consistently, with increasing neighbourhood social capital scores. This was particularly so among men. (**Table 7.17**)

Area deprivation category

As might be expected, the pattern of results for people living in the different types of area was similar to those for people in the different social class and income groups. For both men and women, diet quality was lowest in the more deprived areas, and was higher in the more affluent areas. Among men, for example, 29% had a 'less healthy diet' in the more deprived areas, compared with 19% in the more affluent areas. The corresponding proportions for women were 26% and 10%. (**Table 7. 18**)

Levels of knowledge about diet also tended to be lower in the more deprived areas, particularly among women. (**Table 7.18**)

7.6 Assessing the relative importance of different characteristics associated with diet

The previous sections have shown that a number of variables are associated with respondents' diet and their knowledge about diet, but of course, many of these factors will be inter-related. This section uses logistic regression to look at the relative importance of the different factors.

Odds ratios and logistic regression

Logistic regression is a multivariate technique which can be used to predict the odds of a behaviour occurring for people with different combinations of the characteristics. Odds are the ratio of the probability that an event will occur (for example, having a 'less healthy diet') to the probability that an event will not occur. This technique is valuable because it indicates whether each analysis variable makes a significant contribution to explaining the variation in the outcome variable (the health behaviour in question), having held all of the other analysis variables under consideration constant.

Two sets of logistic regressions relating to the diet measures were carried out. The first included only the demographic and socio-economic variables discussed in Section 7.4, and the second included the new variables discussed in Section 7.5. Once Model 2 had been run to identify significant variables it was re-run to obtain relative odds for only those variables which had been significant (that is, those which had an independent association with the aspect of diet).

The results of the logistic regression analysis are shown in Tables 7.19 and 7.20. The columns headed 'multiplying factors' can be thought of as 'weights'. For example, they represent the factor by which the odds of someone having a 'less healthy diet' increase with the characteristic shown compared with a reference category. For each variable, the reference category (shown with a value of 1.00) was taken to be the first category. The baseline odds shown at the top of each table represent the average odds for the respondents with all of the reference categories shown[12]. For each category of the variable, a 95% confidence interval is also shown. If the interval contains the value 1.00, then the odds ratio is likely to be significantly different from the reference category. Undue weight should not be given to the significance or

Figure 7.6 Logistic Regression Model 1 for the dietary indicators – variables with significant independent effects

	Had a 'less healthy diet'	Had a 'more healthy diet'	Mentioned at least three of the main components of a healthy diet
Demographic and socio-economic variables:			
Sex	*	*	*
Age	*	*	*
Marital status	-	-	-
Social class	-	*	-
Gross household income	*	*	*
Economic activity	-	-	-
Highest qualification level	*	*	*
Housing tenure	*	-	-

* Had an independent affect

- Had no independent effect

otherwise of particular categories, as this depends to some extent on which was chosen as the reference category. A more detailed explanation of logistic regression is given in Appendix C.

Logistic regression model including the demographic and socio-economic variables – Model 1

Table 7.19 gives the details of the first logistic regression model, for the three measures relating to respondents' diet. Figure 7.6 gives a summary, indicating which of the variables had significant independent effects in this model.

Four of the variables – sex, age, income and qualification level - had independent effects on all three of the diet measures. In addition, social class was related to the likelihood of having a 'more healthy diet', and housing tenure to having a 'less healthy diet'. Neither marital status nor economic activity had a significant independent effect on any of the measures.

The model confirms the pattern of results for these variables discussed in Section 7.5 above. Diet quality was higher for women than for men. Holding all other variables constant, the odds of women having a 'more healthy diet' were two-thirds greater than those for men (1.68 compared with 1.00). Diet quality increased with age until the 55–64 age-group and declined among those aged 75 or over. Even so, those aged 75 or over had more than twice the odds of those aged 16–24 to have a 'more healthy diet'. Similarly, diet quality increased with both income and with highest qualification level. For example, the odds of someone in a household with a gross annual income of £20,000 or more having a 'more healthy diet' were twice those of someone in a household with less than £5,000 income a year.

While the pattern of odds is similar for the measure of knowledge about diet, the differences by sex, age and income are somewhat less marked than they were for diet quality. The differences by qualification level, however, are more marked, indicating that, as might be expected, higher levels of qualifications are particularly associated with greater knowledge about diet. Another difference from the pattern for diet quality is a small increase in the odds of those in the lowest income group mentioning at least three of the components of a healthy diet, compared with those in the next highest income group. The reasons for this are not clear. It may be due partly to the association between knowledge and low income only being significant for men, not for women, as shown in Table 7.8. **(Table 7.19)**

Logistic regression model including all the analysis variables – Model 2

Model 2 included the additional variables discussed in Section 7.5. Full details of the logistic regression analysis are shown in Table 7.20. The variables which had significant independent effects are indicated with an asterisk in Figure 7.7.

The four main analysis variables from Model 1 – sex, age, income and qualification level – were retained for all three measures of diet in Model 2. Age had the strongest effects, so that, for example, the odds of those aged 55–64 having a 'more healthy diet' were nearly three times greater than for those aged 16–24. Even so, after controlling for all other factors, the odds of having a 'more healthy diet' were twice as high for those in the highest household income group as for those in the lowest income group. Similar differences were found for the highest and lowest qualification-level groups. In addition, tenure was retained in the model for having a 'less healthy diet'. Social class was not retained in the model for having a 'more healthy diet'.

Figure 7.7 Logistic Regression Model 2 for the dietary indicators – variables with significant independent effects

	Had a 'less healthy diet'	Had a 'more healthy diet'	Mentioned at least three of the main components of a healthy diet
Demographic and socio–economic variables:			
Sex	*	*	*
Age	*	*	*
Marital status	-	-	-
Social class	-	-	-
Gross household income	*	*	*
Economic activity	-	-	-
Highest qualification level	*	*	*
Housing tenure	*	-	-
Household type	-	-	-
Social environment variables:			
Personal support group	-	-	*
Community activity	-	*	*
Satisfaction with control over own life decisions	-	*	-
Influence over decisions affecting neighbourhood	-	-	-
Neighbourhood social capital score	*	-	-
Area deprivation category	-	-	*

* Had an independent affect

\- Had no independent effect

None of the variables which were new in Model 2 were significant for all three measures of diet, though involvement in community activity had an independent effect on two of the measures – having a 'more healthy diet' and the knowledge measure. Most of the variables had independent effects on one of the measures. The new variables were more likely to be significant in the model for knowledge about diet than for diet quality. Three of them – personal support group, community activity and area deprivation category – had independent effects on this measure. Generally therefore the social environment variables had only limited independent effects on the three measures of diet. **(Table 7.20)**

Notes and references

1.   Department of Health. *Saving Lives: Our healthier nation.* TSO (London: 1999).

2.   Department of Health. *The Health of the Nation: a strategy for health in England.* HMSO (London: 1992).

3.   Health Education Authority. *Enjoy healthy eating: the balance of good health.* HEA (London: 1995).

4.   Bridgwood et al. *Health in England in 1995: what people know, what people think, what people do.* HMSO (London: 1996), and Hansbro J el al, *Health in England 1996.* TSO (London: 1997).

5.   Dowler E and Calvert C. *Nutrition and diet in lone parent families in London.* Family Policy Study Centre (London: 1995).

6.   Cooper H et al. The influence of social support and social capital on health: a review and analysis of British data. HEA (London: 1999).

7.   An accurate measure would require a weighed dietary record to be kept by respondents, as is done for the programme of national dietary surveys, as reported, for example, in *The Dietary and Nutritional Survey of British Adults,* Gregory *et al,* HMSO (London: 1990). This was beyond the scope of the present survey. (This 1990 report includes a chapter on the classification of diets using principal component analysis. It identifies five main types based on the different groups of foods eaten by people.)

8.   This HEMS coding list is broadly in line with the range of answers given in response to questions about people's understanding of 'healthy eating' in a study involving in–depth interviews. Keane A and Willetts A, *Concepts of healthy eating: an anthropological investigation in South East London. Goldsmith's* College (London: 1996).

9.   Hansbro J et al. *Health in England 1996.* TSO (London: 1997), Pg 41, 'Annex to Chapter 4' describes the changes made for the 1996 survey. The method used in the 1995 HEMS suggested that knowledge about what constitutes a healthy diet was high, in that, when asked specifically about different types of food, the vast majority of people could say whether it was best to eat plenty of these or to cut down on them. For the 1996 and subsequent surveys, the questions to ascertain knowledge about diet were revised. This was to obtain a survey indicator which discriminates more between different levels of knowledge.

10.   Cooper H et al. *The influence of social support and social capital on health: a review and analysis of British data.* HEA (London: 1999), Chapter 7.

11.   Hansbro J et al. *Health in England 1996.* TSO (London: 1997), Pg 41, 'Annex to Chapter 4' describes the changes made for the 1996 survey.

12.   For example, in Model 2, the odds of having a less healthy diet for people with different characteristics can be calculated by multiplying the baseline odds shown at the top of the table by the appropriate factors. So, for example, a male aged 16–24, whose household has an income of less than £5,000 and who has no educational qualifications, is in LA housing and has a low social capital score would have odds calculated as shown below:

        0.243 x 1.00 x 1.00 x 1.96 x 1.69 x 1.49 x 1.27= 1.52

        This would give odds of 1.52 to 1 that a person with these characteristics would have a 'less healthy diet'.

Table 7.1 Diet quality by age and sex
Adults aged 16 and over

Age	16-24	25-34	35-44	45-54	55-64	65-74	75 and over	Total
*Diet quality (based on a survey diet score)**	%	%	%	%	%	%	%	%
Men								
A - 'less healthy diet'	31	24	18	16	16	16	25	21
B -	36	42	42	39	32	35	34	38
C -	26	24	27	27	35	34	32	28
D - 'more healthy diet'	6	9	13	18	17	14	9	12
Base = 100%	*232*	*426*	*463*	*428*	*384*	*349*	*253*	*2535*
Women								
A - 'less healthy diet'	23	19	16	11	10	14	19	16
B -	39	35	32	32	30	29	36	33
C -	27	32	35	35	39	39	33	34
D - 'more healthy diet'	11	15	18	22	22	18	12	17
Base = 100%	*270*	*627*	*568*	*462*	*402*	*444*	*454*	*3227*
All								
A - 'less healthy diet'	27	22	17	14	13	15	21	18
B -	37	38	37	35	31	32	36	36
C -	27	28	31	31	37	37	32	31
D - 'more healthy diet'	9	12	15	20	19	16	11	15
Base = 100%	*502*	*1053*	*1031*	*890*	*786*	*793*	*707*	*5762*

*These groups are derived from the survey diet score grouped in to four groups (see Section 7.4).

Table 7.2 Aspects of usual diet by age

Adults aged 16 and over

Age	16-24	25-34	35-44	45-54	55-64	65-74	75 and over	Total
Aspects of usual diet				Percentage consuming each food				
Men								
Aspects with positive diet score								
Eats brown, granary, wholemeal, wheatmeal or S.Asian breads	19	32	38	42	45	45	38	36
Has skimmed or semi-skimmed milk	69	71	74	77	69	66	51	70
Eats bread or rolls daily*	80	81	81	86	8:	93	94	85
Eats potatoes, rice or pasta daily*	38	46	52	53	60	63	63	52
Eats fruit or vegetables or salads daily*	44	49	56	64	71	76	75	59
Aspects with negative diet score								
Spreads butter or hard margarine on bread	24	20	18	20	28	29	34	23
Has fried foods fried in solid fat	5	6	9	10	12	15	22	10
Eats chips and other fried food daily*	7	5	2	1	2	2	2	3
Eats biscuits, cakes or confectionery daily*	36	30	34	33	39	54	60	37
Base = 100%†	*233*	*432*	*464*	*432*	*390*	*350*	*254*	*2555*
Women								
Aspects with positive diet score								
Eats brown, granary, wholemeal, wheatmeal or S.Asian breads	34	42	43	57	54	57	52	48
Has skimmed or semi-skimmed milk	6:	75	75	78	77	69	53	72
Eats bread or rolls daily*	78	74	79	79	83	92	94	81
Eats potatoes, rice or pasta daily*	38	49	57	61	61	65	66	56
Eats fruit or vegetables or salads daily*	63	63	72	80	84	86	83	74
Aspects with negative diet score								
Spreads butter or hard margarine on bread	23	19	20	23	30	35	44	26
Has fried foods fried in solid fat	7	6	9	8	9	18	20	10
Eats chips and other fried food daily*	3	1	1	1	1	0	1	1
Eats biscuits, cakes or confectionery daily*	38	32	35	33	31	50	54	38
Base = 100%†	*272*	*631*	*572*	*463*	*406*	*447*	*456*	*3247*
All								
Aspects with positive diet score								
Eats brown, granary, wholemeal, wheatmeal or S.Asian breads	26	37	41	49	50	51	47	42
Has skimmed or semi-skimmed milk	69	73	75	78	73	68	52	71
Eats bread or rolls daily*	79	78	80	82	86	92	94	83
Eats potatoes, rice or pasta daily*	38	48	54	57	61	64	65	54
Eats fruit or vegetables or salads daily*	53	56	64	72	78	81	80	67
Aspects with negative diet score								
Spreads butter or hard margarine on bread	24	20	19	21	29	32	41	25
Has fried foods fried in solid fat	6	6	9	9	11	17	21	10
Eats chips and other fried food daily*	5	3	2	1	1	1	1	2
Eats biscuits, cakes or confectionery daily*	37	31	34	33	35	52	56	38
Base = 100%†	*505*	*1063*	*1036*	*895*	*796*	*797*	*710*	*5802*

* Frequency of eating foods 'daily' means at least once every day.

† Bases are shown from 'eats potatoes, rice or pasta daily'. Bases may vary slightly for other items.

Table 7.3 Knowledge about diet by age and sex
Adults aged 16 and over

Age	16-24	25-34	35-44	45-54	55-64	65-74	75 and over	Total
*Components of a healthy diet mentioned**			Percentage giving each answer					
Men								
Eat lots of fruit, vegetables or salad	59	59	65	66	69	62	53	62
Cut down on fatty or fried foods, eat grilled food	37	43	44	44	34	36	24	39
Eat lots of fibre, cereals, wholemeal food	23	23	24	31	2:	23	19	25
Eat lots of starch, carbohydrates, potatoes, pasta or rice	26	25	24	18	15	13	8	20
Mentioned at least three of the four main components above	11	16	16	17	14	10	4	14
Base†	*229*	*429*	*460*	*429*	*384*	*347*	*251*	*2529*
Women								
Eat lots of fruit, vegetables or salad	68	72	75	78	79	78	67	74
Cut down on fatty or fried foods, eat grilled food	39	44	46	42	36	36	23	39
Eat lots of fibre, cereals, wholemeal food	23	27	2:	30	24	25	16	26
Eat lots of starch, carbohydrates, potatoes, pasta or rice	22	26	27	22	20	14	10	21
Mentioned at least three of the four main components above	11	19	20	19	13	14	6	16
Base†	*270*	*626*	*571*	*460*	*405*	*444*	*445*	*3221*
All								
Eat lots of fruit, vegetables or salad	63	65	70	72	74	70	62	68
Cut down on fatty or fried foods, eat grilled food	38	44	45	43	35	36	24	39
Eat lots of fibre, cereals, wholemeal food	23	25	27	31	27	24	17	26
Eat lots of starch, carbohydrates, potatoes, pasta or rice	24	26	26	20	17	14	9	21
Mentioned at least three of the four main components above	11	17	18	18	14	12	5	15
Base†	*499*	*1055*	*1031*	*889*	*789*	*791*	*696*	*5750*

* Respondents answers were recorded verbatim, then coded into the eleven precodes or as 'other'. (For further detail see Table B.7.4).

† Percentages total to more than 100% because more than one answer could be given.

Table 7.4 Selected aspects of people's usual diets by year and sex
Adults aged 16-74

Year	Men			Women			All		
	1995	1996	1998	1995	1996	1998	1995	1996	1998
Aspects of usual diet	*Percentage consuming each food*								
Has skimmed or semi-skimmed milk	67	67	74	73	74	76	71	71	75
Eats bread or rolls daily*	85	84	84	80	81	80	83	83	82
Eats potatoes, pasta or rice daily*	43	53	51	50	56	55	47	55	53
Eats fruit, vegetables and salad daily*	54	59	58	71	72	74	62	66	66
Has fried foods fried in solid fat	12	10	9	11	10	9	11	10	9
Base = 100%†	*2118*	*1934*	*2301*	*2545*	*2474*	*2791*	*4663*	*4408*	*5092*

* Frequency of eating foods 'daily' means at least once every day.

† Percentage total to more than 100% because more than one answer could be given

Table 7.5 Knowledge about diet by year and sex
Adults aged 16-74

Year	Men		Women		All	
	1996	1998	1996	1998	1996	1998
Knowledge of what constitutes a healthy diet*	*Percentage giving each answer*					
Eat lots of fruit, vegetables or salad	60	63	73	75	67	69
Cut down on fatty or fried foods, eat grilled food	44	40	46	41	45	41
Eat lots of fibre, cereals, wholemeal food	27	26	27	27	27	26
Eat lots of starch, carbohydrates, potatoes, pasta or rice	19	21	20	23	20	22
Mentioned at least three of the four main components above	14	15	17	17	16	16
Base†	*2013*	*2278*	*2568*	*2776*	*4582*	*5054*

* Respondents answers were recorded verbatim, then coded into the eleven precodes or as 'other'. (For further detail see Table B.7.4).

† Percentages total to more than 100% because more than one answer could be given.

Table 7.6 Dietary indicators by marital status and sex
Adults aged 16-74

Dietary indicators	Had a less healthy diet			Had a more healthy diet			Mentioned at least three of four components of a healthy diet			Base = 100%
	Observed %*	Expected %†	Obs/exp (%)†	Observed %*	Expected %†	Obs/exp (%)†	Observed %*	Expected %†	Obs/exp (%)†	
Marital status										
Men										
Single	**29**	27	107	**8**	9	89	**12**	13	94	*495*
Married/cohabiting	**18**	19	91 **	**14**	13	104	**15**	15	103	*1628*
Widowed/divorced/ separated	**28**	19	147 **	**11**	13	82	**10**	12	83	*412*
Total	*21*	*21*	*100*	*12*	*12*	*100*	*14*	*14*	*100*	2535
Women										
Single	**23**	20	111	**13**	13	96	**13**	14	94	*547*
Married/cohabiting	**13**	15	86 **	**19**	18	107 **	**18**	17	103	*1659*
Widowed/divorced/ separated	**19**	15	127 **	**13**	17	78 **	**12**	13	94	*1021*
Total	*16*	*16*	*100*	*17*	*17*	*100*	*16*	*16*	*100*	3227

* The percentages refer to the proportions of the subgroups reporting each dietary indicator, so do not add to 100.

† See Appendix C for a full explanation of age-standardisation.

** Age-standardised ratio is significantly different from 100, at the 95% level.

Table 7.7 Dietary indicators by social class based on own current or last job and sex
Adults aged 16 and over

Dietary indicators	Had a less healthy diet			Had a more healthy diet			Mentioned at least three of four components of a healthy diet			Base = 100%
	Observed %*	Expected %†	Obs/exp (%)†	Observed %*	Expected %†	Obs/exp (%)†	Observed %*	Expected %†	Obs/exp (%)†	
Social class										
Men										
I & II	**16**	20	79 **	**18**	13	135 **	**19**	15	127 **	*940*
III (Non-manual)	**24**	22	107	**11**	11	95	**14**	14	104	*273*
III (Manual)	**21**	20	104	**9**	13	73 **	**12**	14	83 **	*788*
IV & V	**28**	22	127 **	**8**	12	73 **	**9**	13	66 **	*462*
Total	*21*	*21*	*100*	*13*	*13*	*100*	*14*	*14*	*100*	2477
Women										
I & II	**11**	15	75 **	**22**	18	127 **	**18**	17	108	*824*
III (Non-manual)	**14**	16	88	**16**	17	96	**17**	16	105	*1055*
III (Manual)	**16**	16	104	**19**	17	115	**17**	15	111	*290*
IV & V	**21**	15	135 **	**13**	17	75 **	**13**	15	82 **	*928*
Total	*16*	*16*	*100*	*17*	*17*	*100*	*16*	*16*	*100*	3099

* The percentages refer to the proportions of the subgroups reporting each dietary indicator, so do not add to 100.

† See Appendix C for a full explanation of age-standardisation.

** Age-standardised ratio is significantly different from 100, at the 95% level.

†† Members of the Armed Forces, persons in inadequately described occupations and persons who have never worked are excluded from this analysis and from the bases shown.

Table 7.8 Dietary indicators by gross household income and sex
Adults aged 16 and over

Dietary indicators	Had a less healthy diet			Had a more healthy diet			Mentioned at least three of four components of a healthy diet			Base = 100%
	Observed %*	Expected %†	Obs/exp (%)†	Observed %*	Expected %†	Obs/exp (%)†	Observed %*	Expected %†	Obs/exp (%)†	
Gross household income										
Men										
£20,000 or more	17	21	82 **	15	12	124 **	19	15	124 **	196
£10,000-£19,999	20	20	101	10	13	80 **	10	14	75 **	436
£5,000-£9,999	28	20	138 **	10	13	76	6	11	57 **	682
Under £5,000	37	20	182 **	4	13	34 **	6	13	46 **	1084
Total	*21*	*21*	*100*	*13*	*13*	*100*	*14*	*14*	*100*	*2398*
Women										
£20,000 or more	11	16	70 **	21	17	122 **	20	17	113 **	537
£10,000-£19,999	16	16	99	17	17	98	14	16	86	735
£5,000-£9,999	20	16	130 **	12	17	72 **	13	14	92	722
Under £5,000	27	17	152 **	11	16	72 **	12	13	91	978
Total	*16*	*16*	*100*	*17*	*17*	*100*	*16*	*16*	*100*	*2972*

* The percentages refer to the proportions of the subgroups reporting each dietary indicator, so do not add to 100.

† See Appendix C for a full explanation of age-standardisation.

** Age-standardised ratio is significantly different from 100, at the 95% level.

Table 7.9 Dietary indicators by economic activity and sex
Adults aged 16 and over

Dietary indicators	Had a less healthy diet			Had a more healthy diet			Mentioned at least three of four components of a healthy diet			Base = 100%
	Observed %*	Expected %†	Obs/exp (%)†	Observed %*	Expected %†	Obs/exp (%)†	Observed %*	Expected %†	Obs/exp (%)†	
Economic activity status										
Men										
Employed	20	21	98	13	12	104	16	15	105 **	1559
Unemployed	40	23	174 **	5	11	43 **	7	15	42 **	91
Economically inactive	20	21	95	12	12	97	9	10	91	882
Total	*21*	*21*	*100*	*12*	*12*	*100*	*14*	*14*	*100*	*2532*
Women										
Employed	14	16	90 **	18	18	104	18	17	101	1776
Unemployed	30	18	167 **	9	16	58	15	17	88	81
Economically inactive	18	16	111 **	15	16	96	12	13	98	1368
Total	*16*	*16*	*100*	*17*	*17*	*100*	*16*	*16*	*100*	*3225*

* The percentages refer to the proportions of the subgroups reporting each dietary indicator, so do not add to 100.

† See Appendix C for a full explanation of age-standardisation.

** Age-standardised ratio is significantly different from 100, at the 95% level.

Health in England 1998: investigating the links between social inequalities and health

Table 7.10 Dietary indicators by highest qualification level and sex
Adults aged 16 and over

Dietary indicators	Had a less healthy diet			Had a more healthy diet			Mentioned at least three of four components of a healthy diet			Base = 100%
	Observed %*	Expected %†	Obs/exp (%)†	Observed %*	Expected %†	Obs/exp (%)†	Observed %*	Expected %†	Obs/exp (%)†	
Highest qualification level										
Men										
'A' Level or above	16	21	79 **	16	12	132 **	18	15	119 **	998
GCSE A-G or below	22	22	103	10	12	81 **	13	14	94	902
No qualifications	28	20	139 **	9	13	70 **	8	12	66 **	634
Total	21	21	100	12	12	100	14	14	100	2534
Women										
'A' Level or above	11	16	67 **	23	17	137 **	22	17	131 **	887
GCSE A-G or below	15	16	94	16	17	94	15	16	90	1275
No qualifications	21	15	143 **	13	17	74 **	11	14	78 **	1061
Total	16	16	100	17	17	100	16	16	100	3223

* The percentages refer to the proportions of the subgroups reporting each dietary indicator, so do not add to 100.

† See Appendix C for a full explanation of age-standardisation.

** Age-standardised ratio is significantly different from 100, at the 95% level.

Table 7.11 Dietary indicators by housing tenure and sex
Adults aged 16 and over

Dietary indicators	Had a less healthy diet			Had a more healthy diet			Mentioned at least three of four components of a healthy diet			Base = 100%
	Observed %*	Expected %†	Obs/exp (%)†	Observed %*	Expected %†	Obs/exp (%)†	Observed %*	Expected %†	Obs/exp (%)†	
Housing tenure										
Men										
Owner-occupier	18	21	86 **	14	13	111 **	15	14	107 **	1877
Rents from local authority	33	22	154 **	6	12	47 **	8	13	64 **	362
Rents privately	29	23	126 **	9	11	79	12	14	88	291
Total	21	21	100	12	12	100	14	14	100	2530
Women										
Owner-occupier	13	16	81 **	19	17	109 **	17	16	106 **	2155
Rents from local authority	26	16	161 **	11	16	67 **	11	15	77 **	613
Rents privately	21	18	120	13	16	86	14	15	91	455
Total	16	16	100	17	17	100	16	16	100	3223

* The percentages refer to the proportions of the subgroups reporting each dietary indicator, so do not add to 100.

† See Appendix C for a full explanation of age-standardisation.

** Age-standardised ratio is significantly different from 100, at the 95% level.

Table 7.12 Dietary indicators by household type and sex
Adults aged 16 and over

Dietary indicators	Had a less healthy diet			Had a more healthy diet			Mentioned at least three of four components of a healthy diet			Base = 100%
	Observed %*	Expected %†	Obs/exp (%)†	Observed %*	Expected %†	Obs/exp (%)†	Observed %*	Expected %†	Obs/exp (%)†	
Household type										
Men										
One person household	25	20	123	12	13	94	12	13	97	581
Living with others (no dependent children)	21	21	99	13	13	107	12	13	95	1302
Living with others (with dependent children)	20	21	92	11	12	90	17	16	111	631
Lone adult (with dependent children)	[8]	-	-	-	-	-	-	-	-	21
Total	21	21	100	12	12	100	14	14	100	2535
Women										
One person household	18	17	101	17	22	76 **	11	16	69 **	953
Living with others (no dependent children)	14	15	97	18	18	102	15	15	101	1234
Living with others (with dependent children)	16	17	89	17	16	102	19	18	102	762
Lone adult (with dependent children)	28	18	154 **	9	15	57 **	18	18	99	278
Total	16	16	100	17	17	100	16	16	100	3227

* The percentages refer to the proportions of the subgroups reporting each dietary indicator, so do not add to 100.

† See Appendix C for a full explanation of age-standardisation.

** Age-standardised ratio is significantly different from 100, at the 95% level.

Table 7.13 Dietary indicators by size of personal support group and sex
Adults aged 16 and over

Dietary indicators	Had a less healthy diet			Had a more healthy diet			Mentioned at least three of four components of a healthy diet			Base = 100%
	Observed %*	Expected %†	Obs/exp (%)†	Observed %*	Expected %†	Obs/exp (%)†	Observed %*	Expected %†	Obs/exp (%)†	
Personal support group										
Men										
9 or more people	18	21	82 **	13	12	110	16	14	113	574
4 - 8 people	22	21	102	13	12	105	15	14	105	1094
1 - 3 people	22	21	108	11	13	87	12	14	87	801
No support	31	20	146	8	13	66	2	14	16 **	54
Total	21	21	100	12	12	100	14	14	100	2523
Women										
9 or more people	16	15	104	20	18	114	18	16	114	686
4 - 8 people	13	16	82 **	18	17	106	15	16	97	1511
1 - 3 people	20	16	124 **	13	17	80 **	14	15	94	989
No support	20	14	142	8	19	52	12	16	72	33
Total	16	16	100	17	17	100	16	16	100	3219

* The percentages refer to the proportions of the subgroups reporting each dietary indicator, so do not add to 100.

† See Appendix C for a full explanation of age-standardisation.

** Age-standardised ratio is significantly different from 100, at the 95% level.

Table 7.14 Dietary indicators by community activity and sex
Adults aged 16 and over

Dietary indicators	Had a less healthy diet			Had a more healthy diet			Mentioned at least three of four components of a healthy diet			Base = 100%
	Observed %*	Expected %†	Obs/exp (%)†	Observed %*	Expected %†	Obs/exp (%)†	Observed %*	Expected %†	Obs/exp (%)†	
Community activity										
Men										
Some community activity	18	21	86	17	13	131 **	16	14	117	*570*
No community activity	22	21	104	11	12	91 **	13	14	95	*1965*
Total	*21*	*21*	*100*	*12*	*12*	*100*	*14*	*14*	*100*	2535
Women										
Some community activity	13	16	82 **	22	17	128 **	20	16	124 **	*1082*
No community activity	17	16	108 **	14	17	86 **	14	16	88 **	*2145*
Total	*16*	*16*	*100*	*17*	*17*	*100*	*16*	*16*	*100*	3227

* The percentages refer to the proportions of the subgroups reporting each dietary indicator, so do not add to 100.

† See Appendix C for a full explanation of age-standardisation.

** Age-standardised ratio is significantly different from 100, at the 95% level.

Table 7.15 Dietary indicators by whether agrees with the statement 'I am satisfied with the amount of control I have over decisions that affect my life' and sex
Adults aged 16 and over

Dietary indicators	Had a less healthy diet			Had a more healthy diet			Mentioned at least three of four components of a healthy diet			Base = 100%
	Observed %*	Expected %†	Obs/exp (%)†	Observed %*	Expected %†	Obs/exp (%)†	Observed %*	Expected %†	Obs/exp (%)†	
Whether satisfied with the amount of control over decisions that affect life										
Men										
Agree	20	21	97	13	12	103	13	14	94	*1881*
Neither agree nor disagree	25	20	121	13	13	100	16	14	112	*247*
Disagree	21	20	104	11	13	85	17	15	118	*395*
Total	*21*	*21*	*100*	*12*	*12*	*100*	*14*	*14*	*100*	2523
Women										
Agree	16	16	100	18	17	103	16	16	100	*2552*
Neither agree nor disagree	14	16	88	15	17	90	15	16	93	*294*
Disagree	17	15	112	15	18	85	18	16	106	*364*
Total	*16*	*16*	*100*	*17*	*17*	*100*	*16*	*16*	*100*	3210

* The percentages refer to the proportions of the subgroups reporting each dietary indicator, so do not add to 100.

† See Appendix C for a full explanation of age-standardisation.

** Age-standardised ratio is significantly different from 100, at the 95% level.

Table 7.16 Dietary indicators by whether agrees with the statement 'I can influence decisions that affect my neighbourhood' and sex
Adults aged 16 and over

Dietary indicators	Had a less healthy diet			Had a more healthy diet			Mentioned at least three of four components of a healthy diet			Base = 100%
	Observed %*	Expected %†	Obs/exp (%)†	Observed %*	Expected %†	Obs/exp (%)†	Observed %*	Expected %†	Obs/exp (%)†	
Whether can influence decisions that affect neighbourhood										
Men										
Agree	**20**	20	102	**16**	13	123	**15**	14	107	*579*
Neither agree nor disagree	**18**	22	84 **	**13**	12	108	**16**	14	111	*645*
Disagree	**23**	21	108	**11**	13	86 **	**13**	14	91	*1290*
Total	*21*	*21*	*100*	*12*	*12*	*100*	*14*	*14*	*100*	*2514*
Women										
Agree	**13**	15	83 **	**19**	18	109	**20**	16	122 **	*769*
Neither agree nor disagree	**14**	16	88	**18**	17	110	**14**	16	85	*815*
Disagree	**18**	16	115 **	**15**	17	90 **	**15**	15	97	*1608*
Total	*16*	*16*	*100*	*17*	*17*	*100*	*16*	*16*	*100*	*3192*

* The percentages refer to the proportions of the subgroups reporting each dietary indicator, so do not add to 100.

† See Appendix C for a full explanation of age-standardisation.

** Age-standardised ratio is significantly different from 100, at the 95% level.

Table 7.17 Dietary indicators by neighbourhood social capital score and sex
Adults aged 16 and over

Dietary indicators	Had a less healthy diet			Had a more healthy diet			Mentioned at least three of four components of a healthy diet			Base = 100%
	Observed %*	Expected %†	Obs/exp (%)†	Observed %*	Expected %†	Obs/exp (%)†	Observed %*	Expected %†	Obs/exp (%)†	
Neighbourhood social capital score										
Men										
Very high	**20**	21	95	**13**	12	103	**21**	14	149 **	*448*
High	**18**	21	88	**14**	13	115	**11**	14	79 **	*733*
Medium	**22**	21	105	**12**	12	102	**16**	14	112	*690*
Low	**24**	21	111	**:**	12	79 **	**11**	14	78 **	*654*
Total	*21*	*21*	*100*	*12*	*12*	*100*	*14*	*14*	*100*	*2525*
Women										
Very high	**12**	16	79 **	**19**	17	109	**19**	16	118	*576*
High	**12**	16	86	**18**	17	109	**17**	16	105	*896*
Medium	**17**	16	105	**15**	17	90	**14**	15	91	*881*
Low	**1:**	16	122 **	**16**	17	94	**14**	16	92	*862*
Total	*16*	*16*	*100*	*17*	*17*	*100*	*16*	*16*	*100*	*3215*

* The percentages refer to the proportions of the subgroups reporting each dietary indicator, so do not add to 100.

† See Appendix C for a full explanation of age-standardisation.

** Age-standardised ratio is significantly different from 100, at the 95% level.

Health in England 1998: investigating the links between social inequalities and health

Table 7.18 Dietary indicators by area deprivation category and sex
Adults aged 16 and over

Dietary indicators	Had a less healthy diet			Had a more healthy diet			Mentioned at least three of four components of a healthy diet			*Base = 100%*
	Observed %*	Expected %†	Obs/exp (%)†	Observed %*	Expected %†	Obs/exp (%)†	Observed %*	Expected %†	Obs/exp (%)†	
Area deprivation category										
Men										
1 More Affluent	**19**	21	89	**16**	12	130 **	**16**	14	115	*487*
2	**19**	21	90	**15**	13	120	**17**	14	121	*455*
3	**19**	21	89	**13**	12	105	**13**	14	90	*650*
4	**23**	21	107	**9**	12	72 **	**12**	14	90	*558*
5 More Deprived	**29**	21	137 **	**8**	12	64 **	**12**	14	85	*385*
Total	*21*	*21*	*100*	*12*	*12*	*100*	*14*	*14*	*100*	*2535*
Women										
1 More Affluent	**10**	15	66 **	**19**	18	107	**19**	15	122 **	*568*
2	**14**	16	86	**1:**	17	115	**18**	16	109	*634*
3	**15**	16	96	**17**	17	102	**15**	15	97	*799*
4	**18**	16	108	**15**	17	92	**16**	15	103	*716*
5 More Deprived	**26**	17	154 **	**13**	16	77 **	**9**	16	60 **	*510*
Total	*16*	*16*	*100*	*17*	*17*	*100*	*16*	*16*	*100*	*3227*

* The percentages refer to the proportions of the subgroups reporting each dietary indicator, so do not add to 100.

† See Appendix C for a full explanation of age-standardisation.

** Age-standardised ratio is significantly different from 100, at the 95% level.

Table 7.19 Logistic regression for dietary indicators - model 1
Adults aged 16 and over

Characteristics	Number of cases	Less healthy diet		More healthy diet		Mentioned at least three of the components of a healthy diet	
		Multiplying factors	95% Confidence intervals	Multiplying factors	95% Confidence intervals	Multiplying factors	95% Confidence intervals
Baseline odds		0.260		0.117		0.151	
Sex							
Male (R)	2342	1.00		1.00		1.00	
Female	2860	0.63 *	0.54 - 0.73	1.68 *	1.41 - 2.00	1.37 *	1.17 - 1.61
Age							
16-24 (R)	346	1.00		1.00		1.00	
25-34	994	0.86	0.65 - 1.15	1.34	0.87 - 2.08	1.63 *	1.11 - 2.38
35-44	983	0.65 *	0.48 - 0.88	1.72 *	1.12 - 2.65	1.85 *	1.27 - 2.71
45-54	831	0.47 *	0.35 - 0.65	2.67 *	1.74 - 4.10	1.89 *	1.28 - 2.78
55-64	720	0.39 *	0.28 - 0.55	3.06 *	1.97 - 4.76	1.63 *	1.13 - 2.54
65-74	718	0.36 *	0.25 - 0.50	2.92 *	1.85 - 4.61	1.63 *	1.07 - 2.48
75 and over	610	0.52 *	0.37 - 0.73	2.37 *	1.47 - 3.82	0.65	0.39 - 1.09
Social class							
I&II (R)	1687	-	- -	1.00	-	-	- -
III (Non-manual)	1227	-	- -	0.85 *	0.68 - 1.06	-	- -
III (Manual)	1010	-	- -	0.87	0.67 - 1.12	-	- -
IV&V	1278	-	- -	0.72	0.55 - 0.93	-	- -
Gross household income							
£20,000 or more (R)	2019	1.00		1.00		1.00	
£10,000 - £19,999	1366	1.30 *	1.06 - 1.58	0.82	0.67 - 1.00	0.70 *	0.57 - 0.86
£5,000 - £9,999	1131	1.57 *	1.23 - 2.00	0.62 *	0.48 - 0.81	0.68 *	0.53 - 0.88
Under £5,000	686	1.90 *	1.44 - 2.50	0.49 *	0.35 - 0.68	0.78	0.58 - 1.04
Highest qualification level							
'A'Level or above (R)	1772	1.00		1.00		1.00	
GCSE A-G or below	1952	1.27 *	1.06 - 1.54	0.70 *	0.58 - 0.86	0.71 *	0.60 - 0.85
No qualifications	1478	1.71 *	1.37 - 2.13	0.57 *	0.44 - 0.74	0.50 *	0.39 - 0.65
Housing tenure							
Owner-occupier (R)	3654	1.00		-	- -	-	- -
Rents local authority	892	1.54 *	1.26 - 1.89	-	- -	-	- -
Rents privately	656	1.22	0.98 1.53	-	- -	-	- -
Number of cases in the model	5202			5202		5196	

* Significant at the 95% level.

(R) reference category

Table 7.20 Logistic regression for dietary indicators - model 2
Adults aged 16 and over

Characteristics	Number of cases	Less healthy diet		More healthy diet		Mentioned at least three of the components of a healthy diet	
Baseline odds		**0.243**		**0.163**		**0.270**	
		Multiplying factors	95% Confidence intervals	Multiplying factors	95% Confidence intervals	Multiplying factors	95% Confidence intervals
Sex							
Male (R)	2388	1.00		1.00		1.00	
Female	2957	0.63 *	0.54 - 0.73	1.59 *	1.35 - 1.88	1.28 *	1.09 - 1.51
Age							
16-24 (R)	422	1.00		1.00		1.00	
25-34	1015	0.85	0.65 - 1.11	1.24	0.84 - 1.83	1.45 *	1.03 - 2.04
35-44	991	0.65 *	0.49 - 0.85	1.52 *	1.04 - 2.23	1.61 *	1.15 - 2.27
45-54	836	0.47 *	0.35 - 0.64	2.46 *	1.68 - 3.60	1.59 *	1.12 - 2.26
55-64	721	0.38 *	0.28 - 0.53	2.77 *	1.88 - 4.10	1.40	0.97 - 2.02
65-74	727	0.36 *	0.26 - 0.50	2.64 *	1.76 - 3.96	1.25	0.85 - 1.84
75 and over	633	0.51 *	0.37 - 0.69	2.18 *	1.42 - 3.35	0.55 *	0.34 - 0.87
Gross household income							
£20,000 or more (R)	2059	1.00		1.00		1.00	
£10,000 - £19,999	1400	1.31 *	1.07 - 1.60	0.78 *	0.64 - 0.95	0.74 *	0.60 - 0.90
£5,000 - £9,999	1162	1.58 *	1.25 - 2.01	0.59 *	0.46 - 0.76	0.76 *	0.59 - 0.98
Under £5,000	724	1.96 *	1.50 - 2.57	0.48 *	0.35 - 0.65	0.90	0.67 - 1.20
Highest qualification level							
'A'Level or above (R)	1810	1.00		1.00		1.00	
GCSE A-G or below	2000	1.25 *	1.04 - 1.51	0.66 *	0.55 - 0.79	0.75 *	0.63 - 0.90
No qualifications	1535	1.69 *	1.36 - 2.10	0.51 *	0.40 - 0.64	0.57 *	0.45 - 0.74
Housing tenure							
Owner-occupier (R)	3728	1.00		-	- -	-	- -
Rents local authority	926	1.49 *	1.22 - 1.82	-	- -	-	- -
Rents privately	691	1.18	0.95 - 1.47	-	- -	-	- -
Personal support group							
9 or more people (R)	1172	-	- -	-	- -	1.00	
4-8 people	2431	-	- -	-	- -	0.83	0.69 - 1.01
1-3 people	1660	-	- -	-	- -	0.76 *	0.61 - 0.94
No support	80	-	- -	-	- -	0.34 *	0.14 - 0.87
Community activity							
Some community activity(R)	1534	-	- -	1.00		1.00	
No community activity	3807	-	- -	0.74 *	0.63 - 0.87	0.81 *	0.69 - 0.96
Whether satisfied with amount of control over decisions that affect life							
Agree (R)	4119	-	- -	1.00		-	- -
Neither agree nor disagree	503	-	- -	0.87	0.66 - 1.14	-	- -
Disagree	719	-	- -	0.74 *	0.58 - 0.94	-	- -
Neighbourhood social capital score							
Very High (R)	955	1.00		-	- -	-	- -
High	1517	0.97	0.77 - 1.21	-	- -	-	- -
Medium	1469	1.13	0.91 - 1.42	-	- -	-	- -
Low	1404	1.27 *	1.02 - 1.59	-	- -	-	- -
Area deprivation category							
1 More affluent (R)	986	-	- -	-	- -	1.00	
2	1010	-	- -	-	- -	0.94	0.75 - 1.19
3	1331	-	- -	-	- -	0.83	0.66 - 1.04
4	1197	-	- -	-	- -	0.86	0.68 - 1.10
5 More deprived	819	-	- -	-	- -	0.57 *	0.42 - 0.77
Number of cases in the model		**5345**		**5341**		**5343**	

* Significant at the 95% level.

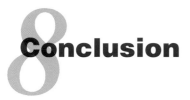

Conclusion

8.1 Introduction

This chapter draws together the results presented in the report to show the personal, social and neighbourhood characteristics associated with various health measures. It aims to give a broad picture of the relative importance of these characteristics and, with some provisos, a view on those groups which appear consistently to have less healthy lifestyles, as defined by the survey. Five areas of health status and behaviour have been discussed in this report: self-reported health status, smoking, drinking, physical activity and diet. For each of these areas, analysis was carried out to show which personal factors and social environment characteristics had significant independent effects on a number of health measures.

The variables in the analysis were divided into two groups: demographic and socio-economic characteristics, and social environment characteristics.

Those variables defined as demographic and socio-economic were:

- Sex
- Age
- Marital status
- Social class
- Gross household income
- Economic activity
- Highest qualification level
- Housing tenure
- Household type

The social environment variables were:
- Personal support group
- Community activity
- Satisfaction with control over own life decisions
- Influence over decisions affecting neighbourhood
- Neighbourhood social capital score (summarising views about the neighbourhood)
- Area deprivation category

Description of the analysis techniques

Several analysis techniques have been presented in this report but for this chapter logistic regression has been used to highlight the main factors associated with health. When looking at the results there are some important provisos to bear in mind about the technique. If a variable did not have a significant effect on a health measure, it does not necessarily mean that there was no association with the variable. The logistic regression analysis identified those variables with a significant effect, *after holding all the other variables in the model constant.* However, if two variables were highly correlated with one another, the logistic regression model would only retain one as significant[1].

It should also be noted that, in some instances, the survey may not have identified a variable as having an independent effect due to small sample numbers: for example, when it was only a small subgroup within a variable which had the particularly strong association with the health measure.

Given these provisos, however, the logistic regression method does enable broad conclusions to be drawn as to the main social and personal characteristics which affect health behaviours.

8.2 Characteristics with independent effects – for all reported health measures

All the measures in the five areas of health discussed in the report, are shown in Figure 8.1 together with the demographic, socio-economic and social environment variables used in the analysis. An asterisk (*) shows where a variable was found to have a significant independent effect on the health measure.

Demographic and socio-economic variables

The age of the informant was an important factor in all of the health measures analysed and this was the only variable which showed a significant effect for all measures. The sex of the informant and their highest qualification level were also important factors in that they were both independently associated with at least one of the measures in each of the areas of health status and behaviour.

Of the other demographic and socio-economic variables, marital status, income, housing tenure and household type were associated with at least one of the health measures in four out of the five areas of health status or behaviour. Social class, however, was only significant in three areas; self-reported health, cigarette smoking and physical activity. Economic activity had independent, but strong affects in just two areas - self-reported health and physical activity.

Social environment variables

The social environment variables had fewer independent effects on the health measures than the demographic and socio-economic variables. As a group, they were more likely to be independently associated with stress levels and with smoking status, than with the other aspects of health and health behaviour. They featured least in relation to the measures of physical activity and diet quality.

The measures of personal support and of community activity were significant factors in explaining variation in four out of the five areas of health status and behaviour. (Personal support was not a significant factor in explaining an individual's level of physical activity, while community activity was not significant in the area of self-reported health status).

Satisfaction with control over life decisions and neighbourhood social capital score were important variables in three of the areas of health status and behaviour (as was the measure of influence over decisions affecting the neighbourhood) but the former two variables appeared to be particularly important in explaining self-reported health status and cigarette smoking. The HEMS measure of area deprivation, which would be correlated to other variables in this survey, was significant only in explaining cigarette smoking status. **(Figure 8.1)**

8.3 Subgroups with the highest odds of reporting particular health measures

Figure 8.1 is a useful summary of the variables which were important in explaining the variation in the health measures, but in order to look at these effects in more detail, this section investigates a subset of the health measures shown in the previous section. In order to summarise the relationship between health behaviour and status, and personal and social characteristics, only a reduced number of the health measures could be explored here. The six health measures were chosen to represent two from the analysis of self-reported health status and, in addition, four measures to represent 'high-risk' behaviour for each health behaviour.

Figure 8.2 shows those groups most likely to report less healthy lifestyles, as defined by the survey. (In several cases, the group with the highest odds was not statistically different from another group so, in order not to mislead, the other group is shown in parenthesis in the Figure.)

The measures of health status and behaviour selected, are as follows:

The proportions of adults who reported having:
 • 'less than good' general health,
 • a large amount of stress in the last 12 months,
and the proportions who:
 • were current cigarette smokers,
 • usually drank over 21 units of alcohol a week (men), or over 14 units (women)
 • were classified as having a 'sedentary' level of physical activity,
 • were classified as having a 'less healthy diet' (based on a survey diet score).

Despite the provisos mentioned in this report, the results enable some broad conclusions to be drawn as to the effect of personal and social circumstances on health status and behaviour. The ability to be able to identify particular groups who consistently displayed less healthy lifestyles would be useful, but the picture is not altogether clear.

For a number of variables, very different subgroups emerged with the highest odds of having all of the 'less healthy' behaviours. For household income, for example, it was generally the lower income groups who had the highest odds across the health measures, but the exception was for drinking where the highest income group had the highest odds.

For age, there was even more variation. The youngest groups had the highest odds of being current smokers, of drinking over 21/14 units and of having a 'less healthy diet', but the oldest group had the highest odds of being 'sedentary'. Those in the middle age-groups had the highest odds of having a large amount of stress, while those aged 55–64 had the highest odds of reporting 'less than good' general health. **(Figure 8.2)**

One of the main aims of HEMS 1998 has been to explore how personal, social and neighbourhood characteristics affect health status and behaviour. Clearly, the relationship is complex. Some characteristics, such as age, income and household type are strongly related to health, but the subgroups within these who were most likely to have the less healthy attributes differ for the different aspects of health. However, for other characteristics, particular subgroups do appear consistently across the health measures to be those with less healthy attributes. These include respondents with no educational qualifications, those with no personal support group, those not involved in community activities, those lacking control over decisions affecting their lives, those with low 'neighbourhood social capital', and to some extent, those in local authority housing.

Notes and references

1.   For example, the survey showed that self-reported general health status varied in relation to social class, (- the proportions reporting 'less than good' general health and/or having a limiting long-standing illness were greater in the manual social classes than in the non-manual classes). However, after taking account of all the other variables included in the logistic regression model, social class did not have a significant effect on this health measure. This is probably because it was correlated with other variables retained in the model, such as income, economic activity and housing tenure. Similarly, area deprivation category was correlated with some of the socio-economic variables and therefore may not at first sight appear to be associated with as many of the measures as it may have been if a different set of variables had originally been included in the models.

Figure 8.1 Variables which have significant independent effects, for each health status or health behaviour

Analysis	Self-reported status			Cigarette smoking status		Alcohol consumption (usual weekly units)		
	Less than good good health	Limiting long-standing illness	Large amounts of stress	Current smoker	Never smoked	1–21, men/ 1–4, women	Over 21, men/ over 14 women	Over 36, men/ Over 26, women
Demographic								
Sex	-	-	*	-	*	-	*	*
Age	*	*	*	*	*	*	*	*
Marital status	-	-	*	*	*	*	-	-
Household type	*	*	*	*	*	*	*	*
Socio-economic variables								
Social class	-	-	*	*	-	-	-	-
Gross household income	*	*	*	-	-	-	*	-
Economic activity	*	*	-	-	-	-	-	-
Highest qualification level	*	-	-	*	*	*	-	-
Housing tenure	*	*	*	*	*	*	-	-
Social environment variables								
Personal support group	*	-	*	-	*	*	*	*
Community activity	-	-	-	*	*	-	*	*
Satisfaction with control over decisions affecting own life	*	*	*	*	*	-	-	-
Influence over decisions affecting neighbourhood	-	-	*	*	-	*	-	-
Neighbourhood social capital	*	*	*	*	*	-	-	-
Area deprivation category	-	-	-	*	*	-	-	-

Analysis	Levels of physical activity			Dietary indicators		
	'Sedentary'	'Moderate'	'Vigorous'	'Less healthy diet'	'More healthy diet'	Mentioned at least three main components
Demographic						
Sex	-	*	*	*	*	*
Age	*	*	*	*	*	*
Marital status	-	*	*	-	-	-
Household type	*	-	-	-	-	-
Socio-economic variables						
Social class	*	*	-	-	-	-
Gross household income	*	-	*	*	*	*
Economic activity	*	*	-	-	-	-
Highest qualification level	*	*	-	*	*	*
Housing tenure	-	-	-	*	-	-
Social environment variables						
Personal support group	-	-	-	-	-	*
Community activity	*	*	-	-	*	*
Satisfaction with control over decisions affecting own life	-	-	-	-	*	-
Influence over decisions affecting neighbourhood						
Neighbourhood social capital	-	-	-	*	-	-
Area deprivation category	-	-	-	-	-	*

* Has significant independent effect
- Has no significant independent effect

Figure 8.2 Variables with significant independent effects on six health measures, and the subgroups within those variables with the highest odds

Analysis variables	Self-reported health status		Cigarette smoking status	Alcohol consumption (usual weekly units)	Level of physical activity	Diet quality (based on a survey score)
	Has 'less than good' health	Had large amounts of stress	Was a current smoker	Drank over 21 units (men)/or over 14 units (women)	Was 'sedentary' (did 30 mins or more moderate activity less than once a week)	Had a 'less healthy diet'
Demographic varables						
Sex	-	Women	-	Men	-	Men
Age	55–64 (45–54)	35–44 (25–34, 45–54)	16–24 (25–34)	16–24	75 and over	16–74 (25–34)
Marital status	-	Wid, div, sep (Married)	Wid, div, sep	-	-	-
Household type	One person (Other adults– no dep. children)	Lone parent (One person)	Lone parent (Other adults– no dep. children)	One person	Other adults– no dep. children (All except lone parent)	-
Socio-economic variables						
Social class	-	I/II	III Manual (IV/V)	-	III Non-manual	-
Gross household income	£5,000–9,999 (<£5,000)	£5,000–9,999	-	£20,000+	£5,000–9,999 (<£5,000)	<£5,000 (£5,000–9,999)
Economic activity	Inactive	-	-	-	Inactive	-
Highest qualification level	No qualifications	-	No qualifications	-	No qualifications	No qualifications
Housing tenure	LA	LA	Privately rented	-	-	LA
Social environment variables						
Personal support group	None (1–3, and 9+)	None	-	None (4–8, and 9+)	-	-
Community activity	-	-	Not involved	Not involved	Not involved	-
Whether agrees: satisfied with control over decisions affecting own life	Disagree (Neither agree nor disagree)	Disagree	Disagree	-	-	-
Whether agrees: can influence decisions affecting neighbourhood	-	Disagree (Agree)	Agree (Disagree)	-	-	-
Neighbourhood social capital	Low	Low	Low	-	-	Low (Medium)
Area deprivation category	-	-	Category 4 (Categories 2, 3, and 5 'more deprived')	-	-	-

Notes to table:

Sub-group not in parenthesis - Variable has significant independent effect, and sub-group within with highest odds.

(Sub-group in parenthesis with highest odds). - Variable has significant independent effect, (and sub-group with odds not significantly different from those for the sub-group

- No sub-group shown - Variable has no significant independent effect.

Health in England 1998: investigating the links between social inequalities and health

Part B - *Supplementary tables*

This section presents tables on aspects of general health status, smoking, drinking, physical activity and diet which are outside of the main focus of Chapters 3 to 7 of the report. These include:

- **Trend tables**

    Trend tables are included on topics presented in previous HEMS reports. These tables compare available results from HEMS 1995 and 1996 with those for 1998. In previous HEMS there was an upper age limit of 74 years, so to ensure comparability, trend tables in this report include only respondents aged 16–74.

- **New aspects**

    1998 tables are presented for some of the new topics included in the 1998 survey but not discussed within Chapters 3 to 7. These tables include respondents aged 16 and over.

Table B.3.1 Self-reported effect of stress on health by age and sex

Adults aged 16 and over

Age	16-24	25-34	35-44	45-54	55-64	65-74	75 and over	Total
Self-reported effect of stress on health	%	%	%	%	%	%	%	%
Men								
Very harmful	2	5	7	6	6	6	8	5
Quite harmful	15	29	30	30	26	20	24	26
Not harmful	75	59	59	58	52	50	38	58
Completely free of stress	7	4	2	4	11	20	26	8
Don't know	1	3	2	2	4	4	4	3
Base = 100%	*233*	*432*	*466*	*433*	*390*	*350*	*253*	*2557*
Women								
Very harmful	6	7	6	9	6	8	9	7
Quite harmful	29	29	38	35	36	26	26	32
Not harmful	62	58	51	50	48	52	43	52
Completely free of stress	2	4	3	3	8	14	16	6
Don't know	0	3	2	3	2	1	6	2
Base = 100%	*272*	*630*	*571*	*464*	*406*	*447*	*460*	*3250*
All								
Very harmful	4	6	6	7	6	7	9	6
Quite harmful	22	29	34	33	31	23	25	29
Not harmful	69	58	55	54	50	51	41	55
Completely free of stress	5	4	3	4	10	16	20	7
Don't know	1	3	2	2	3	2	5	2
Base = 100%	*505*	*1062*	*1037*	*897*	*796*	*797*	*713*	*5807*

Table B.3.2   Self-reported effect of stress on health by year and sex

Adults aged 16–74

Year	1996	1998
Self-reported effect of stress on health	%	%
Men		
Very harmful	6	5
Quite harmful	35	26
Not harmful	51	60
Completely free of stress	7	7
Don't know	2	2
Base = 100%	*2039*	*2304*
Women		
Very harmful	10	7
Quite harmful	43	33
Not harmful	41	54
Completely free of stress	5	5
Don't know	1	2
Base = 100%	*2594*	*2790*
All		
Very harmful	8	6
Quite harmful	39	29
Not harmful	46	56
Completely free of stress	6	6
Don't know	1	2
Base = 100%	*4633*	*5094*

1996 - 1998

Table B.3.3   Whether agrees that 'generally health is a matter of luck' by age and sex
Adults aged 16 and over

Age	16-24	25-34	35-44	45-54	55-64	65-74	75 and over	Total
Whether agrees that 'generally health is a matter of luck'	%	%	%	%	%	%	%	%
Men								
Agree	18	22	24	34	38	41	48	30
Neither agrees nor disagrees	19	13	14	15	12	14	16	14
Disagree	63	65	61	51	50	45	36	56
Base = 100%	*232*	*433*	*466*	*431*	*387*	*349*	*249*	*2547*
Women								
Agree	24	25	27	33	40	44	53	33
Neither agrees nor disagrees	18	15	14	14	15	15	15	15
Disagree	58	60	59	54	45	42	32	52
Base = 100%	*272*	*629*	*572*	*462*	*405*	*444*	*456*	*3240*
All								
Agree	21	24	26	33	39	42	51	32
Neither agrees nor disagrees	18	14	14	15	13	14	16	15
Disagree	60	62	60	52	48	43	33	54
Base = 100%	*504*	*1062*	*1038*	*893*	*792*	*793*	*705*	*5787*

Table B.3.4   Whether agrees that 'generally health is a matter of luck' by year and sex
Adults aged 16–74

Year	1995	1996	1998
Whether agrees that 'generally health is a matter of luck'	%	%	%
Men			
Strongly agrees	2	2	2
Agrees	24	22	26
Neither agrees nor disagrees	10*	16	14
Disagrees	54	52	48
Strongly disagrees	10	8	9
Base = 100%	*2121*	*2039*	*2298*
Women			
Strongly agrees	2	2	3
Agrees	24	23	28
Neither agrees nor disagrees	14*	19	15
Disagrees	55	50	48
Strongly disagrees	6	6	6
Base = 100%	*2548*	*2589*	*2784*
All			
Strongly agrees	2	2	3
Agrees	24	23	27
Neither agrees nor disagrees	12*	17	15
Disagrees	54	51	48
Strongly disagrees	8	7	8
Base = 100%	*4669*	*4628*	*5082*

* 'Don't know' in 1995.

Table B.3.5   Whether agrees that 'I don't really have time to think about my health' by age and sex
Adults aged 16 and over

Age	16-24	25-34	35-44	45-54	55-64	65-74	75 and over	Total
Whether agrees that 'I don't really have time to think about my health'	%	%	%	%	%	%	%	%
Men								
Agree	15	20	18	19	24	26	31	20
Neither agrees nor disagrees	14	16	12	11	11	10	14	13
Disagree	71	64	69	70	65	63	56	67
Base = 100%	*232*	*433*	*466*	*433*	*389*	*346*	*248*	*2547*
Women								
Agree	20	22	28	28	32	36	32	28
Neither agrees nor disagrees	16	11	12	8	9	15	14	12
Disagree	64	67	60	64	59	49	54	60
Base = 100%	*272*	*628*	*571*	*464*	*406*	*443*	*454*	*3238*
All								
Agree	17	21	23	24	28	31	31	24
Neither agrees nor disagrees	15	14	12	10	10	13	14	12
Disagree	67	66	64	67	62	56	55	63
Base = 100%	*504*	*1061*	*1037*	*897*	*795*	*789*	*702*	*5785*

Table B.3.6   Whether agrees that 'I don't really have time to think about my health' by year and sex
Adults aged 16–74

Year	1995	1996	1998
Whether agrees that 'I don't really have time to think about my health'	%	%	%
Men			
Strongly agrees	2	2	1
Agrees	24	25	19
Neither agrees nor disagrees	9*	19	13
Disagrees	60	51	58
Strongly disagrees	6	4	9
Base = 100%	*2120*	*2036*	*2299*
Women			
Strongly agrees	4	4	3
Agrees	32	31	24
Neither agrees nor disagrees	8*	18	12
Disagrees	52	45	54
Strongly disagrees	4	2	8
Base = 100%	*2546*	*2594*	*2784*
All			
Strongly agrees	3	3	2
Agrees	28	28	21
Neither agrees nor disagrees	8*	19	12
Disagrees	55	48	56
Strongly disagrees	5	3	8
Base = 100%	*4666*	*4630*	*5083*

* 'Don't know' in 1995.

Table B.3.7   Respondents' assessment of factors which have a bad effect on their health by age and sex

Age	16-24	25-34	35-44	45-54	55-64	65-74	75 and over	Total
Factors which are bad for health	%	%	%	%	%	%	%	%
Men								
Stress	16	29	34	28	19	10	14	24
My weight	10	26	29	25	24	24	11	23
The amount I smoke	29	28	19	21	12	10	5	20
Eating a poor diet	32	26	20	11	9	4	3	18
Environmental pollution	18	18	19	16	17	11	9	17
Road traffic in this area	6	8	14	11	15	11	12	11
The amount of alcohol I drink	20	15	10	8	6	1	2	10
Being unemployed	5	5	5	8	8	2	0	5
Violent crime in this area	4	4	3	5	5	4	4	4
Living on my own	1	2	2	3	4	4	11	3
The quality of local health services	2	2	2	2	6	4	4	3
The quality of my housing	4	2	2	2	3	2	1	2
My sexual behaviour	0	1	2	1	0	1		1
None of these	24	24	24	29	34	45	48	30
*Base**	*233*	*433*	*465*	*433*	*389*	*350*	*252*	*2555*
Women								
Stress	32	32	35	34	24	12	15	28
My weight	23	31	32	36	33	27	13	29
The amount I smoke	28	20	16	15	11	6	2	15
Eating a poor diet	37	23	17	12	5	5	4	16
Environmental pollution	16	16	17	15	13	12	7	14
Road traffic in this area	10	9	13	10	10	11	10	10
The amount of alcohol I drink	12	5	4	5	0	1	0	4
Being unemployed	5	5	6	5	2	0	0	4
Violent crime in this area	6	5	4	4	7	8	7	6
Living on my own	3	4	4	3	6	11	16	6
The quality of local health services	2	4	6	5	5	4	4	4
The quality of my housing	5	5	5	2	4	2	3	4
My sexual behaviour	2	1	2	1	0	-	-	1
None of these	26	25	26	24	32	42	47	30
*Base**	*272*	*631*	*572*	*464*	*406*	*447*	*457*	*3249*
All								
Stress	24	31	35	32	22	11	15	26
My weight	16	28	30	31	29	26	12	26
The amount I smoke	28	24	17	18	11	8	3	17
Eating a poor diet	34	24	19	11	7	5	4	17
Environmental pollution	18	17	18	16	15	11	8	16
Road traffic in this area	8	8	14	10	12	11	11	11
The amount of alcohol I drink	16	10	7	6	3	1	1	7
Being unemployed	5	5	5	6	5	1	0	4
Violent crime in this area	5	4	4	4	6	6	6	5
Living on my own	2	3	3	3	5	8	14	4
The quality of local health services	2	3	4	4	5	4	4	4
The quality of my housing	4	4	4	2	3	2	2	3
My sexual behaviour	1	1	2	1	0	0		1
None of these	25	24	25	26	33	43	47	30
*Base**	*505*	*1064*	*1037*	*897*	*795*	*797*	*709*	*5804*

* Percentages total to more than 100% because more than one answer could be given.

Table B.4.1 Mean and median cigarette consumption per smoker by age and sex
Current cigarette smokers aged 16 and over

Age		16-24	25-34	35-44	45-54	55-64	65-74	75 and over	Total
		Mean and median consumption per smoker							
Men									
Daily cigarette consumption	- mean	10.9	15.3	17.7	18.7	15.0	16.2	13.8	15.4
	- standard deviation	7.7	8.7	11.0	9.4	8.6	10.6	7.6	9.5
	- median	10.0	15.0	18.6	20.0	16.0	15.0	11.1	15.0
Weekly cigarette consumption	- mean	76.2	106.9	123.8	130.6	105.2	113.5	96.3	107.8
	- standard deviation	53.7	60.7	77.1	65.6	60.1	74.5	53.1	66.7
	- median	70.0	105.0	130.0	140.0	112.0	105.0	77.6	105.0
Base = 100%		*97*	*163*	*137*	*120*	*101*	*67*	*33*	*718*
Women									
Daily cigarette consumption	- mean	10.4	11.9	15.1	15.2	15.1	13.2	10.8	13.2
	- standard deviation	7.1	8.3	9.3	9.2	10.1	8.6	6.5	8.8
	- median	10.0	11.4	15.0	15.0	14.3	10.6	10.0	11.4
Weekly cigarette consumption	- mean	72.6	83.3	106.0	106.7	105.5	92.2	75.7	92.1
	- standard deviation	49.9	58.3	65.2	64.3	70.7	59.9	45.7	61.8
	- median	70.0	80.0	105.0	105.0	100.4	74.0	70.0	80.0
Base = 100%		*118*	*228*	*170*	*134*	*96*	*68*	*43*	*857*
All									
Daily cigarette consumption	- mean	10.6	13.8	16.4	17.0	15.0	14.8	12.1	14.3
	- standard deviation	7.4	8.7	10.3	9.4	9.3	9.8	7.1	9.3
	- median	10.0	13.6	16.4	16.4	15.0	13.3	10.0	14.1
Weekly cigarette consumption	- mean	74.4	96.5	114.8	118.9	105.3	103.3	84.7	100.2
	- standard deviation	51.8	60.7	71.9	66.1	65.4	68.6	49.8	64.8
	- median	70.0	95.0	115.0	115.0	105.0	92.9	70.0	99.0
Base = 100%		*215*	*391*	*307*	*254*	*197*	*135*	*76*	*1575*

Table B.4.2   Mean and median cigarette consumption per smoker by year and sex
Current cigarette smokers aged 16-74

Year		1995	1996	1998
		Mean and median consumption per smoker		
Men				
Daily cigarette consumption	- mean	15.5	15.3	15.4
	- standard deviation	10.1	8.9	9.6
	- median	15.0	15.0	15.0
Weekly cigarette consumption	- mean	108.6	107.3	108.1
	- standard deviation	70.6	62.4	67.0
	- median	105.0	105.0	105.0
Base = 100%		*651*	*636*	*685*
Women				
Daily cigarette consumption	- mean	13.8	12.9	13.2
	- standard deviation	9.6	8.0	8.9
	- median	12.1	11.4	11.4
Weekly cigarette consumption	- mean	96.9	90.5	92.8
	- standard deviation	67.5	56.1	62.3
	- median	85.0	80.0	80.0
Base = 100%		*748*	*761*	*814*
All				
Daily cigarette consumption	- mean	14.7	14.2	14.4
	- standard deviation	9.9	8.6	9.3
	- median	14.0	13.6	14.3
Weekly cigarette consumption	- mean	103.0	99.1	100.7
	- standard deviation	69.3	60.0	65.2
	- median	98.0	95.0	100.0
Base = 100%		*1399*	*1397*	*1499*

Table B.4.3   Cigarette smoking status by standard region of residence and sex
Adults aged 16 and over

Region	North	Yorkshire & Humberside	North West	East Midlands	West Midlands	East Anglia	Greater London	Outer Metropolitan & SE	South West	Total England
Smoking status	%	%	%	%	%	%	%	%	%	%
Men										
Current cigarette smokers:										
Less than 10 a day	7	4	5	7	7	13	10	9	6	8
10, less than 20 a day	9	9	12	10	10	16	10	11	12	11
20 or more per day	12	12	11	11	12	6	12	9	10	11
Total current cigarette smokers*	28	25	29	28	28	35	32	30	29	29
Ex-regular cigarette smokers	24	30	32	31	30	27	25	31	35	30
Never or only occasionally smoked cigarettes	48	45	39	41	42	38	43	40	36	41
Base = 100%	*181*	*287*	*294*	*215*	*295*	*144*	*300*	*561*	*277*	*2554*
Women										
Current cigarette smokers:										
Less than 10 a day	8	7	9	10	6	10	10	8	9	8
10, less than 20 a day	7	11	12	13	11	12	9	10	7	10
20 or more per day	8	10	12	8	5	5	8	3	5	7
Total current cigarette smokers*	24	29	33	31	22	26	26	22	21	26
Ex-regular cigarette smokers	25	20	20	18	18	19	18	23	20	20
Never or only occasionally smoked cigarettes	51	51	46	51	60	54	55	55	59	54
Base = 100%	*221*	*348*	*452*	*305*	*338*	*158*	*377*	*694*	*356*	*3249*
All										
Current cigarette smokers:										
Less than 10 a day	8	6	7	8	6	11	10	9	8	8
10, less than 20 a day	8	10	12	12	11	14	9	11	10	11
20 or more per day	10	11	12	9	8	5	10	6	8	9
Total current cigarette smokers*	26	27	32	30	25	31	29	26	25	27
Ex-regular cigarette smokers	25	25	25	24	24	23	22	27	27	25
Never or only occasionally smoked cigarettes	50	48	43	47	51	46	50	48	48	48
Base = 100%	*402*	*635*	*746*	*520*	*633*	*302*	*677*	*1255*	*633*	*5803*

* Includes those for whom number of cigarettes was not known.

Table B.4.4   Whether current smokers would like to give up smoking altogether by year and sex
Current cigarette smokers aged 16-74

1995 - 1998

Year	1995	1996	1998
Whether current smokers would like to give up smoking altogether	%	%	%
Men			
Yes	68	67	70
No	25	29	25
Don't know	7	4	5
Base = 100%	*658*	*642*	*689*
Women			
Yes	68	64	69
No	24	31	26
Don't know	8	5	6
Base = 100%	*749*	*762*	*814*
All			
Yes	68	65	69
No	25	30	25
Don't know	7	5	6
Base = 100%	*1407*	*1404*	*1503*

Table B.4.5   Length of time ex-smokers have stopped smoking by age and sex
Ex-smokers aged 16 and over

Age	16-24	25-34	35-44	45-54	55-64	65-74	75 and over	Total
Length of time ex-smokers have stopped	%	%	%	%	%	%	%	%
Men								
Less than 6 months	24	26	5	2	4	2	-	6
6 months, less than 1 year	24	6	2	2	1	0	-	2
One year but less than 2 years	6	5	8	2	1	2	1	3
Two years but less than 5 years	46	27	4	7	6	5	2	9
Five years or more	-	37	81	87	89	91	97	81
Base = 100%	*10*	*77*	*105*	*140*	*171*	*198*	*149*	*850*
Women								
Less than 6 months	45	10	2	1	4	2	1	5
6 months, less than 1 year	15	12	2	2	2	2	2	4
One year but less than 2 years	11	15	3	2	3	3	1	4
Two years but less than 5 years	19	27	9	8	7	7	2	10
Five years or more	11	35	84	88	85	86	94	78
Base = 100%	*19*	*87*	*101*	*103*	*107*	*148*	*144*	*709*
All								
Less than 6 months	36	19	4	1	4	2	0	6
6 months, less than 1 year	19	9	2	2	1	1	1	3
One year but less than 2 years	8	9	6	2	1	2	1	3
Two years but less than 5 years	30	27	6	8	6	6	2	9
Five years or more	6	36	82	88	88	89	96	79
Base = 100%	*29*	*164*	*206*	*243*	*278*	*346*	*293*	*1559*

Table B.4.6   Length of time ex-smokers have stopped smoking by year and sex
Ex-smokers aged 16-74

1995 - 1998

Year	1995	1996	1998
Length of time ex-smokers have stopped	%	%	%
Men			
Less than 6 months	3	5	7
6 months, less than 1 year	2	3	2
One year but less than 2 years	3	4	3
Two years but less than 5 years	13	11	10
Five years or more	79	76	78
Base = 100%	*635*	*600*	*701*
Women			
Less than 6 months	6	6	6
6 months, less than 1 year	4	4	4
One year but less than 2 years	5	4	5
Two years but less than 5 years	18	14	11
Five years or more	67	72	74
Base = 100%	*520*	*537*	*565*
All			
Less than 6 months	4	6	6
6 months, less than 1 year	3	3	3
One year but less than 2 years	4	4	4
Two years but less than 5 years	15	12	10
Five years or more	74	74	77
Base = 100%	*1155*	*1137*	*1266*

Table B.4.7   Main reason why ex-smokers stopped smoking by age and sex

Ex-smokers aged 16 and over

Age	16-24	25-34	35-44	45-54	55-64	65-74	75 and over	Total
Main reason for stopping smoking	%	%	%	%	%	%	%	%
Men								
Health reasons	44	60	68	56	64	66	59	62
Cost	38	15	8	21	15	14	21	16
Family reasons	12	20	14	16	7	8	8	12
Advised to by health professional	-	1	1	0	5	6	4	3
Did not like it/enjoy it	6	-	10	6	5	6	7	6
Other/None of these	-	4	-	1	3	1	1	2
Base = 100%	*10*	*68*	*97*	*132*	*161*	*184*	*135*	*787*
Women								
Health reasons	35	46	49	51	52	58	51	51
Cost	13	6	13	11	15	19	16	14
Family reasons	6	13	10	6	15	9	12	10
Pregnant	22	22	23	18	5	2	1	12
Advised to by health professional	-	-	1	-	2	3	4	2
Did not like it/enjoy it	20	12	3	13	9	6	12	10
Other/None of these	4	1	1	2	2	2	3	2
Base = 100%	*18*	*83*	*87*	*100*	*101*	*140*	*138*	*667*
All								
Health reasons	39	54	60	54	60	62	55	57
Cost	24	11	10	17	15	16	18	15
Family reasons	9	17	12	12	10	8	10	11
Pregnant	12	11	10	7	3	1	1	5
Advised to by health professional	-	-	1	0	4	5	4	2
Did not like it/enjoy it	14	5	7	9	7	6	10	7
Other/None of these	2	3	1	2	2	2	2	2
Base = 100%	*28*	*151*	*184*	*232*	*262*	*324*	*273*	*1454*

Table B.4.8 Main reason why ex-smokers stopped smoking by year and sex

Ex-smokers aged 16-74

1995 - 1998

Year	1995	1996	1998
Main reason for stopping smoking	%	%	%
Men			
Health reasons	62	60	62
Cost	14	18	15
Family reasons	7	10	12
Advised to by health professional	1	1	2
Did not like it/enjoy it*	-	9	6
Other/None of these	15	2	2
Base = 100%	*634*	*576*	*652*
Women			
Health reasons	49	49	51
Cost	12	15	13
Family reasons	10	11	10
Pregnant	12	13	14
Advised to by health professional	1	2	1
Did not like it/enjoy it*	-	9	9
Other/None of these	14	2	2
Base = 100%	*519*	*517*	*529*
All			
Health reasons	57	55	57
Cost	14	16	14
Family reasons	8	11	11
Pregnant	6	5	6
Advised to by health professional	1	1	2
Did not like it/enjoy it*	-	9	7
Other/None of these	15	2	2
Base = 100%	*1153*	*1093*	*1181*

* 'Did not enjoy it/like it' was not used as a code in 1995.

Table B.5.1   Percentage who have heard about measuring alcohol in units by age and sex
Adults aged 16 and over

Age	16-24	25-34	35-44	45-54	55-64	65-74	75 and over	Total
Whether heard of units	Percentage who have heard about measuring alcohol in units							
Men	89	91	89	88	81	71	48	84
Base=100%	233	431	464	432	390	350	254	2554
Women	89	86	88	86	77	65	40	78
Base=100%	272	631	572	463	406	447	457	3248
All	89	89	88	87	79	68	43	81
Base=100%	505	1062	1,036	895	796	797	711	5802

Table B.5.2   Percentage who have heard about measuring alcohol in units by year and sex
Adults aged 16-74

1995-1998

Year	1995	1996	1998
Whether heard of units	%	%	%
Men	83	84	86
Base=100%	2120	2042	2300
Women	77	81	83
Base=100%	2545	2600	2791
All	80	83	85
Base=100%	4665	4642	5091

Table B.5.3 Percentage who had heard of alcohol units and correctly identified the number in specified drinks by age and sex

Adults aged 16 and over who had heard of alcohol units

Age	16-24	25-34	35-44	45-54	55-64	65-74	75 and over	Total
Type of drink	Percentage correctly identifying the number of units							
Men								
Glass of wine	43	62	56	54	41	34	19	49
Pint of beer*	50	70	64	62	50	34	22	56
Single pub measure of spirits	35	57	46	42	37	26	18	41
Base=100%	*196*	*358*	*363*	*327*	*277*	*241*	*190*	*1952*
Women								
Glass of wine	40	56	56	50	36	26	11	43
Pint of beer*	45	61	57	46	32	24	7	43
Single pub measure of spirits	31	44	42	40	26	22	8	33
Base=100%	*211*	*498*	*445*	*331*	*279*	*295*	*350*	*2409*
All								
Glass of wine	42	59	56	52	38	30	14	46
Pint of beer*	48	66	61	55	42	29	12	50
Single pub measure of spirits	33	51	44	41	32	24	12	37
Base=100%	*407*	*856*	*808*	*658*	*556*	*536*	*540*	*4361*

* In 1995 and 1996, this question referred to a pint of beer. In 1998 the question asked about the number of units in half a pint of beer.

Table B.5.4 Percentage who had heard of alcohol units and correctly identified the number in specified drinks by year and sex

Adults aged 16-74 who had heard of alcohol units

1995-1998

Year	1995	1996	1998
Type of drink	%	%	%
Men			
Glass of wine	44	45	51
Pint of beer*	50	51	58
Single pub measure of spirits	35	37	43
Base=100%	*1742*	*1705*	*1762*
Women			
Glass of wine	38	41	47
Pint of beer*	30	34	47
Single pub measure of spirits	27	30	36
Base=100%	*1925*	*2072*	*2059*
All			
Glass of wine	41	43	49
Pint of beer*	40	43	53
Single pub measure of spirits	31	34	40
Base=100%	*3667*	*3777*	*3821*

* In 1995 and 1996, this question referred to a pint of beer. In 1998 the question asked about the number of units in half a pint of beer.

Table B.5.5 Respondent's opinion on how many units of alcohol a day a man can regularly drink without risking his health by age and sex

Adults aged 16 and over

Age	16-24	25-34	35-44	45-54	55-64	65-74	75 and over	Total
Number of units of alcohol that can be drunk without risk (men)	%	%	%	%	%	%	%	%
Men								
None/ No safe limit	1	1	1	2	1	1	1	1
Below daily benchmark for men*	22	25	23	20	16	14	10	20
Equivalent of daily benchmark*	30	45	43	43	36	30	22	38
Over daily benchmark for men	23	17	17	19	20	16	10	18
Don't know	24	12	15	16	26	38	57	22
Base=100%	*230*	*426*	*458*	*422*	*377*	*335*	*245*	*2493*
Women								
None/ No safe limit	2	3	2	1	1	0	0	2
Below daily benchmark for men*	22	31	28	26	25	16	11	24
Equivalent of daily benchmark*	33	36	36	42	30	25	11	32
Over daily benchmark for men	24	12	15	10	11	6	6	12
Don't know	20	18	18	21	34	52	71	30
Base=100%	*268*	*622*	*563*	*452*	*392*	*432*	*433*	*3162*
All								
None/ No safe limit	2	2	2	1	1	1	1	1
Below daily benchmark for men*	22	28	26	23	21	15	10	22
Equivalent of daily benchmark*	31	41	40	42	33	28	15	35
Over daily benchmark for men	23	15	16	14	15	11	8	15
Don't know	22	15	16	19	30	46	66	26
Base=100%	*498*	*1048*	*1021*	*874*	*769*	*767*	*678*	*5655*

* Daily benchmark is 3-4 units per day for men.

Table B.5.6 Respondent's opinion on how many units of alcohol a day a woman can regularly drink without risking her health by age and sex
Adults aged 16 and over

Age	16-24	25-34	35-44	45-54	55-64	65-74	75 and over	Total
Number of units of alcohol that can be drunk without risk (women)	%	%	%	%	%	%	%	%
Men								
None/ No safe limit	2	2	2	1	2	1	1	2
Below daily benchmark for women*	15	17	17	12	11	8	5	14
Equivalent of daily benchmark*	39	53	48	48	40	34	22	44
Over daily benchmark for women	21	16	17	18	19	14	8	17
Don't know	24	13	16	20	29	43	64	24
Base=100%	*229*	*424*	*457*	*421*	*376*	*328*	*241*	*2476*
Women								
None/ No safe limit	3	4	2	2	2	1	2	2
Below daily benchmark for women*	16	25	23	17	18	12	6	18
Equivalent of daily benchmark*	40	45	48	52	38	30	19	41
Over daily benchmark for women	23	8	9	8	10	6	4	10
Don't know	18	17	17	21	33	51	70	29
Base=100%	*268*	*619*	*566*	*453*	*390*	*428*	*436*	*3160*
All								
None/ No safe limit	2	3	2	2	2	1	2	2
Below daily benchmark for women*	16	21	20	15	14	10	6	16
Equivalent of daily benchmark*	40	49	48	50	38	32	20	42
Over daily benchmark for women	22	12	13	13	14	10	6	13
Don't know	21	15	16	20	31	47	67	27
Base=100%	*497*	*497*	*1023*	*874*	*766*	*756*	*677*	*5636*

* Daily benchmark is 2 - 3 units per day for women.

Table B.6.1 Whether respondent thinks that they are getting enough exercise to keep fit by year and sex
Adults aged 16-74

1995-1998

Year	Men			Women			All		
	1995	1996	1998	1995	1996	1998	1995	1996	1998
Whether getting enough exercise to keep fit	%	%	%	%	%	%	%	%	%
Yes	52	54	51	48	49	47	50	52	49
No	46	44	46	49	48	51	47	46	48
Can't take exercise	2	2	2	2	2	2	2	2	2
Base = 100%	*2113*	*2039*	*2293*	*2542*	*2529*	*2785*	*4655*	*4631*	*5078*

Table B.6.2 Whether would like to take more exercise and when intends to do so by year and sex
Adults aged 16-74

1996-1998

Year	Men		Women		All	
	1996	1998	1996	1998	1996	1998
Percentage who would like to take more exercise:	66	69	69	71	68	70
Base = 100%	*1976*	*2220*	*2508*	*2697*	*4484*	*4917*
When intends to take more exercise	%	%	%	%	%	%
Within the next month	25	30	25	29	25	30
Within the next six months	19	20	22	24	20	22
Within the next year	10	8	9	9	10	8
Intends to take more exercise but not in the next year	3	3	4	4	4	4
Unlikely to take more exercise	43	38	39	34	41	36
Base = 100%	*1984*	*2211*	*2515*	*2689*	*4499*	*4900*

Table B.7.1   Aspects of usual diet by diet quality and sex
Adults aged 16 and over

Diet quality*	'Less healthy diet'	'More healthy diet'	Total
Usual diet	Percentage consuming each food		
Men			
Aspects with positive diet score			
Eats brown, granary, wholemeal, wheatmeal or S.Asian breads	11	76	36
Has skimmed or semi-skimmed milk	41	92	71
Eats bread or rolls daily†	67	96	85
Eats potatoes, rice or pasta daily†	24	76	52
Eats fruit or vegetables or salads daily†	22	97	59
Aspects with negative diet score			
Spreads butter or hard margarine on bread	47	4	23
Has fried foods fried in solid fat	24	1	10
Eats chips and other fried food daily†	8	1	3
Eats biscuits, cakes or confectionery daily†	54	21	38
Base = 100%	*531*	*323*	*2535*
Women			
Aspects with positive diet score			
Eats brown, granary, wholemeal, wheatmeal or S.Asian breads	15	81	48
Has skimmed or semi-skimmed milk	38	91	72
Eats bread or rolls daily†	60	91	82
Eats potatoes, rice or pasta daily†	28	78	56
Eats fruit or vegetables or salads daily†	33	97	74
Aspects with negative diet score			
Spreads butter or hard margarine on bread	55	4	26
Has fried foods fried in solid fat	32	1	10
Eats chips and other fried food daily†	5	0	1
Eats biscuits, cakes or confectionery daily†	59	19	38
Base = 100%	*534*	*543*	*3227*
All			
Aspects with positive diet score			
Eats brown, granary, wholemeal, wheatmeal or S.Asian breads	13	79	42
Has skimmed or semi-skimmed milk	40	92	71
Eats bread or rolls daily†	64	93	83
Eats potatoes, rice or pasta daily†	26	77	54
Eats fruit or vegetables or salads daily†	27	97	67
Aspects with negative diet score			
Spreads butter or hard margarine on bread	51	4	25
Has fried foods fried in solid fat	28	1	10
Eats chips and other fried food daily†	7	0	2
Eats biscuits, cakes or confectionery daily†	56	20	38
Base = 100%	*1065*	*866*	*5762*

* These groups are derived from a diet score grouped into four groups (see Chapter 7 and Appendix C).

† Frequency of eating foods 'daily' means at least once every day.

Table B.7.2 Consumption of fats by age and sex

Adults aged 16 and over

Age	16-24	25-34	35-44	45-54	55-64	65-74 over	75 and	Total
Food				Percentage consuming each food				
Men								
Drinks skimmed, semi-skimmed milk	71	73	77	80	70	67	52	72
Eats chips less than once a week	19	32	36	39	47	42	46	36
Does not use solid fat for cooking	95	94	90	90	87	84	77	90
Uses no, low, reduced fat spread	56	65	65	67	60	59	49	62
Uses low-fat varieties of milk, cooking fat and spread,* and eats chips less than once a week	12	19	19	24	23	22	14	19
Base = 100%†	*233*	*432*	*464*	*432*	*390*	*350*	*254*	*2555*
Women								
Drinks skimmed, semi-skimmed milk	72	76	77	79	81	70	54	74
Eats chips less than once a week	36	53	56	59	64	60	56	55
Does not use solid fat for cooking	93	94	91	92	90	82	79	90
Uses no, low, reduced fat spread	58	63	64	65	61	54	44	60
Uses low-fat varieties of milk, cooking fat and spread,* and eats chips less than once a week	22	32	32	34	36	24	19	29
Base = 100%†	*272*	*631*	*572*	*463*	*406*	*447*	*455*	*3246*
All								
Drinks skimmed, semi-skimmed milk	71	75	77	79	76	69	53	73
Eats chips less than once a week	27	42	46	49	56	52	52	45
Does not use solid fat for cooking	94	94	91	91	89	83	78	90
Uses no, low, reduced fat spread	57	64	64	66	61	56	46	60
Uses low-fat varieties of milk, cooking fat and spread,* and eats chips less than once a week	17	25	26	29	30	24	17	24
Base = 100%†	*505*	*1063*	*1036*	*895*	*796*	*797*	*709*	*5801*

* Skimmed or semi-skimmed milk, low- or reduced-fat spread and cooking oil.

† Bases are shown from 'eats chips less than once a week'. Bases may vary slightly for other items.

Table B.7.3   Consumption of fats by year and sex
Adults aged 16-74

1995-1998

Year	Men			Women			All		
	1995	1996	1998	1995	1996	1998	1995	1996	1998
Food	Percentage consuming each food								
Drinks skimmed, semi-skimmed milk	67	67	74	73	74	76	71	71	75
Eats chips less than once a week	31	35	35	48	53	55	40	44	45
Does not use solid fat for cooking	88	90	91	89	90	91	89	90	91
Uses no, low, reduced fat spread	49	52	62	59	56	61	54	54	62
Uses low-fat varieties of milk, cooking fat and spread,* and eats chips less than once a week	14	17	20	25	27	30	20	22	25
Base = 100%†	*2118*	*1934*	*2301*	*2545*	*2474*	*2791*	*4663*	*4408*	*5092*

* Skimmed or semi-skimmed milk, low- or reduced-fat spread and cooking oil.

† Bases are shown from 'eats chips less than once a week'. Bases may vary slightly for other items.

Health in England 1998: investigating the links between social inequalities and health

Table B.7.4 Knowledge about diet by age and sex
Adults aged 16 and over

Age	16-24	25-34	35-44	45-54	55-64	65-74 over	75 and	Total
Components of a healthy diet mentioned*				*Percentage giving each answer*				
Men								
Eat lots of fruit, vegetables or salad	59	59	65	66	69	62	53	62
Cut down on fatty or fried foods, eat grilled food	37	43	44	44	34	36	24	39
Eat lots of fibre, cereals, wholemeal food	23	23	24	31	30	23	19	25
Eat lots of starch, carbohydrates, potatoes, pasta or rice	26	25	24	18	15	13	8	20
Mentioned at least three of the four main components above	11	16	16	17	14	10	4	14
Eat a balanced diet	35	35	29	24	24	14	22	28
Eat everything in moderation	10	15	15	14	14	13	22	14
Avoid red meat, eat white meat, fish	8	14	16	19	15	20	15	15
Cut down on sugar, cakes and confectionery	11	7	6	6	6	8	4	7
Eat lots of meat, eggs, cheese, drink lots of milk	11	8	7	9	10	11	14	9
Drink lots of water, fruit juice, liquid	7	4	5	6	2	4	2	5
Cut down on salt	1	2	4	2	2	2	2	2
Other	26	20	23	27	22	31	35	25
Including:								
Food which is full of vitamins and minerals	8	4	4	2	1	0	-	3
Eat regularly, 3 meals a day, not between meals	0	2	1	1	2	1	5	1
Eat fresh food, avoid convenience foods and takeaways	-	0	0	3	1	2	2	1
Eat whatever you like	0	0	0	2	3	3	3	1
Alcohol (changing types of drink or cutting down)	-	1	1	2	1	2	1	1
No meat, meat free diet	0	1	1	1	-	-	0	1
Don't know	2	0	0	2	2	3	5	2
Base+	*229*	*429*	*460*	*429*	*384*	*347*	*251*	*2529*
Women								
Eat lots of fruit, vegetables or salad	68	72	75	78	79	78	67	74
Cut down on fatty or fried foods, eat grilled food	39	44	46	42	36	36	23	39
Eat lots of fibre, cereals, wholemeal food	23	27	30	30	24	25	16	26
Eat lots of starch, carbohydrates, potatoes, pasta or rice	22	26	27	22	20	14	10	21
Mentioned at least three of the four main components above	11	19	20	19	13	14	6	16
Eat a balanced diet	38	26	24	22	17	14	16	23
Eat everything in moderation	9	13	12	13	10	12	15	12
Avoid red meat, eat white meat, fish	6	16	21	25	29	24	20	20
Cut down on sugar, cakes and confectionery	13	11	13	13	11	11	8	12
Eat lots of meat, eggs, cheese, drink lots of milk	5	5	6	5	11	10	9	7
Drink lots of water, fruit juice, liquid	10	7	8	4	6	7	7	7
Cut down on salt	4	3	3	3	1	1	1	2
Other	20	19	19	22	23	22	29	22
Including:								
Food which is full of vitamins and minerals	5	4	1	5	2	2	1	3
Eat regularly, 3 meals a day, not between meals	2	1	1	2	1	2	3	2
Eat fresh food, avoid convenience foods and takeaways	1	1	2	2	1	3	2	2
Eat whatever you like	-	0	1	0	0	1	3	1
Alcohol (changing types of drink or cutting down)	1	-	-	1	1	0	1	1
No meat, meat free diet	-	1	1	2	2	1	0	1
Don't know	1	1	1	0	1	2	2	1
Base†	*270*	*626*	*571*	*460*	*405*	*444*	*445*	*3221*

continued

Table B.7.4 - continued
Adults aged 16 and over

Age	16-24	25-34	35-44	45-54	55-64	65-74 over	75 and	Total
Components of a healthy diet mentioned*				Percentage giving each answer				
All								
Eat lots of fruit, vegetables or salad	63	65	70	72	74	70	62	68
Cut down on fatty or fried foods, eat grilled food	38	44	45	43	35	36	24	39
Eat lots of fibre, cereals, wholemeal food	23	25	27	31	27	24	17	26
Eat lots of starch, carbohydrates, potatoes, pasta or rice	24	26	26	20	17	14	9	21
Mentioned at least three of the four main components above	11	17	18	18	14	12	5	15
Eat a balanced diet	36	31	26	23	21	14	18	25
Eat everything in moderation	10	14	14	13	12	13	17	13
Avoid red meat, eat white meat, fish	7	15	18	22	22	22	18	18
Cut down on sugar, cakes and confectionery	12	9	9	10	8	10	6	9
Eat lots of meat, eggs, cheese, drink lots of milk	8	7	6	7	11	10	11	8
Drink lots of water, fruit juice, liquid	8	6	6	5	4	5	5	6
Cut down on salt	3	2	4	2	2	1	2	2
Other	23	20	21	25	22	27	31	23
Including:								
Food which is full of vitamins and minerals	7	4	2	3	1	1	0	3
Eat regularly, 3 meals a day, not between meals	1	2	1	1	2	2	4	2
Eat fresh food, avoid convenience foods and takeaways	0	0	1	3	1	3	2	1
Eat whatever you like	0	0	0	1	1	2	3	1
Alcohol (changing types of drink or cutting down)	1	0	1	2	1	1	1	1
No meat, meat free diet	0	1	1	1	1	1	0	1
Don't know	1	1	0	1	1	2	3	1
Base†	*499*	*1055*	*1031*	*889*	*789*	*791*	*696*	*5750*

* Respondents' answers were recorded verbatim, then coded into the eleven precodes or as 'other'. 'Other' answers mentioned by at least 1% of respondents are listed here.

† Percentages total to more than 100% because more than one answer could be given.

Table B.7.5   Knowledge about diet by year and sex
Adults aged 16-74

Year	Men		Women		All	
	1996	1998	1996	1998	1996	1998
*Components of a healthy diet mentioned**	Percentage giving each answer					
Eat lots of fruit, vegetables or salad	60	63	73	75	67	69
Cut down on fatty or fried foods, eat grilled food	44	40	46	41	45	41
Eat lots of fibre, cereals, wholemeal food	27	26	27	27	27	26
Eat lots of starch, carbohydrates, potatoes, pasta or rice	19	21	20	23	20	22
Mentioned at least three of the four main components above	14	15	17	17	16	16
Eat a balanced diet	29	28	23	24	26	26
Eat everything in moderation	19	14	16	12	18	13
Avoid red meat, eat white meat, fish	14	15	18	20	16	18
Cut down on sugar, cakes and confectionery	9	7	14	12	12	10
Eat lots of meat, eggs, cheese, drink lots of milk	7	9	7	7	7	8
Drink lots of water, fruit juice, liquid	4	5	6	7	5	6
Cut down on salt	3	2	4	3	3	2
Other	11	24	11	21	11	22
Including:						
Food which is full of vitamins and minerals	-	3	-	3	-	3
Eat regularly, 3 meals a day, not between meals	-	1	-	1	-	1
Eat fresh food, avoid convenience foods and takeaways	-	1	-	2	-	1
Eat whatever you like	-	1	-	0	-	1
Alcohol (changing types of drink or cutting down)	-	1	-	1	-	1
No meat, meat free diet	-	1	-	1	-	1
Don't know	1	1	1	1	1	1
Base†	*2013*	*2278*	*2568*	*2776*	*4582*	*5054*

* Respondents' answers were recorded verbatim, then coded into the eleven precodes or as 'other'. 'Other' answers mentioned by at least 1% of respondents are listed here. In 1996, the answers given as 'other' were coded but the proportions in each category were too small to show separately.

† Percentages total to more than 100% because more than one answer could be given.

Table B.7.6 Whether agrees that 'I get confused over what's supposed to be healthy and what isn't' by age and sex
Adults aged 16 and over

Age	16-24	25-34	35-44	45-54	55-64	65-74	75 and over	Total
Whether agrees that 'I get confused over what's supposed to be healthy and what isn't	%	%	%	%	%	%	%	%
Men								
Strongly agree	2	3	3	3	6	8	2	4
Agree	26	31	32	33	31	34	29	31
Neither agree nor disagree	20	10	12	10	10	9	17	12
Disagree	42	47	47	50	50	48	48	47
Strongly disagree	9	9	6	4	4	2	4	6
Base = 100%	*232*	*432*	*464*	*431*	*387*	*349*	*250*	*2545*
Women								
Strongly agree	1	1	2	2	2	5	3	2
Agree	23	21	24	21	27	26	28	24
Neither agree nor disagree	16	9	8	11	9	9	11	10
Disagree	53	60	56	57	56	54	54	56
Strongly disagree	6	9	9	9	6	5	4	7
Base = 100%	*272*	*631*	*570*	*462*	*406*	*445*	*447*	*3233*
All								
Strongly agree	2	2	3	2	4	6	3	3
Agree	24	26	28	27	29	30	28	27
Neither agree nor disagree	18	10	10	10	9	9	14	11
Disagree	48	53	52	54	53	51	52	52
Strongly disagree	8	9	7	7	5	4	4	7
Base = 100%	*504*	*1063*	*1034*	*893*	*793*	*794*	*697*	*5778*

Table B.7.7 Whether agrees that 'I get confused over what's supposed to be healthy and what isn't' by year and sex
Adults aged 16-74

1995-1998

	Men			Women			All		
Year	1995	1996	1998	1995	1996	1998	1995	1996	1998
Whether agrees that 'I get confused over what's supposed to be healthy and what isn't'									
Strongly agree	5	3	4	3	3	2	4	3	3
Agree	39	31	31	33	27	24	36	29	27
Neither agree nor disagree	9*	15	12	7*	10	10	8*	13	11
Disagree	43	45	47	50	53	56	47	49	52
Strongly disagree	4	6	6	6	7	8	5	6	7
Base = 100%	*2119*	*2035*	*2295*	*2544*	*2595*	*2786*	*4663*	*4630*	*5081*

* 'Don't know' in 1995.

Table B.7.8 Whether agrees that 'experts never agree about what foods are good for you' by age
Adults aged 16 and over

Age	16-24	25-34	35-44	45-54	55-64	65-74 over	75 and	Total
Whether agrees that 'experts never agree what foods are good for you'	%	%	%	%	%	%	%	%
Strongly agree	5	12	12	10	15	13	10	11
Agree	45	50	54	60	62	67	60	56
Neither agree nor disagree	27	18	16	14	11	9	18	16
Disagree	20	19	17	15	12	10	11	16
Strongly disagree	2	1	1	1	1	1	1	1
Base = 100%	*502*	*1058*	*1,029*	*893*	*790*	*788*	*680*	*5740*

Table B.7.9 Whether agrees that 'experts never agree about what foods are good for you' by year
Adults aged 16-74

1995-1998

Year	1995	1996	1998
Whether agrees that 'experts never agree what foods are good for you'			
Strongly agree	11	13	11
Agree	59	55	55
Neither agree nor disagree	12*	16	16
Disagree	16	14	16
Strongly disagree	1	1	1
Base = 100%	*4658*	*4611*	*5060*

* 'Don't know' in 1995.

Table B.7.10   Whether agrees that 'eating healthy food is expensive' by age and sex
Adults aged 16 and over

Age Whether agrees that 'eating healthy food is expensive'	16-24	25-34	35-44	45-54	55-64	65-74 over	75 and	Total
	%	%	%	%	%	%	%	%
Men								
Strongly agree	5	4	6	3	6	6	5	5
Agree	21	28	25	30	32	31	36	28
Neither agree nor disagree	20	14	14	12	15	13	11	14
Disagree	50	47	50	50	44	48	44	48
Strongly disagree	4	6	5	4	4	2	3	4
Base = 100%	*232*	*431*	*464*	*430*	*386*	*348*	*249*	*2540*
Women								
Strongly agree	3	6	6	3	5	5	5	5
Agree	22	32	29	23	30	35	38	30
Neither agree nor disagree	16	15	14	10	10	10	10	12
Disagree	53	42	47	57	51	47	44	49
Strongly disagree	7	4	4	7	4	3	3	5
Base = 100%	*272*	*629*	*570*	*462*	*405*	*446*	*443*	*3227*
All								
Strongly agree	4	5	6	3	6	5	5	5
Agree	22	30	27	27	31	33	37	29
Neither agree nor disagree	18	15	14	11	12	12	10	13
Disagree	52	45	49	54	48	48	44	48
Strongly disagree	6	5	4	6	4	3	3	4
Base = 100%	*504*	*1,060*	*1,034*	*892*	*791*	*794*	*692*	*5767*

Table B.7.11 Percentage 'strongly agreeing' or 'agreeing' that 'eating healthy food is expensive' by year
Adults aged 16-74

1995-1998

| Year | 1995 | 1996 | 1998 | Base=100% | | |
				1995	1996	1998
	Percentage 'strongly agreeing' or 'agreeing' that 'eating healthy food is expensive'					
Age						
16-24	32	30	25	515	485	504
25-34	41	39	35	1039	1020	1060
35-44	37	37	33	900	925	1034
45-54	38	36	30	789	758	892
55-64	41	41	36	716	667	791
65-74	49	42	38	704	766	794
All aged 16-74	39	37	33	4663	4564	5075

Table B.7.12 Whether agrees that 'healthy foods are enjoyable' by age and sex
Adults aged 16 and over

Age	16-24	25-34	35-44	45-54	55-64	65-74 over	75 and	Total
Whether agrees that 'healthy foods are enjoyable'	%	%	%	%	%	%	%	%
Men								
Strongly agree	11	10	10	14	10	12	13	11
Agree	55	62	61	62	71	71	73	64
Neither agree nor disagree	25	21	20	16	14	12	7	18
Disagree	8	6	7	6	5	5	6	6
Strongly disagree	1	1	1	1	0	-	-	1
Base = 100%	233	432	464	431	384	349	250	2543
Women								
Strongly agree	12	13	15	15	14	12	16	14
Agree	62	69	70	72	72	70	74	70
Neither agree nor disagree	16	12	11	8	9	12	9	11
Disagree	8	6	4	4	5	5	2	5
Strongly disagree	1	0	0	0	0	0	-	0
Base = 100%	272	630	572	462	405	446	448	3235
All								
Strongly agree	12	11	12	15	12	12	15	13
Agree	58	66	65	67	72	70	74	67
Neither agree nor disagree	21	16	16	12	11	12	8	14
Disagree	8	6	6	5	5	5	3	6
Strongly disagree	1	1	1	0	0	0	-	0
Base = 100%	505	1062	1036	893	789	795	698	5778

Table B.7.13 Whether agrees that 'healthy foods are enjoyable' by year and sex
Adults aged 16-74

	Men			Women			All		
Year	**1995**	**1996**	**1998**	**1995**	**1996**	**1998**	**1995**	**1996**	**1998**
Whether agrees that 'healthy foods are enjoyable'	%	%	%	%	%	%	%	%	%
Strongly agree	9	9	11	11	10	14	10	9	12
Agree	66	61	63	75	69	69	71	65	66
Neither agree nor disagree	14*	24	19	8*	15	11	11*	19	15
Disagree	10	6	6	7	5	5	8	6	6
Strongly disagree	1	0	1	0	0	0	0	0	1
Base = 100%	*2119*	*2036*	*2293*	*2543*	*2595*	*2787*	*4662*	*4631*	*5080*

* 'Don't know' in 1995.

Part C - *Supplementary topics - tables only*

As in previous HEMS, the 1998 survey included questions on sexual health and behaviour in the sun. The results are not reported on in the main body of the report but, for completeness, tables are included showing the data for 1998. These are as follows:

■ **C.1 Sexual health tables**

These tables include both trend data and data from questions asked for the first time in HEMS 1998. The new questions were asked as part of a European Commission funded research project and were also asked in a number of other European countries.

As the module on sexual health was only addressed to respondents aged 16–54, results for the sexual health data are shown for these age-groups alone.

■ **C.2 Behaviour in the sun tables**

These tables include both trend data and data from questions asked for the first time in 1998. In previous HEMS there was an upper age limit of 74 years, so to ensure comparability, trend tables in this section include only those respondents aged 16–74. Tables for topics new in 1998 include respondents aged 16 and over.

Table C.1.1 Age at first intercourse by current age and sex
Adults aged 16-54

Age at interview	16-19	20-24	25-34	35-44	45-54	Total	HEMS 1995 Total
Age at first intercourse	%	%	%	%	%	%	%
Men							
Never had a sexual partner	42	7	2	3	2	7	15
Under 16	21	25	34	22	20	25	21
16-17	33	38	34	35	28	33	29
18-19	5	25	19	22	24	20	19
20-24	-	4	8	14	19	11	13
25 or over	-	2	3	4	7	4	3
Base = 100%	*105*	*114*	*419*	*448*	*414*	*1500*	*1369*
Mean (average) age	15.7	16.8	16.7	17.6	18.2	17.3	17.4
Standard error of the mean	0.1	0.2	0.1	0.1	0.1	0.1	0.1
5th percentile	12	14	13	14	13	13	14
10th percentile	14	14	14	15	14	14	14
Median age	16	17	16	17	18	17	17
90th percentile	17	19	20	21	23	21	21
95th percentile	18	20	22	24	27	24	24
*Base = 100%**	*63*	*106*	*409*	*432*	*404*	*1414*	*1191*
Women							
Never had a sexual partner	29	12	3	2	2	6	13
Under 16	33	24	18	12	9	16	14
16-17	36	45	39	37	25	35	31
18-19	3	12	26	29	34	25	24
20-24	-	7	12	17	26	15	17
25 or over	-	-	2	3	4	2	2
Base = 100%	*114*	*145*	*609*	*545*	*434*	*1847*	*1662*
Mean (average) age	15.4	16.5	17.4	18.0	18.8	17.7	17.7
Standard error of the mean	0.1	0.1	0.1	0.1	0.1	0.1	0.1
5th percentile	13	13	14	14	15	14	14
10th percentile	14	14	15	15	16	15	15
Median age	16	16	17	18	18	17	17
90th percentile	17	19	20	22	22	21	21
95th percentile	17	22	23	23	24	23	23
*Base = 100%**	*85*	*131*	*591*	*534*	*423*	*1764*	*1474*

continued

Table C.1.1 *Continued*

Age at interview	16-19	20-24	25-34	35-44	45-54	Total	HEMS 1995 Total
All	%	%	%	%	%	%	%
Never had a sexual partner	36	10	3	3	2	7	14
Under 16	27	24	26	17	15	21	17
16-17	34	41	37	36	26	34	30
18-19	4	18	22	26	29	22	21
20-24	-	6	10	15	23	13	15
25 or over	-	1	3	4	6	3	3
Base = 100%	*219*	*259*	*1028*	*993*	*848*	*3347*	*3031*
Mean (average) age	15.5	16.6	17.0	17.8	18.5	17.5	17.6
Standard error of the mean	0.1	0.1	0.1	0.1	0.1	0.0	0.0
5th percentile	13	13	13	14	14	14	14
10th percentile	14	14	14	15	15	14	15
Median age	16	16	17	17	18	17	17
90th percentile	17	19	20	21	22	21	21
95th percentile	18	21	22	24	25	23	23
Base = 100%*	*148*	*237*	*1000*	*966*	*827*	*3178*	*2665*

* Excludes those reporting no sexual partner.

Table C.1.2 Method of contraception used at first intercourse by age and sex
Adults aged 16-54, who first had intercourse in the last five years

Age	16-19	20-24	25 and over	Total*	HEMS 1995 Total
Method of contraception	%	%	%	%	%
Men					
Male condom\sheath	71	73	[6]	68	71
Contraceptive pill	25	43	[3]	31	12
Emergency morning after pill	2	2	-	2	4
Female condom	-	-	-	-	1
Other, including sterilisation	0	2	-	1	2
None of these	9	4	[6]	12	10
Can't remember	4	0	[1]	2	5
Percentage using at least one method	87	96	[9]	86	84
Base = 100%	*61*	*45*	*14*	*120*	*119*
Women					
Male condom\sheath	72	71	[12]	70	67
Contraceptive pill	26	22	[3]	24	26
Emergency morning after pill	9	6	-	7	4
Female condom	1	3	-	2	-
Other, including sterilisation	0	1	[3]	0	0
None of these	8	6	-	9	10
Can't remember	-	-	-	-	1
Percentage using at least one method	92	94	[15]	91	88
Base = 100%	*83*	*57*	*18*	*158*	*159*
All					
Male condom\sheath	71	72	44	69	69
Contraceptive pill	26	32	15	27	19
Emergency morning after pill	6	4	0	5	4
Female condom	1	2	0	1	0
Other, including sterilisation	0	1	0	0	1
None of these	9	5	44	10	10
Can't remember	2	0	1	1	3
Percentage using at least one method	90	95	55	88	86
Base = 100%	*144*	*102*	*32*	*278*	*278*

*   Totals add to more than 100% because respondents may have used more than one method.

Table C.1.3 Number of sexual partners in the last 12 months by age and sex
Adults aged 16-54

Age	16-19	20-24	25-34	35-44	45-54	Total*	HEMS 1995 Total*	HEMS 1996 Total
Number of sexual partners in the last 12 months	%	%	%	%	%	%	%	%
Men								
None	48	14	7	8	11	13	16	14
One	24	49	78	80	82	71	67	69
Two	12	9	6	7	3	7	7	7
Three to four	11	17	6	3	1	5	6	5
Five to nine	5	8	3	2	0	3	2	2
Ten or more	-	4	2	1	3	2	2	1
Base = 100%	*105*	*114*	*418*	*450*	*414*	*1501*	*1341*	*1375*
Median	2	3	2	2	3	1	1	1
95th percentile	7	8	4	3	2	4	5	4
Base = 100%†	*56*	*99*	*386*	*402*	*352*	*1295*	*1114*	*1173*
Women								
None	30	17	9	10	13	13	14	12
One	37	53	81	86	85	76	77	78
Two	19	14	6	3	2	6	6	5
Three to four	6	15	3	1	0	3	2	3
Five to nine	6	1	0	0	0	1	0	1
Ten or more	2	1	1	0	0	1	0	0
Base = 100%	*114*	*146*	*611*	*549*	*436*	*1856*	*1596*	*1716*
Median	2	2	2	1	1	1	1	1
95th percentile	6	3	2	1	1	3	2	2
Base = 100%†	*84*	*124*	*550*	*481*	*358*	*1597*	*1353*	*1484*
All								
None	40	16	8	9	12	13	15	13
One	30	51	79	83	83	73	72	74
Two	15	12	6	5	3	6	7	6
Three to four	9	16	4	2	1	4	4	4
Five to nine	6	5	2	1	0	2	1	1
Ten or more	1	2	1	1	2	1	1	1
Base = 100%	*219*	*260*	*1029*	*999*	*850*	*3357*	*3078*	*3091*
Median	2	2	2	1	2	1	1	1
95th percentile	6	6	3	2	2	3	3	3
Base = 100%†	*140*	*223*	*936*	*883*	*710*	*2892*	*2467*	*2657*

* Proportions differ from those shown in the 1995 report because they exclude married, cohabiting, widowed, divorced and separated respondents who said they had never had a sexual partner.

† Excludes respondents who did not report a sexual partner in the last year.

Table C.1.4 Number of sexual partners in the last 12 months by social class based on own current or last job, age and sex
Adults aged 16-54

Social class	Men					Women				
	I and II	III (NM)	III (M)	IV & V	Total*	I and II	III (NM)	III (M)	IV & V	Total*
Age and number of sexual partners in the last 12 months	%	%	%	%	%	%	%	%	%	%
16-34										
None	4	22	7	27	13	9	15	7	14	13
One	76	59	70	50	65	78	66	69	62	68
Two or more	20	19	24	23	22	13	19	24	24	19
35-54										
None	8	15	10	8	9	9	14	14	10	11
One	84	73	80	78	81	88	84	82	86	86
Two or more	9	12	10	15	10	3	3	3	4	3
All										
None	6	19	8	19	11	9	14	10	12	12
One	81	66	76	61	74	84	75	75	75	78
Two or more	13	16	16	19	16	7	10	14	13	10
Bases = 100%										
16-34	189	89	176	126	584	224	302	79	204	809
35-54	384	97	252	126	863	309	349	68	251	978
All	573	186	428	252	1447	533	651	147	455	1787
Median	1	1	1	1	1	1	1	1	1	1
95th percentile	5	4	4	6	4	2	2	2	3	3
Base = 100%†	525	151	383	202	1267	475	547	129	395	1547

* Members of the Armed Forces, persons in inadequately described occupations and persons who have never worked are not shown as separate categories but are included in the figures for all persons.

† Excludes respondents who did not report a sexual partner in the last year.

Table C.1.5 Number of partners in the last year and whether used a condom on the last occasion of intercourse by age and sex
Adults aged 16-54

Age	16-24	25-34	35-44	45-54	Total	HEMS 1995 Total
Number of partners in the last year and whether used a condom on the last occasion of intercourse	%	%	%	%	%	%
Men						
No partner	32	6	8	11	13	21
One partner	35	78	80	82	71	63
Two or more partners, used a condom on last occasion of intercourse	18	7	4	1	7	8
Two or more partners, did not use a condom on last occasion of intercourse	13	8	7	6	8	7
Two or more partners, never used a condom	2	0	2	0	1	1
Base = 100%	*219*	*418*	*450*	*414*	*1501*	*1392*
Women						
No partner	24	9	10	13	13	19
One partner	45	81	86	85	76	72
Two or more partners, used a condom on last occasion of intercourse	15	3	1	0	4	3
Two or more partners, did not use a condom on last occasion of intercourse	14	6	2	2	6	5
Two or more partners, never used a condom	3	0	1	0	1	1
Base = 100%	*260*	*611*	*549*	*436*	*1856*	*1685*
All						
No partner	28	8	9	12	13	20
One partner	40	79	83	83	73	67
Two or more partners, used a condom on last occasion of intercourse	16	5	2	1	6	6
Two or more partners, did not use a condom on last occasion of intercourse	13	7	5	4	7	6
Two or more partners, never used a condom	2	0	1	0	1	1
Base = 100%	*479*	*1029*	*999*	*850*	*3357*	*3077*

Table C.1.6 Whether had a new sexual partner in the last year and whether used a condom on the first occasion of intercourse by age and sex
Adults aged 16-54

Age	16-24	25-34	35-44	45-54	Total
Whether new sexual partner in the last year and whether used a condom on the first occasion of intercourse	%	%	%	%	%
Men					
No new sexual partner	37	81	88	93	79
Had a new sexual partner, used a condom on first occasion of intercourse	43	12	6	4	13
Had a new sexual partner, did not use a condom on first occasion of intercourse	20	7	6	4	8
Base = 100%	*154*	*384*	*399*	*350*	*1287*
Women					
No new sexual partner	45	84	90	93	81
Had a new sexual partner, used a condom on first occasion of intercourse	43	9	5	4	13
Had a new sexual partner, did not use a condom on first occasion of intercourse	12	6	5	3	6
Base = 100%	*204*	*546*	*478*	*355*	*1583*
All					
No new sexual partner	41	83	89	93	80
Had a new sexual partner, used a condom on first occasion of intercourse	43	11	6	4	13
Had a new sexual partner, did not use a condom on first occasion of intercourse	16	7	6	4	7
Base = 100%	*358*	*930*	*877*	*705*	*2870*

Table C.1.7 Percentage who had changed their behaviour because of concern about AIDS by age and sex
Adults aged 16-54

Age	16-24	25-34	35-44	45-54	Total*	HEMS 1995 Total*
Percentage who had changed their behaviour because of concern about AIDS	%	%	%	%	%	%
Men						
Using a condom	18	14	6	2	10	15
Sticking to one partner	10	14	11	4	10	12
Finding out more about someone	18	9	5	2	8	10
Having fewer partners	5	7	2	1	4	5
Not having sex	3	1	1	1	1	2
Avoiding some sexual practices	1	4	1	1	2	3
Other changes	1	1	0	0	0	1
Not changed behaviour	62	64	76	89	73	64
Changed, but not because of AIDS	4	8	5	3	5	6
Base = 100%	*226*	*425*	*455*	*418*	*1524*	*1427*
Women						
Using a condom	17	11	5	2	8	11
Sticking to one partner	12	13	8	5	9	11
Finding out more about someone	14	8	3	1	6	9
Having fewer partners	8	4	2	1	4	3
Not having sex	2	1	2	2	2	3
Avoiding some sexual practices	1	1	1	-	1	2
Other changes	2	0	0	0	1	1
Not changed behaviour	63	69	80	87	75	70
Changed, but not because of AIDS	4	7	7	4	5	7
Base = 100%	*265*	*614*	*555*	*437*	*1871*	*1720*
All						
Using a condom	17	13	6	2	9	13
Sticking to one partner	11	13	9	5	10	12
Finding out more about someone	16	9	4	2	7	10
Having fewer partners	6	6	2	1	4	4
Not having sex	2	1	1	1	2	2
Avoiding some sexual practices	1	3	1	0	1	2
Other changes	2	0	0	0	1	1
Not changed behaviour	63	66	78	88	74	67
Changed, but not because of AIDS	4	7	6	4	5	6
Base = 100%	*491*	*1039*	*1010*	*855*	*3395*	*3147*

* Totals add to more than 100% because respondents may have changed in more than one way.

Table C.1.8 Respondents' assessment of their risk of getting HIV/AIDS compared to other people in this country by age and sex
Adults aged 16-54

Age	16-24	25-34	35-44	45-54	Total*
Risk of getting HIV/AIDS 'compared to other people in this country'	%	%	%	%	%
Men					
A greater risk of gettng HIV/AIDS	3	3	2	2	3
The same risk of gettng HIV/AIDS	46	22	14	9	21
Less risk of gettng HIV/AIDS	35	66	73	77	64
Don't know	16	9	10	12	11
Base = 100%	*226*	*425*	*456*	*418*	*1525*
Women					
A greater risk of gettng HIV/AIDS	2	2	2	1	2
The same risk of gettng HIV/AIDS	49	23	15	12	23
Less risk of gettng HIV/AIDS	33	67	70	79	64
Don't know	16	8	13	8	11
Base = 100%	*265*	*616*	*555*	*436*	*1872*
All					
A greater risk of gettng HIV/AIDS	2	3	2	2	2
The same risk of gettng HIV/AIDS	47	22	14	10	22
Less risk of gettng HIV/AIDS	34	67	72	78	64
Don't know	16	8	12	10	11
Base = 100%	*491*	*1041*	*1011*	*854*	*3397*

* This question is different to those asked in 1995 and 1996, which referred to the likelihood of 'someone like me getting HIV (the AIDS virus)'.

Table C.1.9 Respondents' assessment of the likelihood of 'someone like me getting a sexually transmitted infection'
by age and sex
Adults aged 16-54

Age	16-24	25-34	35-44	45-54	Total	HEMS 1995 Total	HEMS 1996 Total
Likelihood of 'someone like me getting a sexually transmitted infection'	%	%	%	%	%	%	%
Men							
Very high	2	1	1	1	1	3	2
Quite high	16	4	2	2	5	7	7
Low	57	64	66	51	60	61	53
No risk	7	24	25	44	26	26	33
Don't know	16	6	6	3	7	3	5
Base = 100%	*226*	*425*	*456*	*418*	*1525*	*1431*	*1399*
Women							
Very high	3	2	1	0	2	2	2
Quite high	18	3	2	2	6	6	5
Low	53	59	62	51	57	58	56
No risk	11	28	31	43	29	31	34
Don't know	15	8	4	4	7	4	4
Base = 100%	*265*	*616*	*555*	*436*	*1872*	*1722*	*1738*
All							
Very high	3	1	1	0	1	2	2
Quite high	18	4	2	2	6	6	6
Low	55	62	64	51	58	60	54
No risk	9	26	28	44	27	28	34
Don't know	16	7	5	4	7	3	4
Base = 100%	*491*	*1041*	*1011*	*854*	*3397*	*3153*	*3137*

Table C.1.10 Whether would find it difficult to raise the subject of using a condom with a new partner by age and sex
Adults aged 16-54

Age	16-24	25-34	35-44	45-54	Total	HEMS 1995 Total	HEMS 1996 Total
Whether would find it difficult	%	%	%	%	%	%	%
Men							
Strongly agree	3	5	5	7	5	5	6
Agree	13	6	7	9	8	12	10
Neither agree nor disagree	15	12	16	20	16	22	19
Disagree	39	48	50	47	46	53	47
Strongly disagree	29	29	22	17	24	9	18
Base = 100%	*226*	*422*	*454*	*416*	*1518*	*1428*	*1388*
Women							
Strongly agree	6	5	10	9	8	6	7
Agree	8	7	7	9	8	11	12
Neither agree nor disagree	6	11	14	14	12	21	13
Disagree	42	41	43	47	43	50	45
Strongly disagree	37	36	26	23	30	12	23
Base = 100%	*264*	*615*	*554*	*436*	*1869*	*1718*	*1720*
All							
Strongly agree	5	5	8	8	6	5	7
Agree	11	6	7	9	8	12	11
Neither agree nor disagree	11	12	15	17	14	21	16
Disagree	41	44	46	46	45	51	46
Strongly disagree	33	32	24	20	27	10	20
Base = 100%	*490*	*1037*	*1008*	*852*	*3387*	*3146*	*3108*

Table C.1.11 Whether would use a condom if 'in the near future they did have sex with a new partner' by age and sex
Adults aged 16-54

Age	16-24	25-34	35-44	45-54	Total	HEMS 1995 Total	HEMS 1996 Total
Whether would use a condom	%	%	%	%	%	%	%
Men							
Would always use a condom	68	60	56	51	58	54	58
It would depend	27	32	33	32	31	34	31
Would never use a condom	2	1	2	1	1	2	1
Wouldn't contemplate having sex	4	7	10	16	9	11	10
Base = 100%	*226*	*424*	*455*	*416*	*1521*	*1421*	*1392*
Women							
Would always use a condom	78	73	70	63	71	64	67
It would depend	17	15	14	11	14	18	17
Would never use a condom		1	1	0	1	1	
Wouldn't contemplate having sex	5	12	15	26	15	18	15
Base = 100%	*265*	*614*	*553*	*435*	*1867*	*1716*	*1729*
All							
Would always use a condom	73	66	63	57	64	59	62
It would depend	22	24	24	21	23	25	24
Would never use a condom	1	0	1	1	1	1	1
Wouldn't contemplate having sex	4	10	12	21	12	14	13
Base = 100%	*491*	*1038*	*1008*	*851*	*3388*	*3137*	*3121*

Table C.1.12 Percentage agreeing with statements about condom use by age and sex
Adults aged 16-54

Age	16-24	25-34	35-44	45-54	Total
Whether agrees	%	%	%	%	%
Men					
Using condoms would protect against being infected with HIV/AIDS					
Agree	86	88	89	88	88
Disagree	6	8	5	7	6
Neither agree nor disagree	8	4	6	5	6
Using condoms would protect against being infected with other sexually transmitted infections					
Agree	82	88	90	92	88
Disagree	8	6	5	5	6
Neither agree nor disagree	10	6	6	3	6
Base = 100%*	*226*	*425*	*456*	*417*	*1524*
Women					
Using condoms would protect against being infected with HIV/AIDS					
Agree	87	89	89	91	89
Disagree	7	7	7	4	6
Neither agree nor disagree	6	4	4	5	5
Using condoms would protect against being infected with other sexually transmitted infections					
Agree	84	91	90	92	89
Disagree	6	6	6	4	5
Neither agree nor disagree	10	3	4	4	5
Base = 100%*	*265*	*615*	*554*	*436*	*1870*
All					
Using condoms would protect against being infected with HIV/AIDS					
Agree	87	88	89	90	89
Disagree	6	7	6	5	6
Neither agree nor disagree	7	4	5	5	5
Using condoms would protect against being infected with other sexually transmitted infections					
Agree	83	89	90	92	89
Disagree	7	6	5	5	6
Neither agree nor disagree	10	5	5	4	6
Base = 100%*	*491*	*1040*	*1010*	*853*	*3394*

* Bases are taken from statement about sexually transmitted infections - bases may vary slightly for other items.

Table C.1.13 When thinks that a vaccine against HIV/AIDS will be available by age and sex
Adults aged 16-54

Age	16-24	25-34	35-44	45-54	Total
When respondent thinks a vaccine against HIV/AIDS will be available	%	%	%	%	%
Men					
Available right now	2	2	4	3	3
Available in next 5 years	24	25	28	27	26
Available in next 10 years	33	37	37	37	36
Available at some time but more than					
10 years away	26	25	26	26	26
Never available	14	10	6	6	9
Base = 100%	*224*	*419*	*452*	*410*	*1505*
Women					
Available right now	4	2	2	2	2
Available in next 5 years	20	18	26	27	23
Available in next 10 years	33	34	29	29	31
Available at some time but more than					
10 years away	32	36	32	33	33
Never available	11	11	10	8	10
Base = 100%	*262*	*605*	*547*	*425*	*1839*
All					
Available right now	4	2	3	3	3
Available in next 5 years	22	22	27	27	24
Available in next 10 years	33	36	33	33	34
Available at some time but more than					
10 years away	29	30	29	30	30
Never available	12	10	8	7	9
Base = 100%	*486*	*1024*	*999*	*835*	*3344*

Table C.1.14 Whether heard of the new treatments for HIV/AIDS by age and sex
Adults aged 16-54

Age	16-24	25-34	35-44	45-54	Total
Whether heard of new treatments for HIV/AIDS	%	%	%	%	%
Men					
Yes, heard of new treatments	23	36	32	30	31
Not heard	66	52	57	59	58
Not sure	11	11	11	11	11
Base = 100%	*226*	*425*	*456*	*417*	*1524*
Women					
Yes, heard of new treatments	14	28	25	32	25
Not heard	70	56	59	50	58
Not sure	16	16	15	19	16
Base = 100%	*265*	*616*	*556*	*436*	*1873*
All					
Yes, heard of new treatments	19	32	29	30	28
Not heard	68	54	58	54	58
Not sure	13	14	13	15	14
Base = 100%	*491*	*1041*	*1012*	*853*	*3397*

Table C.1.15 Percentage agreeing with statements about HIV/AIDS by age and sex
Adults aged 16-54, who had heard of new treatments for HIV/AIDS

Age	16-24	25-34	35-44	45-54	Total
Whether agrees	%	%	%	%	%
Men					
With the new treatments, it is possible to be cured of HIV/AIDS					
Agree	5	5	5	3	5
Disagree	70	82	76	79	78
Neither agree nor disagree	25	14	19	18	18
With the new treatments, it is possible for HIV positive people not to transmit the virus					
Agree	4	6	4	4	5
Disagree	69	79	81	78	77
Neither agree nor disagree	27	16	15	18	18
Base = 100%*	*80*	*198*	*201*	*163*	*642*
Women					
With the new treatments, it is possible to be cured of HIV/AIDS					
Agree	5	6	10	10	8
Disagree	63	72	67	70	69
Neither agree nor disagree	32	22	23	20	23
With the new treatments, it is possible for HIV positive people not to transmit the virus					
Agree	9	7	11	8	9
Disagree	71	70	70	77	72
Neither agree nor disagree	20	23	19	14	19
Base = 100%*	*85*	*266*	*223*	*213*	*787*
All					
With the new treatments, it is possible to be cured of HIV/AIDS					
Agree	5	6	7	7	6
Disagree	67	77	72	74	73
Neither agree nor disagree	28	17	21	19	20
With the new treatments, it is possible for HIV positive people not to transmit the virus					
Agree	6	6	7	6	7
Disagree	70	75	76	77	75
Neither agree nor disagree	24	19	17	16	18
Base = 100%*	*165*	*464*	*424*	*376*	*1429*

* Bases are taken from statement about curing HIV/AIDS - bases may vary slightly for other items.

Table C.1.16 Characteristics of new partner and respondent's opinions on new partner by age and sex of respondent
Adults aged 16-54, reporting a new partner in the last year

Age	Men			Women			All		
	16-34	35-54	Total	16-34	35-54	Total	16-34	35-54	Total
Respondent's opinions on new sexual partner	%	%	%	%	%	%	%	%	%
Age of new partner									
Under 16	4	-	3	4	1	3	4	1	3
16-19	38	14	32	26	3	20	33	8	26
20-24	30	8	24	28	8	23	29	8	24
25-34	24	33	27	32	21	30	28	28	28
35-44	2	29	9	9	26	13	5	28	11
45+	1	16	5	1	41	11	1	28	8
Whether it was new partner's first time									
Yes	14	17	14	12	11	12	13	14	13
No	75	79	76	82	86	83	78	82	79
Don't know	12	5	10	6	3	5	9	4	8
How well knew new partner									
Very well	36	41	38	48	65	52	42	52	45
Fairly well	43	39	42	40	22	36	42	32	39
Not very well	10	14	11	8	11	8	9	12	10
Not at all	11	5	9	4	2	3	7	4	6
Respondents' view of role of prospective new partner at time of first having sex with them									
Possible spouse, fiancé or steady partner	37	37	37	51	68	55	44	51	45
Casual partner	35	41	37	26	14	23	31	29	30
One-night stand	19	6	16	8	1	6	14	4	11
Other	3	2	3	4	1	3	3	2	3
Not sure	6	12	8	11	16	13	9	14	10
Whether respondent thought of HIV risk at time of first sexual intercourse with new partner									
Yes	43	40	42	51	36	47	47	38	45
No	57	60	58	49	64	53	53	62	55
Base = 100%*	*172*	*99*	*271*	*213*	*89*	*302*	*385*	*188*	*573*

* Bases are taken from 'How well knew new partner' - bases may vary slightly for other items.

Table C.1.17 Whether respondent thought of HIV risk by respondents' view of role of prospective new partner at time of first having sex with them by sex of respondent

Adults aged 16-54, reporting a new partner in the last year

Respondents' view of role of prospective new partner	Possible spouse, fiance or steady partner	Casual partner	One-night stand	Other	Not sure	Total
Whether respondent thought of HIV risk at time of first sexual intercourse with new partner	%	%	%	%	%	%
Men						
Yes	37	43	47	[1]	[14]	42
No	63	57	53	[5]	[7]	58
Base = 100%	*97*	*106*	*41*	*6*	*21*	*271*
Women						
Yes	50	43	[9]	[3]	36	47
No	50	57	[7]	[1]	64	53
Base = 100%	*172*	*73*	*16*	*4*	*37*	*302*

**Table C.1.18 Whether has ever had a sexually trans-
mitted infection or ever paid for sex by age and sex**
Adults aged 16-54

Age	16-34	35-54	Total
Whether ever had a sexually transmitted infection or ever paid for sex	%	%	%
Men			
Ever had a sexually transmitted infection			
Yes	6	8	7
No	93	92	92
Don't want to answer	0	0	0
Ever paid for sex			
Yes	4	6	5
No	95	94	94
Don't want to answer	1	0	0
Base = 100%	*578*	*841*	*1419*
Women			
Ever had a sexually transmitted infection			
Yes	8	4	6
No	91	96	93
Don't want to answer	1	1	1
Ever paid for sex			
Yes	0	-	0
No	100	100	100
Don't want to answer	0	0	0
Base = 100%	*810*	*963*	*1773*

Table C.1.19 Knowledge of 'safer' sex by age and sex
Adults aged 16-54

Age	16-24	25-34	35-44	45-54	Total*	HEMS 1995 Total*
Knowledge of safer sex	%	%	%	%	%	%
Men						
Using condoms	51	64	63	64	61	54
Having one partner	15	22	18	18	19	29
Taking precautions	42	23	21	18	25	25
Other	16	18	15	15	16	19
Not heard of safe sex	3	4	3	4	4	3
Don't know	-	0	1	0	0	1
Base = 100%	*225*	*424*	*455*	*412*	*1516*	*1338*
Women						
Using condoms	53	69	68	72	66	62
Having one partner	13	23	21	16	18	29
Taking precautions	48	19	20	18	25	23
Other	12	15	13	15	14	14
Not heard of safe sex	4	3	4	4	4	3
Don't know	0	0	2	0	1	1
Base = 100%	*264*	*612*	*554*	*432*	*1862*	*1652*
All						
Using condoms	52	66	65	68	63	58
Having one partner	14	23	20	16	19	29
Taking precautions	45	21	21	18	25	24
Other	14	17	14	15	15	16
Not heard of safe sex	4	4	3	4	4	3
Don't know	0	0	1	0	1	1
Base = 100%	*489*	*1036*	*1009*	*844*	*3378*	*2990*

* Totals add to more than 100% because respondents may have given more than one definition.

Table C.2.1 Number of occasions of sunburn in the 12 months prior to interview by year and sex

Adults aged 16-74

Year	1995*	1996	1995-1998 1998
Number of occasions of sunburn in last 12 months	%	%	%
Men			
Sunburnt in last 12 months	26	29	28
Once	17	17	17
Twice	5	7	7
Three times	2	2	1
Four or more	2	2	2
Not sunburnt	73	71	72
Can't remember	0	0	0
Base = 100%	*2120*	*2042*	*2300*
Women			
Sunburnt in last 12 months	22	23	20
Once	17	15	14
Twice	4	5	4
Three times	1	1	1
Four or more	1	2	1
Not sunburnt	78	77	79
Can't remember	0	0	0
Base = 100%	*2548*	*2599*	*2791*
All			
Sunburnt in last 12 months	24	26	24
Once	17	16	15
Twice	4	6	6
Three times	2	2	1
Four or more	1	2	2
Not sunburnt	75	74	76
Can't remember	0	0	0
Base = 100%	*4668*	*4641*	*5091*

* HEMS 1995 data was presented differently in the 1995 report.

Table C.2.2 Number of occasions of sunburn in the 12 months prior to interview by age and sex
Adults aged 16 and over

Age	16-24	25-34	35-44	45-54	55-64	65-74	75 and over	Total
Number of occasions of sunburn in last 12 months	%	%	%	%	%	%	%	%
Men								
Sunburnt in last 12 months	35	39	31	22	19	10	5	26
Once	20	24	19	14	12	5	2	16
Twice	9	11	8	5	4	4	1	7
Three times	2	1	2	2	0	1	1	1
Four or more	4	3	3	1	3	0	1	2
Not sunburnt	65	61	69	78	81	90	95	74
Can't remember	1	-	-	-	-	0	-	0
Base = 100%	*233*	*431*	*464*	*432*	*390*	*350*	*254*	*2554*
Women								
Sunburnt in last 12 months	38	28	20	18	10	5	3	19
Once	22	19	15	13	8	4	2	13
Twice	9	6	4	3	1	1	0	4
Three times	3	1	1	1	-	-	-	1
Four or more	3	2	1	0	1	1	-	1
Not sunburnt	62	72	80	82	90	95	97	81
Can't remember	-	0	-	1	-	-	0	0
Base = 100%	*272*	*631*	*572*	*463*	*406*	*447*	*458*	*3249*
All								
Sunburnt in last 12 months	36	34	26	20	14	7	3	22
Once	21	22	17	13	10	5	2	14
Twice	9	8	6	4	2	2	1	5
Three times	2	1	1	1	0	0	0	1
Four or more	3	2	2	1	2	0	0	2
None	64	66	74	80	86	93	97	78
Can't remember	0	0	-	0	-	0	0	0
Base = 100%	*505*	*1062*	*1036*	*895*	*796*	*797*	*712*	*5803*

Table C.2.3 Knowldege of ways of reducing risk of skin cancer by age and sex
Adults aged 16 and over

Age	16-24	25-34	35-44	45-54	55-64	65-74	75 and over	Total
Ways of reducing risk of skin cancer	%	%	%	%	%	%	%	%
Men								
Using sun cream	49	48	42	40	37	32	21	42
Staying in the shade	39	34	39	39	40	42	44	39
Wearing cover-up clothing	40	41	42	40	36	44	24	40
Staying out of the mid-day sun	33	37	31	34	35	30	37	34
Using high factor sun cream / block	37	36	31	27	22	21	11	29
Wearing a (wide brimmed) hat	11	15	18	12	14	18	11	14
Staying indoors	13	13	16	18	18	15	17	16
Don't use sunbeds	14	9	8	6	4	2	2	8
*Base = 100%**	*209*	*402*	*434*	*395*	*344*	*305*	*182*	*2271*
Women								
Using sun cream	61	48	46	41	36	34	22	43
Staying in the shade	43	34	41	47	44	50	50	43
Wearing cover-up clothing	37	40	39	38	35	26	21	36
Staying out of the mid-day sun	33	39	41	42	37	43	42	39
Using high factor sun cream / block	26	39	38	39	28	20	11	31
Wearing a (wide brimmed) hat	15	21	22	18	19	20	11	19
Staying indoors	13	16	15	16	18	16	14	15
Don't use sunbeds	23	18	19	13	11	6	4	15
*Base = 100%**	*248*	*596*	*541*	*437*	*372*	*393*	*337*	*2924*
All								
Using sun cream	55	48	44	41	37	33	22	42
Staying in the shade	41	34	40	43	42	46	48	41
Wearing cover-up clothing	39	40	40	39	35	35	22	38
Staying out of the mid-day sun	33	38	36	38	36	37	40	37
Using high factor sun cream / block	32	38	34	33	25	21	11	30
Wearing a (wide brimmed) hat	13	18	20	15	17	20	11	17
Staying indoors	13	15	16	17	18	16	15	16
Don't use sunbeds	19	14	14	10	8	4	3	11
*Base = 100%**	*457*	*998*	*975*	*832*	*716*	*698*	*519*	*5195*

* Totals add to more than 100 because respondents could have given more than one answer.

Table C.2.4 Knowledge of ways of reducing risk of skin cancer by social class based on own current or last job and sex

Adults aged 16 and over

Social class	I and II	III (non-manual)	III (manual)	IV and V	Total*
Ways of reducing risk of skin cancer	%	%	%	%	%
Men					
Using sun cream	41	36	40	47	41
Staying in the shade	41	42	35	35	38
Wearing cover-up clothing	39	35	40	43	40
Staying out of the mid-day sun	36	39	32	29	34
Using high factor sun cream / block	31	29	28	24	29
Wearing a (wide brimmed) hat	16	13	14	15	15
Staying indoors	18	16	16	12	16
Don't use sunbeds	7	11	6	7	7
Base = 100%†	*879*	*250*	*678*	*403*	*2219*
Women					
Using sun cream	43	44	40	42	43
Staying in the shade	42	43	46	42	43
Wearing cover-up clothing	40	36	30	31	36
Staying out of the mid-day sun	44	38	36	37	39
Using high factor sun cream / block	38	33	27	25	32
Wearing a (wide brimmed) hat	24	21	11	15	19
Staying indoors	16	16	12	14	15
Don't use sunbeds	15	14	15	16	15
Base = 100%†	*782*	*986*	*264*	*788*	*2822*
All					
Using sun cream	42	42	40	44	42
Staying in the shade	41	43	38	39	41
Wearing cover-up clothing	40	36	38	36	37
Staying out of the mid-day sun	39	38	33	34	37
Using high factor sun cream / block	34	32	28	25	30
Wearing a (wide brimmed) hat	19	19	13	15	17
Staying indoors	17	16	15	13	16
Don't use sunbeds	10	13	8	13	11
Base = 100%†	*1661*	*1236*	*942*	*1191*	*5041*

* Members of the Armed Forces, persons in inadequately described occupations and persons who have never worked are not shown as separate categories but are included in the figures for all persons.

† Totals add to more than 100 because respondents could have given more than one answer.

Table C.2.5 Occasions on which respondents use suncream by year and sex
Adults aged 16-74

	Men			Women		
Year	**1995**	**1996**	**1998**	**1995**	**1996**	**1998**
Occasions on which respondents use suncream	Percentage using a suncream					
Uses suncream	61	61	66	76	74	79
Sunbathing abroad	39	41	48	44	47	53
Outdoors abroad, but not sunbathing	32	27	37	41	35	46
Sunbathing in this country	25	32	38	43	49	55
Outdoors in this country doing something else	26	26	36	43	38	52
Does not use suncream	38	38	33	21	23	18
Never goes out in the sun	1	1	1	3	2	3
*Base = 100%**	*2115*	*2041*	*2300*	*2547*	*2600*	*2790*

* Totals add to more than 100 because respondents could have given more than one answer.

Table C.2.6 Occasions on which respondents use suncream by age and sex
Adults aged 16 and over

Age	16-24	25-34	35-44	45-54	55-64	65-74	75 and over	Total
Occasions on which respondents use suncream				Percentage using a suncream				
Men								
Uses suncream	69	73	74	68	55	43	24	63
Sunbathing abroad	55	58	56	48	33	19	8	45
Outdoors abroad, but not sunbathing	37	44	43	37	28	22	8	35
Sunbathing in this country	42	48	46	35	28	16	8	36
Outdoors in this country doing something else	30	43	39	36	33	27	16	34
Does not use suncream	30	26	25	29	44	55	70	35
Never goes out in the sun	1	1	1	3	1	2	6	2
*Base = 100%**	*233*	*431*	*464*	*432*	*390*	*350*	*254*	*2554*
Women								
Uses suncream	81	86	84	82	78	59	34	75
Sunbathing abroad	63	62	58	54	47	23	8	48
Outdoors abroad, but not sunbathing	51	52	48	49	44	25	10	42
Sunbathing in this country	62	64	62	56	47	26	11	50
Outdoors in this country doing something else	47	57	54	55	54	42	24	50
Does not use suncream	18	14	14	16	19	33	54	22
Never goes out in the sun	2	1	2	2	3	8	12	4
*Base = 100%**	*272*	*631*	*572*	*463*	*405*	*447*	*458*	*3248*
All								
Uses suncream	75	79	79	75	67	51	30	69
Sunbathing abroad	59	60	57	51	40	21	8	47
Outdoors abroad, but not sunbathing	44	48	46	43	36	23	9	39
Sunbathing in this country	52	56	54	46	38	22	10	44
Outdoors in this country doing something else	38	50	47	45	44	35	21	42
Does not use suncream	24	20	19	23	31	43	60	28
Never goes out in the sun	1	1	1	3	2	5	10	3
*Base = 100%**	*505*	*1062*	*1036*	*895*	*795*	*797*	*712*	*5802*

* Totals add to more than 100 because respondents could have given more than one answer.

Table C.2.7 Factor level of suncream used by year and sex

Adults aged 16-74

Year	1995*	1996	1995 - 1998 1998
Factor levels of suncream used	%	%	%
Men			
2-5	11	9	7
6-10	22	22	16
11-16	13	14	9
17 or over	6	8	23
Don't know	10	9	11
Does not use suncream	38	38	33
Never goes out in the sun	1	1	1
Base = 100%	*2107*	*2026*	*2299*
Women			
2-5	12	12	9
6-10	29	27	17
11-16	18	20	12
17 or over	10	10	34
Don't know	7	5	7
Does not use suncream	21	23	18
Never goes out in the sun	3	3	3
Base = 100%	*2545*	*2590*	*2790*
All			
2-5	11	10	8
6-10	25	24	16
11-16	15	17	11
17 or over	8	9	29
Don't know	8	7	9
Does not use suncream	29	31	25
Never goes out in the sun	2	2	2
Base = 100%	*4652*	*4616*	*5089*

* HEMS 1995 data was presented differently in the 1995 report.

Table C.2.8 Factor level of suncream used by age and sex
Adults aged 16 and over

Age	16-24	25-34	35-44	45-54	55-64	65-74	75 and over	Total
Factor levels of suncream used	%	%	%	%	%	%	%	%
Men								
2 - 5	4	8	10	7	5	4	2	6
6 - 10	17	22	16	14	12	7	3	15
11 - 16	10	11	9	10	7	6	2	9
17 or over	24	27	27	22	19	14	8	22
Don't know	15	5	11	15	12	13	8	11
Does not use suncream	30	26	25	29	44	55	70	35
Never goes out in the sun	1	1	1	3	1	2	6	2
Base = 100%	*233*	*431*	*464*	*432*	*390*	*349*	*253*	*2552*
Women								
2 - 5	4	13	9	9	11	6	3	8
6 - 10	18	20	19	17	15	11	3	16
11 - 16	18	12	12	13	8	6	3	11
17 or over	34	37	39	37	33	21	10	32
Don't know	7	4	5	6	11	14	15	8
Does not use suncream	18	14	14	16	19	33	54	22
Never goes out in the sun	2	1	2	2	3	9	13	4
Base = 100%	*272*	*631*	*572*	*463*	*405*	*447*	*458*	*3248*
All								
2 - 5	4	10	10	8	8	5	2	7
6 - 10	17	21	18	15	13	9	3	15
11 - 16	14	12	10	12	8	6	3	10
17 or over	29	32	33	30	26	18	10	27
Don't know	11	4	8	10	12	13	12	10
Does not use suncream	24	20	19	23	31	43	60	28
Never goes out in the sun	1	1	1	3	2	5	10	3
Base = 100%	*505*	*1062*	*1036*	*895*	*795*	*796*	*711*	*5800*

Table C.2.9 Whether checked skin for spots in past year by age and sex
Adults aged 16 and over

Age	16-24	25-34	35-44	45-54	55-64	65-74	75 and over	Total
Whether checked skin for spots in past year	%	%	%	%	%	%	%	%
Men								
Yes	16	22	22	24	24	20	17	21
No	84	78	78	76	76	80	83	79
Base = 100%	*233*	*431*	*464*	*432*	*390*	*350*	*254*	*2554*
Women								
Yes	24	36	36	41	32	24	20	32
No	76	64	64	59	68	76	80	68
Base = 100%	*272*	*630*	*572*	*463*	*406*	*447*	*458*	*3248*
All								
Yes	20	29	29	32	28	22	19	27
No	80	71	71	68	72	78	81	73
Base = 100%	*505*	*1061*	*1036*	*895*	*796*	*797*	*712*	*5802*

Table C.2.10 Whether checked skin for spots in past year by social class based on own current or last job and sex
Adults aged 16 and over

Social class	I and II	III (non-manual)	III (manual)	IV and V	Total*
Whether checked skin for spots in past year	%	%	%	%	%
Men					
Yes	25	23	20	18	22
No	75	77	80	82	78
Base = 100%	*948*	*274*	*791*	*467*	*2494*
Women					
Yes	43	32	27	24	32
No	57	68	73	76	68
Base = 100%	*830*	*1063*	*292*	*930*	*3117*
All					
Yes	32	30	22	22	27
No	68	70	78	78	73
Base = 100%	*1778*	*1337*	*1083*	*1397*	*5611*

* Members of the Armed Forces, persons in inadequately described occupations and persons who have never worked are not shown as separate categories but are included in the figures for all persons .

Table C.2.11 Number of times has used a sunbed in past 12 months by age and sex

Adults aged 16 and over, with white or olive skin

Age	16-24	25-34	35-44	45-54	55-64	65-74	75 and over	Total
Number of times has used a sunbed in past 12 months	%	%	%	%	%	%	%	%
Men								
Not at all	89	91	93	96	99	98	100	94
1 - 10 times	9	6	5	3	1	1	-	4
11 - 20 times	1	1	2	0	-	1	-	1
More than 20 times	-	1	1	0	-	1	-	0
Base = 100%	*201*	*384*	*403*	*385*	*350*	*325*	*243*	*2291*
Women								
Not at all	83	81	89	94	96	98	99	90
1 - 10 times	12	11	7	4	3	1	0	6
11 - 20 times	3	4	3	2	0	0	-	2
More than 20 times	2	4	2	0	1	1	0	2
Base = 100%	*244*	*567*	*514*	*435*	*377*	*422*	*437*	*2996*
All								
Not at all	86	86	91	95	97	98	100	92
1 - 10 times	11	9	6	4	2	1	0	5
11 - 20 times	2	3	2	1	0	0	-	1
More than 20 times	1	2	1	0	0	1	0	1
Base = 100%	*445*	*951*	*917*	*820*	*727*	*747*	*680*	*5287*

Table C.2.12 Whether checked skin for spots in past year by social class based on own current or last job and sex
Adults aged 16 and over, with white or olive skin

Social class	I and II	III (non-manual)	III (manual)	IV and V	Total*
Number of times has used a sunbed in past 12 months	%	%	%	%	%
Men					
Not at all	96	96	92	95	94
1 - 10 times	3	3	6	4	4
11 - 20 times	1	1	1	0	1
More than 20 times	0	1	1	-	0
Base = 100%	*864*	*245*	*702*	*420*	*2245*
Women					
Not at all	89	90	94	91	90
1 - 10 times	8	6	3	5	6
11 - 20 times	2	2	1	2	2
More than 20 times	1	2	1	2	2
Base = 100%	*765*	*984*	*275*	*864*	*2889*
All					
Not at all	93	91	93	93	92
1 - 10 times	5	5	5	5	5
11 - 20 times	2	2	1	2	2
More than 20 times	1	2	1	1	1
Base = 100%	*1629*	*1229*	*977*	*1284*	*5134*

* Members of the Armed Forces, persons in inadequately described occupations and persons who have never worked are not shown as separate categories but are included in the figures for all persons .

Table C.2.13 Whether having a suntan is important by year and sex

Adults aged 16 and over, with white or olive skin

Year	1995	1996	1995-1998 1998
Respondents' attitudes towards the importance of having a suntan	%	%	%
Men			
Important	23	20	16
Not important	77	80	84
Don't know	0	0	0
Base = 100%	*1934*	*1799*	*2048*
Women			
Important	32	31	24
Not important	67	69	75
Don't know	0	0	0
Base = 100%	*2363*	*2347*	*2559*
All			
Important	28	25	20
Not important	72	74	80
Don't know	0	0	0
Base = 100%	*4297*	*4146*	*4607*

Table C.2.14 Whether having a suntan is important by age and sex
Adults aged 16 and over, with white or olive skin

Age	16-24	25-34	35-44	45-54	55-64	65-74	75 and over	Total
Respondents' attitudes towards the importance of having a suntan	%	%	%	%	%	%	%	%
Men								
Important	27	14	15	14	14	7	8	15
Not important	73	85	85	86	85	93	90	85
Don't know	1	0	0	-	0	1	2	0
Base = 100%	*201*	*384*	*403*	*385*	*350*	*325*	*243*	*2291*
Women								
Important	33	30	26	22	20	11	6	22
Not important	67	69	74	78	80	89	94	77
Don't know	-	1	1	-	0	-	-	0
Base = 100%	*244*	*567*	*514*	*435*	*377*	*422*	*437*	*2996*
All								
Important	30	22	21	18	18	9	6	19
Not important	70	77	79	82	82	91	93	81
Don't know	0	0	0	-	0	0	1	0
Base = 100%	*445*	*951*	*917*	*820*	*727*	*747*	*680*	*5287*

**Table C.2.15 Whether agrees that 'having a suntan
makes me feel healthier' by year and sex**
Adults aged 16 and over, with white or olive skin

Year	1996	1998
Whether agrees that 'having a suntan makes me feel healthier'	%	%
Men		
Agree	41	39
Disagree	41	44
Neither agree nor disagree	18	17
Base = 100%	*1798*	*2045*
Women		
Agree	49	43
Disagree	38	45
Neither agree nor disagree	13	12
Base = 100%	*2346*	*2558*
All		
Agree	45	41
Disagree	40	45
Neither agree nor disagree	16	15
Base = 100%	*4144*	*4603*

Table C.2.16 Whether agrees that 'having a suntan makes me feel healthier' by age and sex
Adults aged 16 and over, with white or olive skin

Age	16-24	25-34	35-44	45-54	55-64	65-74	75 and over	Total
Whether agrees that 'having a suntan makes me feel healthier'	%	%	%	%	%	%	%	%
Men								
Agree	38	44	44	37	36	26	22	38
Disagree	49	37	38	46	48	58	61	46
Neither agree nor disagree	14	19	18	17	16	16	18	17
Base = 100%	*201*	*384*	*403*	*383*	*349*	*325*	*243*	*2288*
Women								
Agree	38	53	48	44	39	26	14	40
Disagree	44	36	40	45	51	61	72	48
Neither agree nor disagree	18	11	13	11	10	13	13	13
Base = 100%	*244*	*567*	*514*	*435*	*377*	*421*	*432*	*2990*
All								
Agree	38	48	46	41	38	26	17	39
Disagree	46	36	39	45	50	60	68	47
Neither agree nor disagree	16	15	15	14	13	14	15	15
Base = 100%	*445*	*951*	*917*	*818*	*726*	*746*	*675*	*5278*

Part D – Appendices

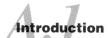

Appendix A Sample design, response to the survey, weighting, and sampling errors

A.1 Introduction

This appendix gives details of the sample design used for the 1998 Health Education Monitoring Survey (HEMS), and of response to the survey. It also describes the weighting procedure applied to the data and presents information on the sampling errors associated with the estimates shown in this report.

A.2 The sample design

The sample design was similar to that used for the 1995 and 1996 surveys; it followed the recommendations of a previous consultancy carried out by ONS for the Health Education Authority (HEA) in Summer 1994 which considered the optimum design for health surveys[1]. It concluded that the Postcode Address File (PAF) is the most complete sampling frame available for general population surveys, and recommended that the sample design incorporate socio-economic as well as regional stratifiers.

A.2.1 Changes made to the sample selection for the 1998 survey

There were two changes made to the sample selection for the 1998 survey from that used in the 1995 and 1996 surveys. As with the previous HEMS surveys, interviews were conducted with one adult in each household. However, instead of restricting interviews to those aged 16–74, interviews were conducted with one adult aged 16 and over. A decision was also taken not to conduct proxy interviews because in previous years these had yielded little information. In past HEMS surveys, proxy interviews had been conducted with another member of the household if the selected person had been unavailable.

A.2.2 Sample size

The sample selection process was designed to yield a representative sample of approximately 5,000 interviews with adults aged 16 and over living in private households in England. One adult was interviewed in each eligible household.

The sample was geographically clustered to give areas of a realistic size for interviewers to cover.

A.2.3 Selection of addresses

Since no suitable frame of households exists, a sample of addresses was selected from the Postcode Address File (PAF). In order to select the appropriate number of addresses a stratified multi-stage random probability design was used. The stages in the selection of the sample were as follows:

(i)   The chosen primary sampling units (PSUs) were postcode sectors, which are similar in size to wards. One hundred and seventy-five were selected by a systematic sampling method from a stratified list of postcode sectors. For this purpose all postcode sectors in England were stratified first by government office region, then according to the proportion of heads of household in socio-economic groups 1 to 5 and 13. Postcode sectors within the resulting strata were ranked by the proportion of households with a car. The stratifying information was based on 1991 Census data.

(ii)   A random selection of postcode sectors was then made, with the chance of selection of each postcode sector being proportional to the total number of delivery points in the sector. From each of the 175 postcode sectors, 51 addresses were randomly selected, to give a total of 8,925 addresses.

A.2.4 Ineligible addresses

Since the requirement was for a sample of adults living in private households, business addresses and institutions were excluded at the sample selection stage as far as possible by using the PAF small users' file as the sampling frame. During fieldwork, 10% (855) of the selected addresses did not contain a private household and were excluded from the sample. These ineligible addresses included demolished or permanently empty addresses, addresses used only on an occasional basis and business premises and institutions where there was no resident private household. (Table A.1)

A.2.5 Conversion of addresses to households

The PAF is a list of delivery points for mail so most households within multi-occupied addresses are separately listed on the frame. It is estimated, however, that a small proportion (less than 2%) of addresses on the PAF contain more than one private household.

Since each address listed on the PAF was given only one chance of selection for the HEMS sample, additional procedures were carried out in the field by interviewers at addresses found to contain more than one household in order to ensure that all households were given a chance of selection. Where the sampled address contained more than one private household, interviewers were asked to interview at all households up to a maximum of three. In the rare event that an address contained more than three households, the interviewer was instructed to list the households systematically and then three were chosen at random by reference to a selection table. In order to limit workloads a maximum of four extra households per quota of addresses was allowed on this survey. In total, 98 extra households were identified in this way for inclusion in the survey, resulting in 8,168 households to be approached by interviewers.

A.3 Sampling individuals within households

As noted above, one adult aged 16 and over was to be interviewed in each eligible household. This was done in preference to interviewing all eligible adults for a number of reasons. It helped interviewers to carry out interviews in private and obtain more reliable information. It ensured that respondents' answers, particularly to the attitudinal questions, were not contaminated by hearing other household members' answers. Finally, individuals in households tend to be similar to one another and where households differ markedly from one another, the resultant clustering can lead to a substantial increase in the standard error around survey estimates. This is particularly true in a topic area such as health behaviours where household members may influence each other.

In households where there was more than one adult aged 16 and over, the interviewer selected one person at random for interview, ensuring that all household members in the eligible age range had the same chance of being selected.

The selection procedure carried out at the household was a standard Social Survey Division procedure and was as follows:

(i)   The interviewers listed everyone in the household on a selection sheet. They then numbered those aged 16 and over in order of age, eldest first.

(ii)   The person to be interviewed was then defined by reference to a selection table which was printed on a set of reference cards.

(iii)   The cards indicated which one of the eligible people should be selected for a given address, depending upon the serial number of the address and the number of eligible people in the household.

The selection table was based on those designed by Kish, which gave a close approximation to the proper fractional representation of each eligible adult in the household for up to six adults[2]. For this survey, selection tables for up to 10 eligible adults were used and a different set of possible selections was shown for each of the 51 addresses in each postcode sector.

In theory this meant that in households with eleven or more eligible people some people would not get a chance of selection. In practice no households as large as this were found on the survey.

Often the person who had been selected for interview was not the person who had given the interviewer the household details, and so interviewers made arrangements to call back and interview the selected person.

A.4 Response to the survey

Table A.2 shows the response of the sample of eligible individuals to the interviewer visit. Seventy one per cent of adults selected agreed to take part in the survey. Twenty per cent refused to take part, either before the interviewer visited the address (1%), at the sampling stage (5%) or at the main interview stage (15%). Interviewers were unable to contact 4% of households, and were not able to contact the sampled person in another 3%. In a further 2% of cases, the selected individual was unable to be interviewed in person, because he or she was too ill, was absent for the whole field period or because of language difficulties. (Table A.2)

Adults aged 16–54 were eligible for the self-completion module on sexual health. Nineteen people had terminated the interview before reaching this module. The majority (97%) of eligible respondents agreed to take part in the self-completion. As the interview was conducted using Computer-Assisted Interviewing (CAI), 88% recorded their own answers on the laptop, while 9% asked the interviewer to key their answers in for them. (Table A.3)

A.5 Weighting procedures

This section describes the re-weighting procedures used to compensate for differing probabilities of selection and non-response bias in the sample.

There were two steps to the weighting. Firstly, weights were applied to take account of the different probabilities of selecting respondents in differently sized households. Secondly, all respondents were weighted up to represent the age-sex-region structure of the total national population of England living in private households.

A.5.1 Weighting for probability of selection within households

Sample weights to allow for the different probabilities of selecting a respondent in differently sized households are shown in Table A.4, and correspond to the number of members of the household aged 16 and over. (Table A.4)

A.5.2 Weighting for non-response bias

As noted above, the response rate for the face-to-face interviews was 71%. The weighting for non-response was applied to the full and partial interviews only, as only these cases were used for analysis.

The age, sex, regional, marital status and ethnic origin distributions of the responding sample on HEMS were compared with the March 1998 to May 1998 quarter of the Labour Force Survey (LFS) for England only, having first been re-weighted for household size. The LFS is a large sample survey carried out quarterly; the data are weighted and grossed to represent the total population.

Tables A.5 to A.8 compare the LFS and HEMS estimates. Only the statistically significant differences will be discussed here.

The HEMS sample under-represented men as a whole. The HEMS sample under-represented people aged 20–29, men aged 30–34, and women aged 80–84. HEMS over-represented men aged 50–54, 60–64 and 70–79 and women aged 35–39. The sample also under-represented people living in Greater London and over-represented men living in East Anglia. (Tables A.5-A.6)

Comparing the proportions of LFS and HEMS respondents in different marital status categories showed that HEMS under-represented single people and over-represented people who were co-habiting. However, it was decided not to re-weight to correct for these small differences. (Table A.7)

With regard to ethnic origin, the HEMS sample slightly under-represented Pakistani women. It was decided not to re-weight for this, however, as the numbers were too small to use for weighting and ethnic origin was not used in the analysis. (Table A.8)

It was decided to re-weight the HEMS sample to give the correct proportions for age, sex and region. When the number of men and women living in London was broken down by age the numbers in some of the cells were too small to use for weighting so it was decided to create a new regional variable; those living in the South East and those not living in the South East and to weight by this. The age-sex-region weights were produced by dividing the population proportion by the sample proportion. The weights are shown in Table A.9. Categories with weights of less than 1.0 were over-represented in the HEMS responding sample and those with weights of more than 1.0 were under-represented. (Table A.9)

A.5.3 The final weighted sample

The final weight applied to the sample is the product of these two sets of weights. For example, applying the product of the two weights would give a weight of 4.16 for a female aged 16–24 living in the South East in a household containing four eligible people (1.04 x 4).

Table A.10 shows the effect of weighting for non-response on the proportions of respondents by sex and age. Table A.11 shows the difference weighting for non-response made to some of the HEMS estimates. It shows that, for some behaviours associated with younger age-groups, such as the proportion of men who drank 51 or more units of alcohol a week, weighting increases the proportion. However, for other variables which are associated with older age-groups, such as the existence of a long-standing limiting illness, the weighting decreases the proportion. (Tables A.10 to A.11)

The tables in the main body of the report present weighted proportions, and unweighted bases.

A.6 Sampling error and the accuracy of the survey results

Like all estimates based on samples, the results of the HEMS survey are subject to variations and errors. The total error associated with any survey estimate is the difference between the estimate derived from the data collected and the true value for the population. The total error can be divided into two main types of error: systematic error and random error.

Systematic error is often referred to as bias. Bias can arise because the sampling frame is incomplete, because of variation in the way interviewers ask questions and record answers, or because non-respondents to the survey have different characteristics to respondents. When designing surveys considerable effort is made to minimise systematic error; these include training interviewers to maximise response rates and to ask questions in a standard way, and carrying out pilot work to test questions and survey procedures and to assess whether the interview and individual questions are understood by and acceptable to respondents. Nonetheless, some systematic error is likely to remain.

Random error occurs because survey estimates are based not on the whole population but only a sample of it. There may be chance variations between such a sample and the whole population. If a number of repeats of the same survey were carried out, this error could be expected to average to zero. The variations depend on both the size of the sample and its design.

Statistical theory, however, enables estimates of random error to be made for each characteristic. A statistical measure of variation, the standard error, can be estimated from the values obtained for the sample, and provides a measure of the statistical precision of the survey estimate. This allows confidence intervals to be calculated around the sample estimate which give an indication of the range in which the true population value is likely to fall. The confidence interval generally used in survey research is the 95% confidence interval; it comprises the range of values from two standard errors below the estimate to two standard errors above the estimate.

For results based on simple random samples, without clustering or stratification, the estimation of standard errors is straightforward. When, as in the case of the HEMS and most other surveys, the sample design is not a simple random sample, a more complex calculation, using a formula which takes account of the random variation of the denominator and the stratification and clustering of the sample design, is necessary[3]. Stratification tends to reduce the standard error, while clustering tends to increase it.

In a complex sample design, the size of the standard error depends on how the characteristic of interest is spread within and between primary sampling units and between strata. So, for example, characteristics likely to be associated with the primary sampling unit, postcode sectors, will tend to have larger standard errors.

Tables A.12–A.19 show the standard error and 95% confidence intervals for selected survey estimates (after weighting). They also show the design factor, or deft; the ratio of the standard error to the standard error that would have resulted had the survey design been a simple random sample of the same size. This is often used to give a broad indication of the degree of clustering. The tables do not cover all the topics discussed in the report; where possible, estimates for attitudes and behaviour are presented for each chapter. **(Tables A.12–A.19)**

A.6.1 Design factors

Design factors of less than 1.2 are considered to be small and indicate that the characteristic is not markedly clustered. However, substantial design factors of 1.2 or more were recorded for a number of characteristics, and this is reflected in being able to make less precise estimates for these characteristics than for other survey measures. A higher design factor indicates that the characteristic is more clustered geographically.

Among the sample characteristics covered in Table A.12, design factors of 1.2 or higher were found for men in the youngest age-

groups, women qualified to 'A' level or above (and all levels of qualification for men) and for single men. The design factors were particularly high for men in Social Classes I and II, and IV and V.

There were also relatively high design factors for a number of diet variables: 'whether eats bread; fruit vegetables and salad; and potatoes, pasta or rice daily' and for women, 'whether heard of folic acid'. The design factors for men who had not used a suncream (and for women with all categories of suncream use) were also high. Very few of the other health-related characteristics covered in the tables had design factors of 1.2 or more and most of the occurrences were for single categories of a variable of interest. **(Tables A.12–A.19)**

Notes and references

1. Elliot D. *Optimising sample designs for surveys of health and related behaviour and attitudes*. Unpublished paper (1994).
2. Kish L. *Survey Sampling*. J Wiley & Sons Ltd (London: 1965).
3. For a full description of the method used to calculate standard errors for complex survey design, see Butcher B and Elliot D. *A Sampling Errors Manual*. HMSO (London: 1992).

Table A.1 The sample of addresses and households

	No.
Selected addresses	8925
Ineligible addresses	855
Demolished or derelict	40
Used solely for business purposes	125
Used for temporary accommodation only	87
Empty	424
Institution	5
Address not traced	115
Other ineligible	59
Addresses at which interviews were sought	8070
Number of extra households sampled at multi-household addresses	98
Total eligible sample of households	8168

Table A.2 Response of adults at interview stage

Response	No.	%
Set sample of households	8168	100
Fully co-operating adults	5801	71
Partially co-operating adults	15	0
Non-responding households/adults	2352	29
Refusal	1601	20
direct to HQ	82	1
at sampling stage	301	5
by sampled person	1218	15
Non-contact	554	7
at sampling stage	338	4
with sampled person	216	3
Selected person unable to be interviewed*	197	2

* Respondents who were unable to be interviewed because of illness, infirmity or language difficulties.

Table A.3 Response of adults aged 16-54 to the self-completion module

Response	No.	%
Adults aged 16-54	3512	100
Co-operated with self-completion	3399	97
Completed by respondent	3073	88
Completed by interviewer	326	9
Self-completion refused	94	3
Did not complete main interview	19	0

Table A.4 Weights for household size

Household size	Weight
1 adult aged 16 and over	1
2 adults aged 16 and over	2
3 adults aged 16 and over	3
4 adults aged 16 and over	4
5 adults aged 16 and over	5
6 adults aged 16 and over	6
7 adults aged 16 and over	7
8 adults aged 16 and over	8
9 adults aged 16 and over	9

Table A.5 Distribution of responders to HEMS compared to Labour Force Survey (LFS) estimates for England by age and sex

Age group	Men HEMS* %	Men LFS† %	Women HEMS* %	Women LFS† %	All HEMS* %	All LFS† %
16-19	7.2	6.2	5.8	5.6	6.4	5.9
20-24	5.9	8.6	5.7	7.7	5.8	8.1
25-29	6.8	10.3	8.2	9.5	7.6	9.9
30-34	9.4	10.9	10.3	10.0	9.9	10.5
35-39	8.7	9.5	10.5	8.9	9.7	9.2
40-44	9.1	8.5	8.5	8.0	8.8	8.2
45-49	9.1	9.2	9.1	8.8	9.1	9.0
50-54	9.0	7.6	8.3	7.3	8.6	7.5
55-59	7.2	6.6	6.2	6.4	6.7	6.5
60-64	7.6	6.0	6.2	5.9	6.8	6.0
65-69	6.4	5.5	5.6	5.9	6.0	5.7
70-74	5.8	4.7	5.5	5.6	5.7	5.2
75-79	4.6	3.2	5.0	4.4	4.8	3.8
80-84	2.0	2.1	2.8	3.6	2.5	2.9
85-89	1.1	0.8	1.5	1.7	1.3	1.3
90 and over	0.3	0.2	0.7	0.7	0.5	0.5
Base = 100%	2,562	18,608,611	3,254	19,581,991	5,816	38,190,602

* HEMS proportions are reweighted for number of adults in household

† LFS survey estimates are weighted and grossed to the population estimates for England.

Table A.6 Distribution of responders to HEMS compared to Labour Force Survey (LFS) estimates for England by standard region and sex

Standard region	Males HEMS* %	Males LFS† %	Females HEMS* %	Females LFS† %	All HEMS* %	All LFS† %
North	7.1	6.3	6.8	6.4	6.9	6.4
Yorkshire and Humberside	11.2	10.3	10.7	10.3	10.9	10.3
North West	11.6	12.9	13.9	13.0	12.9	13.0
East Midlands	8.4	8.5	9.4	8.4	9	8.5
West Midlands	11.6	10.9	10.4	10.7	10.9	10.8
East Anglia	5.6	4.4	4.9	4.4	5.2	4.4
Greater London	11.7	14.2	11.6	14.4	11.7	14.3
South East	21.9	22.4	21.3	22.4	21.6	22.4
South West	10.9	10.0	10.9	10.0	10.9	10.0
Base= 100%	2,562	18,608,613	3,254	19,581,991	5,816	38,190,604

* HEMS proportions are reweighted for number of adults in household

† LFS survey estimates are weighted and grossed to the population estimates for England.

Table A.7 Distribution of responders to HEMS compared to Labour Force Survey (LFS) estimates for England by marital status and sex

Marital status	Men HEMS* %	Men LFS† %	Women HEMS* %	Women LFS† %	All HEMS* %	All LFS† %
Married	61.5	58.5	55.1	53.9	58.1	56.2
Cohabiting	8.9	7.2	7.7	6.3	8.3	6.8
Single	20.3	25.5	17.0	19.0	18.5	22.2
Widowed	3.8	3.6	11.5	12.5	7.9	8.1
Divorced	4.1	3.7	6.5	5.9	5.4	4.8
Separated	1.5	1.5	2.1	2.3	1.8	1.9
Base= 100%	2,562	18,608,612	3,254	19,581,991	5,816	38,190,603

* HEMS proportions are reweighted for number of adults in household.

† LFS survey estimates are weighted and grossed to the population estimates for England.

Table A.8 Distribution of responders to HEMS compared to Labour Force Survey(LFS) by ethnic origin and sex

Ethnic Origin	Men HEMS* %	Men LFS† %	Women HEMS* %	Women LFS† %	All HEMS* %	All LFS† %
White	94.7	94.2	95.1	94.5	94.9	94.3
Indian	1.6	1.7	1.2	1.5	1.4	1.6
Pakistani	0.6	0.9	0.5	0.8	0.5	0.8
Bangladeshi	0.2	0.3	0.2	0.2	0.2	0.3
Black- Caribbean	0.6	0.9	1.1	1.0	0.9	0.9
Other ethnic group	2.4	2.0	1.9	2.0	2.1	2.0
Base	2,555	18,604,202	3,249	19,578,931	5,804	38,183,133

* HEMS proportions are reweighted for number of adults in household.

† LFS survey estimates are weighted and grossed to the population estimates for England.

Table A.9 Age-sex-region weights

	LFS population totals	LFS proportion	Total responding in sample	Sample proportion	Age-sex-region weight
South East					
Men					
16-24	986,922	2.6	81	2.2	1.18
25-39	2,234,842	5.9	236	4.1	1.44
40-54	1,711,435	4.5	220	4.2	1.07
55-74	1,469,791	3.8	246	4.2	0.90
75 and over	416,686	1.1	80	1.2	0.92
Women					
16-24	949,075	2.5	99	2.4	1.04
25-39	2,170,318	5.7	338	5.4	1.06
40-54	1,726,800	4.5	247	4.9	0.92
55-74	1,607,741	4.2	240	3.5	1.20
75 and over	738,290	1.9	148	1.8	1.06
Not South East					
Men					
16-24	1,761,543	4.6	152	3.9	1.18
25-39	3,501,364	9.2	427	7.4	1.24
40-54	3,002,100	7.9	451	8.3	0.95
55-74	2,779,219	7.3	495	8.3	0.88
75 and over	744,711	1.9	174	2.5	0.76
Women					
16-24	1,664,237	4.4	173	3.8	1.16
25-39	3,384,445	8.9	630	10.2	0.87
40-54	2,991,626	7.8	452	9.0	0.87
55-74	3,049,249	8.0	613	9.1	0.88
75 and over	1,300,211	3.4	314	3.6	0.94
Base= 100%	*38,190,605*	*100*	*5816*	*100*	

Table A.10 The effects of weighting for non-response on sex and age

Age	Weighted only for probability of selection within households	Weighted for probability of selection and for non-response*
	%	%
Men		
16-24	13	15
25-34	16	20
35-44	18	19
45-54	18	17
55-64	15	12
65-74	12	10
75 and over	8	6
Women		
16-24	12	13
25-34	19	18
35-44	19	18
45-54	17	16
55-64	12	13
65-74	11	11
75 and over	10	10
Base = 100%	*10945*	*10955*

* Weighted by age, sex and region.

Table A.11 The effects of weighting for non-response on survey estimates of health measures

Survey estimate	Weighted only for probability of selection within households	Weighted for probability of selection and for non-response*
	%	%
General health		
Has 'less than good' general health	25	24
Has limiting long-standing illness	23	22
Has large amount of stress	27	27
Smoking status		
Current cigarette smokers	27	27
Ex-regular cigarette smokers	26	25
Never or only occasionally smoked cigarettes	47	48
Alcohol consumption		
Men		
Non-drinker	3	3
Under one	3	3
1-10	16	16
11-21	11	11
22-35	7	7
36-50	4	4
51 or over	3	4
Women		
Non-drinker	6	6
Under one	9	8
1-7	20	19
8-14	9	9
15-25	6	6
26-35	2	2
36 or over	2	2
Physical activity		
Participates in moderate-intensity activity lasting at least 30 minutes at least five times a week	32	31
Diet		
Eats foods containing fibre and starchy carbohydrates daily	39	38
Eats low-fat varieties of foods	25	24
Base = 100%	*10945*	*10955*

* Weighted by age, sex and region.

Table A.12 Standard errors and 95% confidence intervals for socio-demographic variables

Base	Characteristic	%(p)	Sample size	Standard error of p	95% confidence interval	Deft
	Age					
Men	16-24	14.6	2562	0.97	12.7 – 16.5	1.39
	25-34	20.1	2562	1.01	18.1 – 22.1	1.27
	35-44	19.4	2562	0.90	17.6 – 21.3	1.15
	45-54	17.0	2562	0.79	15.5 – 18.5	1.07
	55-64	12.4	2562	0.63	11.2 – 13.6	0.97
	65-74	10.3	2562	0.66	9.0 – 11.6	1.09
	75 and over	6.1	2562	0.40	5.3 – 6.9	0.84
Women	16-24	13.4	3254	0.67	12.1 – 14.7	1.13
	25-34	18.1	3254	0.75	16.6 – 19.6	1.11
	35-44	18.2	3254	0.79	16.7 – 19.7	1.17
	45-54	16.1	3254	0.76	14.6 – 17.6	1.18
	55-64	12.6	3254	0.65	11.3 – 13.9	1.12
	65-74	11.2	3254	0.62	10.0 – 12.4	1.13
	75 and over	10.3	3254	0.61	9.1 – 11.5	1.14
	Social class of respondent					
Men	I and II	37.7	2495	1.32	35.1 – 40.3	1.36
(excluding armed	III Non-Manual	11.9	2495	0.76	10.4 – 13.4	1.18
forces, never worked	III Manual	31.4	2495	1.12	29.2 – 33.6	1.20
and not known)	IV and V	18.5	2495	1.00	16.5 – 20.5	1.29
Women	I and II	26.4	3118	0.91	24.6 – 28.2	1.15
(excluding armed	III Non-Manual	35.6	3118	0.92	33.8 – 37.4	1.07
forces, never worked	III Manual	8.7	3118	0.50	7.7 – 9.7	0.99
and not known)	IV and V	29.2	3118	0.92	27.4 – 31.0	1.13
	Highest qualification level					
Men	'A' level or above	42.1	2554	1.36	39.4 – 44.8	1.39
	Other qualifications	36.7	2554	1.19	34.4 – 39.0	1.24
	No qualifications	21.2	2554	0.92	19.4 – 23.0	1.31
Women	'A' level or above	28.4	3243	0.95	26.5 – 30.3	1.20
	Other qualifications	41.9	3243	0.96	40.0 – 43.8	1.11
	No qualifications	29.7	3243	0.88	28.0 – 31.4	1.17
	Marital status					
Men	Married	59.0	2562	1.04	57.0 – 61.0	1.07
	Cohabiting	10.1	2562	0.67	8.8 – 11.4	1.12
	Single	22.7	2562	1.05	20.6 – 24.8	1.27
	Widowed/separated/divorced	8.2	2562	0.50	7.2 – 9.2	0.92
Women	Married	53.7	3254	0.98	51.8 – 55.6	1.12
	Cohabiting	7.7	3254	0.52	6.7 – 8.7	1.11
	Single	18.5	3254	0.81	16.9 – 20.1	1.19
	Widowed/separated/divorced	20.1	3254	0.67	18.8 – 21.4	0.96

Table A.13 Standard errors and 95% confidence intervals for general health and social capital variables

Base	Characteristic	%(*p*)	Sample size	Standard error of *p*	95% confidence interval	Deft
	Self-reported effect of stress on health					
Men	Very harmful	5.4	2557	0.40	4.6 – 6.2	0.89
	Quite harmful	25.8	2557	0.86	24.1 – 27.5	1.00
	Not harmful	58.2	2557	1.04	56.2 – 60.2	1.07
	Completely free of stress	8.1	2557	0.63	6.9 – 9.3	1.16
Women	Very harmful	7.1	3250	0.47	6.2 – 8.0	1.05
	Quite harmful	32.0	3250	0.95	30.1 – 33.9	1.16
	Not harmful	52.5	3250	1.05	50.4 – 54.6	1.20
	Completely free of stress	6.2	3250	0.53	5.1 – 7.2	1.25
	How long informant has lived in the area					
Men	Less than 12 months	5.7	2557	0.50	4.7 – 6.7	1.08
	1 year	3.2	2557	0.40	2.4 – 4.0	1.16
	2 years	4.2	2557	0.44	3.3 – 5.0	1.12
	3 years	3.9	2557	0.54	2.8 – 5.0	1.41
	4 years	3.7	2557	0.41	2.9 – 4.5	1.10
	5-9 years	11.5	2557	0.70	10.1 – 12.9	1.11
	6-9 years	11.9	2557	0.73	10.5 – 13.3	1.14
	10-14 years	11.8	2557	0.70	10.4 – 13.2	1.09
	15-19 years	44.1	2557	1.29	41.6 – 46.6	1.32
	20 years or more	0.1	2557	0.09	0.0 – 0.3	1.18
Women	Less than 12 months	5.7	3252	0.48	4.8 – 6.6	1.19
	1 year	3.3	3252	0.33	2.7 – 3.9	1.06
	2 years	4.3	3252	0.38	3.6 – 5.0	1.06
	3 years	3.4	3252	0.40	2.6 – 4.2	1.24
	4 years	3.4	3252	0.31	2.8 – 4.0	0.97
	5-9 years	12.6	3252	0.56	11.5 – 13.7	0.97
	6-9 years	13.8	3252	0.67	12.5 – 15.1	1.11
	10-14 years	11.2	3252	0.62	10.0 – 12.4	1.12
	15-19 years	42.2	3252	1.10	40.0 – 44.4	1.27
	20 years or more	0.2	3252	0.07	0.1 – 0.3	0.94
	Whether seen or spoken to close friends in past two weeks					
Men	Yes	87.3	2556	0.74	85.8 – 88.8	1.12
	No	12.7	2556	0.74	11.2 – 14.2	1.12
Women	Yes	89.2	3251	0.64	87.9 – 90.5	1.18
	No	10.8	3251	0.64	9.5 – 12.1	1.18
	Whether agrees that 'I am satisfied with the amount of control I have over decisions that affect my life'					
Men	Strongly agrees	22.3	2544	1.09	20.2 – 24.4	1.32
	Agrees	52.4	2544	1.34	49.8 – 55.0	1.35
	Neither agrees nor disagrees	9.7	2544	0.59	8.5 – 10.9	1.00
	Strongly disagrees	12.6	2544	0.69	11.2 – 14.0	1.06
	Disagrees	2.9	2544	0.30	2.3 – 3.5	0.90
Women	Strongly agrees	23.6	3230	0.95	21.7 – 25.5	1.27
	Agrees	56.1	3230	1.07	54.0 – 58.2	1.22
	Neither agrees nor disagrees	9.1	3230	0.56	8.0 – 10.2	1.11
	Strongly disagrees	9.9	3230	0.67	8.6 – 11.2	1.29
	Disagrees	1.3	3230	0.21	0.9 – 1.7	1.09

Table A.14 Standard errors and 95% confidence intervals for smoking variables

Base	Characteristic	%(*p*)	Sample size	Standard error of *p*	95% confidence interval	Deft
	Cigarette smoking status					
Men	Heavy smoker	10.5	2554	0.68	9.2 – 11.8	1.12
	Moderate smoker	11.0	2554	0.69	9.6 – 12.4	1.12
	Light smoker	7.6	2554	0.58	6.5 – 8.7	1.10
	Ex-regular smoker	29.7	2554	0.95	27.8 – 31.6	1.05
	Never smoked regularly	41.0	2554	1.06	38.9 – 43.1	1.09
Women	Heavy smoker	6.8	3249	0.44	5.9 – 7.7	1.00
	Moderate smoker	10.4	3249	0.60	9.2 – 11.6	1.12
	Light smoker	8.4	3249	0.60	7.2 – 9.6	1.23
	Ex-regular smoker	20.4	3249	0.77	18.9 – 21.9	1.09
	Never smoked regularly	53.9	3249	0.96	52.0 – 55.8	1.09
	When smokers intend to give up smoking					
Men: smokers	Within the next month	9.2	715	1.25	6.8 – 11.7	1.15
	Within the next six months	14.8	715	1.41	12.0 – 17.6	1.06
	Within the next year	15.6	715	1.51	12.6 – 18.6	1.11
	Intends to give up but not in the next year	21.0	715	1.74	17.6 – 24.4	1.14
	Unlikely to give up smoking	39.4	715	1.92	35.6 – 43.2	1.05
Women: smokers	Within the next month	9.5	845	1.35	6.9 – 12.1	1.34
	Within the next six months	14.2	845	1.50	11.3 – 17.1	1.25
	Within the next year	15.0	845	1.52	12.0 – 18.0	1.24
	Intends to give up but not in the next year	18.8	845	1.53	15.8 – 21.8	1.13
	Unlikely to give up smoking	42.5	845	2.00	38.6 – 46.4	1.18

Health in England 1998: investigating the links between social inequalities and health

Table A.15 Standard errors and 95% confidence intervals for drinking variables

Base	Characteristic	%(*p*)	Sample size	Standard error of *p*	95% confidence interval	Deft
	Alcohol consumption in units per week					
Men	Non-drinker	6.3	2558	0.59	5.1 – 7.5	1.23
	Under one	6.7	2558	0.58	5.6 – 7.8	1.17
	1-10	33.3	2558	1.02	31.3 – 35.3	1.09
	11-21	23.2	2558	0.84	21.6 – 24.8	1.01
	22-35	14.7	2558	0.77	13.2 – 16.2	1.09
	36-50	8.2	2558	0.57	7.1 – 9.3	1.05
	51 and over	7.6	2558	0.60	6.4 – 8.8	1.15
Women	Non-drinker	11.7	3244	0.67	10.4 – 13.0	1.18
	Under one	16.4	3244	0.70	15.0 – 17.8	1.08
	1-7	37.1	3244	1.00	35.1 – 39.1	1.18
	8-14	17.4	3244	0.80	15.8 – 19.0	1.20
	15-25	11.1	3244	0.64	9.8 – 12.4	1.16
	26-35	3.3	3244	0.42	2.5 – 4.1	1.33
	36 and over	3.0	3244	0.37	2.3 – 3.7	1.21
	Whether knows about measuring units of alcohol					
Men	Yes	83.8	2554	0.75	82.3 – 85.3	1.03
	No	14.5	2554	0.75	13.0 – 16.0	1.07
	Don't know	1.6	2554	0.31	1.0 – 2.2	1.23
Women	Yes	78.5	3248	0.85	76.8 – 80.2	1.17
	No	19.9	3248	0.78	18.4 – 21.4	1.12
	Don't know	1.5	3248	0.26	1.0 – 2.0	1.22
	Whether agrees that 'It's OK to get drunk from time to time'					
Men	Strongly agrees	5.8	2549	0.59	4.6 – 7.0	1.27
	Agrees	49.9	2549	1.06	47.8 – 52.0	1.07
	Neither agrees nor disagrees	13.0	2549	0.76	11.5 – 14.5	1.14
	Strongly disagrees	23.2	2549	0.91	21.4 – 25.0	1.08
	Disagrees	8.1	2549	0.63	6.9 – 9.3	1.16
Women	Strongly agrees	3.3	3241	0.34	2.6 – 4.0	1.10
	Agrees	39.8	3241	1.06	37.7 – 41.9	1.23
	Neither agrees nor disagrees	12.8	3241	0.68	11.5 – 14.1	1.16
	Strongly disagrees	31.2	3241	0.93	29.4 – 33.0	1.15
	Disagrees	13.0	3241	0.75	11.5 – 14.5	1.27

Table A.16 Standard errors and 95% confidence intervals for physical activity variables

Base	Characteristic	%(*p*)	Sample size	Standard error of *p*	95% confidence interval	Deft
	When intends to take more exercise					
Men	Within the next month	29.2	2428	1.09	27.1 − 31.3	1.18
	Within the next six months	19.7	2428	0.84	18.1 − 21.3	1.05
	Within the next year	8.0	2428	0.60	6.8 − 9.2	1.10
	Intends to take more exercise but not in the next year	3.2	2428	0.49	2.2 − 4.2	1.37
	Unlikely to take more exercise	39.9	2428	1.14	37.7 − 42.1	1.15
Women	Within the next month	27.2	3050	0.88	25.5 − 28.9	1.09
	Within the next six months	22.6	3050	0.95	20.7 − 24.5	1.25
	Within the next year	8.1	3050	0.55	7.0 − 9.2	1.11
	Intends to take more exercise but not in the next year	3.9	3050	0.44	3.0 − 4.8	1.27
	Unlikely to take more exercise	38.1	3050	1.14	35.9 − 40.4	1.29
	Frequency of moderate-intensity activity for 30 minutes or more					
Men	Less than one day a week (sedentary)	27.1	2555	1.01	25.1 − 29.1	1.15
	1-2 days a week	24.5	2555	0.96	22.6 − 26.4	1.13
	3-4 days a week	12.4	2555	0.73	11.0 − 13.8	1.11
	5 or more days a week	35.9	2555	1.09	33.8 − 38.0	1.15
Women	Less than one day a week (sedentary)	34.8	3247	0.93	33.0 − 36.6	1.12
	1-2 days a week	29.1	3247	0.92	27.3 − 30.9	1.15
	3-4 days a week	12.0	3247	0.69	10.6 − 13.4	1.21
	5 or more days a week	24.1	3247	0.87	22.4 − 25.8	1.16

Table A.17 Standard errors and 95% confidence intervals for diet variables

Base	Characteristic	%(p)	Sample size	Standard error of p	95% confidence interval	Deft
	Eats bread; fruit, vegetables and salad; and potatoes, pasta or rice daily					
Men		33.9	901	1.18	31.6 – 36.2	1.26
Women		41.4	1352	1.00	39.4 – 43.4	1.16
	Uses low-fat varieties of milk, cooking fat and spread, and eats chips less than once a week					
Men		19.3	472	0.89	17.6 – 21.0	1.11
Women		29.1	898	1.05	27.0 – 31.2	1.28
	Whether heard of folic acid					
Men	Yes	-	-	-	- – -	-
	No	-	-	-	- – -	-
	Don't know	-	-	-	- – -	-
Women	Yes	85.8	1714	1.10	83.6 – 88.0	1.31
	No	13.4	1714	1.08	11.3 – 15.5	1.31
	Don't know	0.7	1714	0.22	0.3 – 1.1	1.07
	Whether agrees that 'As long as you take enough exercise you can eat whatever foods you like'					
Men	Strongly agrees	2.4	2545	0.40	1.6 – 3.2	1.32
	Agrees	24.7	2545	1.07	22.6 – 26.8	1.25
	Neither agrees nor disagrees	12.0	2545	0.78	10.5 – 13.5	1.22
	Disagrees	54.0	2545	1.09	51.9 – 56.1	1.11
	Strongly disagrees	6.8	2545	0.54	5.7 – 7.8	1.09
Women	Strongly agrees	1.6	3232	0.33	1.0 – 2.2	1.47
	Agrees	17.0	3232	0.76	15.5 – 18.5	1.15
	Neither agrees nor disagrees	11.0	3232	0.71	9.6 – 12.4	1.28
	Disagrees	64.3	3232	0.98	62.4 – 66.2	1.16
	Strongly disagrees	6.2	3232	0.52	5.2 – 7.2	1.22

Table A.18 Standard errors and 95% confidence intervals for sexual health variables

Base	Characteristic	%(p)	Sample size	Standard error of p	95% confidence interval	Deft
	Number of sexual partners in the last 12 months					
Men	None	13.1	1501	0.96	11.2 – 14.9	1.10
	One	70.7	1501	1.28	68.2 – 73.2	1.09
	Two or more	16.2	1501	1.07	14.1 – 18.3	1.13
Women	None	13.0	1856	0.92	11.2 – 14.8	1.17
	One	76.1	1856	1.12	73.9 – 78.3	1.13
	Two or more	10.9	1856	0.84	9.3 – 12.5	1.16
	Whether would find it difficult to raise the subject of using a condom with a new partner					
Men	Agrees	13.7	1518	1.02	11.7 – 15.7	1.11
	Disagrees	70.6	1518	1.27	68.1 – 73.1	1.08
	Neither agrees nor disagrees	15.8	1518	0.97	13.9 – 17.7	1.04
Women	Agrees	15.3	1869	0.93	13.5 – 17.1	1.11
	Disagrees	73.2	1869	1.12	71.0 – 75.4	1.09
	Neither agrees nor disagrees	11.5	1869	0.87	9.8 – 13.2	1.17
	Used a condom with a new partner					
Men	Yes	61.7	271	3.90	54.1 – 69.3	1.32
	No	38.3	271	3.90	30.7 – 45.9	1.32
Women	Yes	66.7	301	3.07	60.7 – 72.7	1.13
	No	33.3	301	3.07	27.3 – 39.3	1.13

Table A.19 Standard errors and 95% confidence intervals for behaviour in the sun variables

Base	Characteristic	%(*p*)	Sample size	Standard error of *p*	95% confidence interval	Deft
	Whether uses a suncream					
Men	Yes	63.5	2554	1.14	61.3 – 65.7	1.19
	No	34.9	2554	1.15	32.6 – 37.2	1.22
	Never goes out in the sun	1.6	2554	0.30	1.0 – 2.2	1.19
Women	Yes	74.9	3249	0.92	73.1 – 76.7	1.21
	No	21.4	3249	0.93	19.6 – 23.2	1.29
	Never goes out in the sun	3.7	3249	0.45	2.8 – 4.6	1.37
	Whether agrees that 'having a suntan makes me feel healthier'					
Men	Agree	37.6	2288	1.22	35.2 – 40.0	1.21
	Disagree	45.6	2288	1.23	43.2 – 48.0	1.18
	Neither agree nor disagree	16.8	2288	0.87	15.1 – 18.5	1.11
Women	Agree	39.7	2990	0.94	37.9 – 41.5	1.06
	Disagree	47.7	2990	1.08	45.6 – 49.8	1.18
	Neither agree nor disagree	12.6	2990	0.80	11.0 – 14.2	1.31
	Whether has checked skin for spots which could be skin cancer in the last year					
Men	Yes	21.3	2554	0.92	19.5 – 23.1	1.13
	No	78.7	2554	0.92	76.9 – 80.5	1.13
Women	Yes	31.5	2246	0.95	29.6 – 33.4	1.17
	No	68.4	2246	0.95	66.5 – 70.3	1.17

Appendix B Researching social capital for health

B.1 Background

The purpose of this appendix is to provide further details of the HEA's work on social capital since 1996. To date health promotion has concentrated on the individual. As a result there has been an emphasis on psychological approaches to changing health-related behaviour. These involve shifting attitudes, beliefs and intentions and improving knowledge. These efforts have proved successful, if somewhat limited; they have been particularly effective among the better off, better motivated and better educated in society.

However, it is known that health experience and behaviour are affected by the social, cultural, economic, environmental and political contexts in which they occur. These broader determinants of health can also act as barriers to healthy behaviour. The effect of social and environmental factors on health have been subject to scrutiny in developed and developing countries, and the evidence is clear: wealth, occupation, social support, housing and education are related to wide differences in life expectancy, infant mortality and psychosocial wellbeing. However, it is also known that some poorer communities have fewer health problems than others and one concept put forward to explain this is that of social capital.

Although not yet a theory with explanatory power, social capital allows us to examine the processes whereby formal and informal social connections operating through a range of different types of networks can act as a buffer against the worst effects of deprivation. Communities with a high level of social capital are characterised by high levels of trust, positive social norms and many overlapping diverse horizontal networks for communication and exchange of information, ideas and practical help. Social capital is produced within communities, from a diverse range of activities. These connections, networks and associations within any society are important as a means of promoting both social cohesion and health, as well as helping disease.

B.2 Recent HEA research into social capital

Since 1996 the HEA has carried out a wide range of work to investigate the concept of social capital and its links to health. The research commissioned by the HEA since 1996 includes the following studies.

B.2.1 Exploring the empirical relationship between social capital and health – qualitative studies

Social capital and health

The London School of Economics was commissioned by the HEA to carry out a pilot qualitative research study in Luton. Using in-depth interviews and focus groups, the study investigated community networks and relationships in ward-level local communities, focusing on two less-affluent wards; one characterised by relatively low levels of health and the second by relatively high levels of health, in the interests of exploring whether levels of social capital might be higher in the 'high health' ward.

In the report on this phase of the study, Campbell *et al*,[1] identified five aspects of social capital that might be of great relevance to the operationalisation of the concept in the UK:

1. The *existence of community networks* which together constitute the civic community (involving institutions, associated facilities and relationships) – in the voluntary, state and personal spheres – and the density of the networking between these spheres.
2. *Civic identity*: people's sense of belonging to the civic community, together with a sense of solidarity and equality with other community members.
3. *Norms* governing the functioning of networks – in particular norms of co-operation reciprocity (obligating to help others) confidence that others will help oneself); trust (as opposed to fear) of others in the community.
4. *Attitudes* to networks: positive attitudes to the institutions, associated facilities and relationships constituting the civic community.
5. *Civic engagement*: participation in the process of sustaining and/or using such voluntary, state and interpersonal networks – contribution to network functioning; willingness to use them; capacity to use them; frequency of use; contexts of use.

The study hypothesised that social capital, as represented by these factors, may act as a mediator between deprivation and health. In this sense, though a number of communities may be equally deprived, some may have higher social capital and thus better health than others. Given its exploratory nature, the first phase focussed predominantly on community networks and relationships amongst white British people only, in relatively deprived communities.

Social capital as a mediator of health, ethnicity and socio-economic status

The second phase of the study will extend the focus along two dimensions. Firstly, it will take account of a broader array of ethnic groups, exploring issues of health and social capital in members of particular white British, South Asian and African-Caribbean communities in Luton.

Secondly, the study will examine these issues within a broader array of socio-economic contexts, drawing its research sample from members of high/middle income groups (Social Classes I and II), lower income groups (Social Classes IV and V) and extremely deprived groups (totally dependent on state benefits). This extension of focus to include attention to both ethnic and socio-economic variations is particularly important given the broader national interest in health inequalities in Britain, and the belief that variations in health amongst different ethnic and socio-economic groups might relate, in part, to differences in the forms and levels of social capital in these different groups. The research will be qualitative and will include a literature review, focus groups, in-depth interviews, and community consultation workshops.

This is a two-year project and fieldwork is currently underway.

Social capital, gender and health

The research literature and HEA commissioned studies on social capital and health, highlight the potential importance of gender in developing and sustaining social capital. In particular the different roles of men and women in relation to social capital need to be further investigated if we are to develop ways of building it as a community resource. The aim of this study will be to explore the different ways in which men and women develop, sustain and use social capital in their lives, and how it relates to health. This will include consideration of the ways in which people build, sustain and use informal and formal networks in their day to day lives and how they take part in local democratic structures.

The study will look in detail at 'within gender' differences, rather than taking `men' and `women' as homogenous groups. For example, it will be important to distinguish between women of different ages, those who work and those who do not, those with children and those without. This will be a qualitative study involving focus groups, and in-depth interviews.

This is a two-year project and fieldwork is currently underway.

Social capital, age and health

The Luton pilot study,[1] suggested that there is a differential relationship between age (taken here to be the broad age-groups: 15–18; 19–34; 35–55) and perceptions of aspects of social capital and health. Recent policy documents such as the Acheson Report on Health Inequalities[2] endorse an approach to priorities based on stages of the life course (mothers, children and families; young people and adults of working age; older people). Campbell et al, indicated that of the aspects of social capital suggested by Putnam,[3] two factors were more prevalent in areas with higher health status. One was the presence of social networks both at the micro-social level, and outside the local community (defined as being a ward).

The other was the greater level of involvement in local civic issues. The aim of this study will be to investigate the way health promoting social networks are developed, utilised and sustained across different age-groups. A particular focus will be on life transitions such as starting a family and retirement. The study will include consideration of how people in different age-groups (15–18; 19–34; 35–55; over 55) develop, sustain and use formal and informal networks. It will also describe the way in which people in different age-groups engage in local civic issues. Methods will include a literature review, focus groups and in-depth interviews.

This is a two-year project and fieldwork is currently underway.

Social capital and children and families

Following on from the adult-based exploratory study into social capital and health, the HEA, together with the Eleanor Rathbone Trust has funded a fellowship to study social capital in relation to children and young people. Research is being conducted in the same location as the adult study, concentrating in the areas of greatest deprivation, and including a neighbouring rural area. The principal aims of the study are as follows:

1. To explore and develop the concept of 'social capital' as defined by Putnam as it relates to children and young people, using a case study approach.
2. To compare access to social capital among young people and children in a range of different settings.
3. To make recommendations for health promotion efforts at the local community level, as well as explore the implications for local and national policies aimed at promoting health-enabling communities.

The research involves a qualitative school-based study with two age bands of children, 12–13 year olds (Year 8) and 14–15 year-olds (Year 10). A combination of creative and structured methods are being used to explore children's social networks: structured methods involve written autobiographical accounts, and visual methods using photography and map drawing. Group discussions are being used to explore young people's perceptions of, use of, and feelings about neighbourhood and institutions.

Current progress on this research is available in an MSc report.[4]

B.2.2 Exploring the empirical relationship between social capital and health – quantitative studies

The influence of social support and social capital on health

One limitation to quantitative research in this area has been the confusion and considerable diversity in the definition and measurement of social support and social capital. To further our knowledge in this area the HEA commissioned the Sociology Department at the University of surrey to undertake some secondary analysis of an existing dataset, the Health and Lifestyle Survey (HALS),[5] to explore the links between social support and social capital and health and to support the development of improved measures of these concepts.

The secondary analysis, carried out by Cooper et al,[6] examined social support and social capital in relation to health and health-related behaviour. They found that material living conditions and socio-economic position were much stronger predictors of adverse health outcomes than measures of social capital. However, associations were found between health and an individual's perception of their 'neighbourhood social capital'.

The report concluded that quantitative indicators of social capital based on surveys of individuals, complement existing aggregate level analyses of social capital and allow the distribution of social capital to be analysed based on large and representative samples of the population.

Cooper et al, made a number of recommendations for future work in this area:

1. In general, future studies and surveys should include measures of social capital for example, the measure of neighbourhood social capital derived from the HALS.
2. More information should be collected about the extent of community participation in a wider range of activities.
3. In addition, indicators of social capital which relate to perceptions of trust and security should be added to future surveys.
4. Surveys should clearly distinguish between the collection of different types of social support measures. The more important measures relate to perceived closeness of relationships with friends and relatives and the frequency of contact with friends rather than relatives.
5. Measures of social capital are related to an individual's gender, socio-economic circumstances and material living conditions. It is therefore essential that future surveys collect information about all these variables to examine the contribution of social capital to health after adjusting for these structural factors.
6. It is important to measure social capital at both the individual level using surveys and at the aggregate area or community level. Surveys should include area level information based, for example, on ACORN classifications derived from ward or enumeration district data from the population Census. In this way it will be possible to undertake multilevel analysis in order to identify the effects on health of the quality of the area of residence separately from the effects of the individuals perception of their neighbourhood.

Developing a Social Capital Module for the General Household Survey 2000/1

The HEA will work in partnership with the Office for National Statistics and the University of Surrey to develop a social capital module for the General Household Survey (GHS) 2000. This project will develop and validate a module of questions to measure a range of components of social capital. These will include the strength of voluntary organisations, norms of neighbourliness, reciprocity and trust, social cohesiveness and infrastructural resources, community networks, social networks and social support, civic identity, attitudes about neighbourhood and community and civic and community involvement.

In addition, the project will undertake detailed multivariate analysis of the social capital module, creating a range of further social capital indicators, examining their relationship with a range of health measures, and controlling for socio-economic characteristics and measures of material deprivation.

This is a three-year research project, which is currently in its initial year.

Using the Whitehall II study and the Health Survey for England (HSE) to investigate the links between social capital, area and health

The HEA will work with Michael Marmot and colleagues at the Department of Epidemiology and Public Health, University College London on a project, which aims to use two existing studies (Whitehall II and the HSE), to:

1. Collect comprehensive, quantitative measures of the positive and negative aspects of social capital in a range of areas from affluent to deprived.
2. Determine whether the association between social capital and a range of physical and mental health outcomes is independent of the individual characteristics of residents in the area and to investigate interactions between area social capital and individual characteristics in relation to health.
3. Investigate whether the association between area social capital and health is independent of material deprivation.
4. Investigate the biological behavioural mechanisms by which social capital influences health.

In addition, the project will examine the impact of social capital on health in a new Health Action Zone (HAZ).

This is a three-year research project, which is currently in its initial year.

Analysing the British Household Panel Survey (BHPS) to investigate the links between social capital and health

This study has been commissioned by the HEA and is being carried out by the Institute of Social and Economic Research. It will analyse existing and future data from the BHPS in order to examine some of the relationships between social capital and health-related outcomes. The panel design and household basis of the survey will allow the examination of questions that cannot be tackled explicitly with cross-sectional individual level data. These will include looking at health status over time, the possibilities of time lagged effects and multiple levels of analyses between the household and the individuals constituting that household. This study will in particular allow us to assess whether the new National Statistics socio-economic classification is a better predictor of social capital than previous measures of class.

This is a three-year research project, which is currently in its initial year.

B.2.3 Social Action Research Project (SARP) in Two Cities

In addition, the HEA has commissioned two demonstration projects in two cities in England to evaluate the impact of integrated social action research on health inequalities, using social capital as a framework for evaluation. The two cities, Nottingham and Salford are developing models of working based on participation, collaboration and partnerships with local people, statutory and non-statutory agencies and industry.

This 3 year project will involve:

1. Social interventions to promote health and contribute to reductions in inequalities with a focus upon vulnerable groups.
2. The development and implementation of cross-sectoral activities.
3. A formative and process evaluation.
4. An independent scientific evaluation.
5. The setting up of a research network to facilitate information exchange between the two cities and others involved in similar work (see objective 3).

The aims of the SARP programme are twofold:

1. To develop, test and implement reliable measures of social trust, social cohesion, social networking, partnerships and a range of other factors that are hypothesised to be implicated in community health and wellbeing.
2. To develop new methods of lay participation and consultation – through encouraging partnerships across professional boundaries and across sectors and organisations in order to elicit and respond to the needs of the most marginalised and vulnerable to poor health.

Notes and references

1. Campbell C, Wood R and Kelly M. *Social capital and health*. Health Education Authority (London: 1999).

2. Acheson D *et al. Independent Inquiry into Inequalities in Health – Report*. TSO (London: 1998).

3. Putnam R D. *Making Democracy Work. Civic Traditions in Modern Italy*. Princeton University Press (New Jersey: 1995).

4. Morrow V. Searching for social capital in children's accounts of neighbourhood and network: a preliminary analysis in *LSE Gender Institute – discussion paper series*. Issue 7, May 1999.

5. Health Education Authority. *Health and Lifestyles: A Survey of the UK Population, Part 1*. Health Education Authority (London: 1995).

6. Cooper H, Arber S, Fee L and Ginn J. *The influence of social support and social capital on health*. Health Education Authority (1999).

Appendix C Details of analysis methods and derivation of variables

C.1 Age-standardisation

The association between age and health and many health-related behaviours is well-documented. It is therefore important to take age into account when investigating the relationship between health and other characteristics such as social class and marital status. One commonly-used method is the presentation of three-way tables, which tabulate the prevalence of a health measure for a number of age-groups. The resulting tables may, however, be difficult to interpret and suffer from small cell sizes.

An alternative to this is the use of age-standardised tables. The method of standardisation used in this report, in Chapters 3 to 7, is that of indirect standardisation; this is considered more appropriate for survey data than the direct method of standardisation which is used in medical statistics. Direct standardisation involves applying age-specific rates for the whole population of men or women to the age distribution in the sub-group (for example, the social class) of interest. The method does not make use of the rates observed for age-groups within social classes which are likely to be based on small sample totals and to be affected by substantial sampling error.

The age-standardised ratios shown in tables such as Tables 3.5 to 3.17 were calculated by dividing the observed proportions reporting good health by the expected proportion and then multiplying by 100. An age-standardised ratio of more than 100 indicates a greater likelihood of reporting a particular characteristic or behaviour than would be expected in that group on the basis of age distribution alone. Conversely, a ratio of less than 100 indicates that the members of the group are less likely to report the characteristic or behaviour under consideration than would be expected from the age composition of the group. Since standardised ratios are calculated from survey data, they are subject to sampling error and a more precise assessment of their deviation from 100 involves the use of the standard error of the ratio in a conventional test of statistical significance. Although the standard error is not shown in the tables in this report it is possible to give an example. In Table 3.5, the standard error of the ratio for single men with 'less than good' general health is 4.9; multiplying this by 1.96 (the 95% level of significance) gives 9.6; as the difference between 120 (the standardised ratio for this group) and 100 is greater than 9.6, this difference is taken to be significant.

As explained in Appendix A, however, because the sample for the HEMS survey was a multi-stage probability sample involving both stratification and clustering, standard errors assuming a simple random sample will tend to be underestimates. One way of dealing with this is to adjust the standard error by the design

factor (deft) to allow for the complex sample design. For the age-standardised tables presented in this report, an approximation to deft is used (1.2). As shown in Appendix A, only a few of the health-related characteristics covered in Tables A.12–A.19 had design factors of 1.2 or more, and most of the occurrences were for single categories of a variable of interest.

A final stage is needed to take account of the weighting which was applied to the sample to compensate for non-response. The standard error was multiplied by the square root of the mean weight (1.45 for men and 1.31 for women) to allow for the fact that the standardised ratios were calculated on weighted data. In the example for single men with 'less than good' general health discussed above, the final calculation was as follows:

$$4.9 \times 1.96 \times 1.2 \times 1.45 = 16.7$$

The standardised ratio for this group was 120; as the difference between this and 100 is larger than 16.7, it can be concluded that the ratio was higher than expected at the 95% level of significance.

For a more detailed description of the indirect method of standardisation see Foster K. The use of standardisation in survey analysis. OPCS *Survey Methodology Bulletin*, (1993), 33, 19–27.

C.2 Logistic regression

Logistic regression is a multivariate statistical technique which has been used in a number of chapters in this report. It predicts the outcome of a dependent variable which only has two possible outcomes, for example being a current smoker and not being a current smoker, from a set of independent variables. Variables with only two possible outcomes are known as dichotomous or binary variables. Logistic regression was developed specifically for dichotomous variables and makes more appropriate assumptions about the underlying distributions and the range of possible proportions than the multiple linear regression method.

Most of the tables in the HEMS report (for example Table 4.1) are based on crosstabulations. These tables show the proportion of people with a given characteristic who display the behaviour of interest; an example would be the proportion of people aged 16–24 who smoke. What such tables do not show, however, is how much other factors may inter-relate with the independent variable; for example, how much social class and sex may interrelate with age to influence whether or not a person smokes.

Logistic regression looks at how different independent variables interrelate by looking at the odds of the behaviour occurring for different combinations of the independent variables. Odds refers to the ratio of the probability that the event will occur to the probability that the event will not occur. The odds of an event happening are related to its probability (p) in the following way:

$$odds = p/(1-p).$$

To take an example, 29% of men and 26% of women were current cigarette smokers. The odds of doing so are thus 29/71 for men and 26/74 for women, and the odds ratio, or relative odds, of a man being a current cigarette smoker compared with a woman, are (29/71)/(26/74), or about 1.16. The ratio of percentages (29/26) is smaller, 1.12, and the odds ratio is different because it depends on the absolute, as well as the relative size of the percentages (or probabilities).

The odds can be converted into a probability (p) using the following formula:

$$p = \frac{odds}{1 + odds}.$$

Logistic regression can therefore be used to predict the probability of a behaviour occurring given a combination of characteristics, for example, it can be used to model the probability of a person being either a smoker or a non-smoker given their age, sex and social class.

The logistic regression model can be written as

$$Prob(event) = \frac{e^z}{1 + e^z}$$

where e is the base of the natural logarithms. Logistic regression actually models independent variables against the log odds (the natural logarithm of the odds) of an event because this forms a linear relationship.

$$Z = B_0 + B_1X1 + \ldots\ldots B_pX_p.$$

where the Xs are the independent variables, Bs are the model parameters and Bo is the baseline odds. The odds of engaging in behaviour can then be calculated by multiplying the baseline odds by the appropriate factors.

The first category of each of the independent variables is defined as a reference category (with a value of 1). For each of the independent variables included in the regression a coefficient is produced which represents the factor by which the odds of a person taking part in the behaviour increases if the person has that characteristic. The odds produced by the regression are relative odds, that is they are relative to the reference category. Taking the example above, where smoking is the dependent variable, the age group 16–24 is defined as the reference category. The odds given by the model would be relative to this reference category; so it would be possible to say how much greater the odds were of a person aged 65–74 being a smoker than the odds of a person aged 16–24 being a smoker.

There are different methods of including independent variables in the logistic regression model. The method used in the HEMS analysis was forward stepwise selection which is where the model starts off only containing the constant and then at each step the independent variable which is the most highly significant is added in. Variables are then examined and the coefficients which make the observed results 'most likely' are selected while the others are removed using either the Wald statistic or the Likelihood-Ratio test. The Likelihood-Ratio test was used in the HEMS analysis.

When two (or more) independent variables are highly correlated this is referred to as collinearity. If one of the independent variables is fitted in the model, the other will have very little, if any, extra information with which to explain the variation in the dependent variable. Hence SPSS will only fit one of those variables - the one which explains most of the variation in the dependent variable. In Chapter 4, income was not retained as significant in the model 2 for being a current cigarette smoker if area deprivation was excluded. This suggests that income was correlated with area deprivation leading to this variable being dropped from the model.

The odds ratios produced by the regression are presented in the report as 'multiplying factors' and they are shown with the 95% confidence intervals. If the interval contains the value 1.00, then that odds ratio is not significantly different from the reference category. Undue weight should not be given to the significance or otherwise of particular categories, as this depends to some extent on which was chosen as the reference category. The baseline odds shown at the top of each table represent the average odds for the respondents with all of the reference categories shown.

For a more detailed description of logistic regression analysis see Chapter 2 of *SPSS Advanced Statistics User's Guide* (SPSS Inc. 1990).

C.3 Measurement of social class as defined by occupation

Respondents were assigned to a social class on the basis of their own current or last job, using the Standard Occupational Classification[1]. Social class has been presented throughout the report in four categories. Because of the small number of respondents in Social Classes I, II, IV and V, classes I and II, and IV and V have been combined. The four categories used are:

I and II	Professional, managerial and technical occupations
III Non-Manual	Skilled non-manual occupations
III Manual	Skilled manual occupations
IV and V	Unskilled occupations

Respondents who were members of the Armed Forces, whose occupation had been inadequately described or who had never worked were not allocated a social class. The number of respondents in this group in 1998 was much lower than in previous years of HEMS mainly due to a change in the programs which code occupation.

Tables C.3.1–C.3.2 show the distribution by sex and age of respondents' social class. They show that men were more likely than women and men aged 16–24 less likely than other men, to be in Social Classes I and II (i.e. professional and managerial groups). **(Tables C.3.1–C.3.2)**

Table C.3.1 Social class based on own current or last job by age and sex

Age	16-24	25-34	35-44	45-54	55-64	65-74	75 and over	Total
Social class	%	%	%	%	%	%	%	%
Men								
I & II	13	40	44	45	39	37	34	38
III (non-manual)	23	13	12	10	7	9	11	12
III (manual)	26	32	30	31	33	39	30	31
IV & V	38	15	14	13	21	15	25	19
Unclassifiable*	-	1	0	0	0	0	1	0
Base = 100%	*178*	*428*	*463*	*432*	*390*	*350*	*254*	*2495*
Women								
I & II	13	34	32	30	27	19	19	26
III (non-manual)	45	35	34	38	30	35	33	36
III (manual)	11	8	6	7	10	11	11	9
IV & V	31	22	29	25	33	35	36	29
Unclassifiable*	-	-	0	-	-	-	0	0
Base = 100%	*220*	*613*	*565*	*460*	*401*	*431*	*428*	*3118*

* Members of the Armed Forces, persons in inadequately described occupations and persons who had never worked.

Table C.3.2 Age by social class based on own current or last job, and sex

Social class	I & II	III (non-manual)	III (manual)	IV & V	Unclassifiable*	Total
Age	%	%	%	%	%	%
Men						
16-24	4	22	9	24	-	12
25-34	22	22	21	16	33	21
35-44	23	20	19	15	21	20
45-54	21	15	18	13	12	18
55-64	13	7	14	15	12	13
65-74	10	8	13	9	4	11
75 and over	6	6	6	8	17	6
Base = 100%	*948*	*274*	*792*	*467*	*14*	*2495*
Women						
16-24	6	14	14	12	-	11
25-34	24	18	17	14	-	19
35-44	23	18	13	19	67	19
45-54	19	18	14	14	-	17
55-64	13	11	14	15	-	13
65-74	8	11	14	14	-	11
75 and over	7	9	13	12	33	10
Base = 100%	*830*	*1063*	*292*	*931*	*2*	*3118*

* Members of the Armed Forces, persons in inadequately described occupations and persons who had never worked.

Table C.3.3 Social class of HOH based on HOH's current or last job by respondent's social class based on own current or last job, and sex

Respondent's social class	I & II	III (non-manual)	III (manual)	IV & V	Unclassifiable*	Total
Social class of HOH	%	%	%	%	%	%
Men						
I & II	90	6	2	1	-	38
III (non-manual)	4	87	2	4	-	12
III (manual)	3	4	92	4	-	31
IV & V	4	3	5	90	8	18
Unclassifiable*					92	0
Base = 100%	*981*	*261*	*788*	*441*	*15*	*2486*
Women						
I & II	51	14	15	8	9	27
III (non-manual)	31	73	34	18	68	36
III (manual)	5	4	19	6	9	9
IV & V	13	9	31	68	-	29
Unclassifiable*					14	0
Base = 100%	*1058*	*569*	*718*	*746*	*12*	*3103*

* Members of the Armed Forces, persons in inadequately described occupations and persons who had never worked.

The tables in the report show respondents' own social class. Just over half (53%) of respondents were classified as the 'head of household' according to SSD's current definition[2], where this was not the case, information regarding occupation was also collected for the head of household. The majority (76%) of male respondents were themselves the head of household; only 24% of female respondents were the head of household. Table C.3.3 shows the relationship between respondents' own social class and that of the head of household.

The overwhelming majority of men were, of course, classified to the same social class as the head of household. The proportion of women belonging to the same social class as the head of household varied from 19% of women in Social Class III (Manual) to 73% of those categorised as belonging to Social Class III (Non-Manual). **(Table C.3.3)**

Measurement of area deprivation - HEMS Area Deprivation Score, based on the Carstairs Index

The Carstairs index[3] is an area-based measure which was developed to explore deprivation and health in Scotland. The measure has been adapted for use in this report. The HEMS index was created using 1991 Census small area statistics for England. Like the Carstairs index, it was derived from measures of overcrowding, male unemployment, social class and car ownership for each postcode sector. The index is the sum of these four variables, each standardised across all sectors to have zero mean and unit variance. The variables are defined as:

Overcrowding:	Persons in private households living at a density of >1 person per room as a proportion of all persons in private households
Male Unemployment:	Proportion of economically active males who are seeking work
Semi & Unskilled social class:	Proportion of all persons in private households with head of household in Social Class IV or V
No car:	Proportion of all persons in private households with no car

The scores for England ranged from -5.47 to +19.30 with a mean of zero. The distribution of the scores for England was skewed and is shown in Figure C.4.1. Although, there were a very few postcode sectors that were classified as very deprived (i.e with a positive score), the majority of areas were classified as affluent. There were 61% of cases below the mean (more affluent) and 39% of cases above the mean (more deprived). The second stage in developing the score for use in this report was to match the scores for England to the sectors used in the HEMS 1998 sample. This gave an area deprivation score for each of the respondents. For the HEMS sample, the deprivation score ranged from -4.58 to +9.26 and the mean was 0.27. There were 66% of cases below the mean (more affluent) and 34% of cases above the mean (more deprived). **(Figure C.4.1)**

Although Carstairs and Morris calculated a version of their index for England and Wales, the calculation of the HEMS deprivation score differs from the Carstairs index[3] in two respects. First, HEMS used 1991 Census small area statistics for postcode sectors whereas the Carstairs index for England and Wales is

Figure C.4.1 Distribution of HEMS area deprivation score for postcode sectors in England

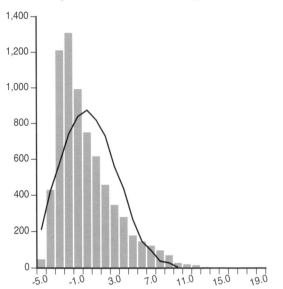

HEMS area deprivation score (postcode sectors in England)

based on 1981 ward-level data. Second, the HEMS score does not include an adjustment to the overcrowding measure needed by Carstairs to make a valid comparison between the index for England and Wales and that for Scotland. Because of these two factors some differences would be expected in the distributions of the HEMS deprivation score and the Carstairs index. However, both indices discriminate between different health measures in a similar way.

For some of their analysis, Carstairs and Morris collapsed their index into seven categories. However, partly because of the differences in derivation outlined above, the HEMS 1998 report used an index collapsed into five approximately equal groups.

Figure C.4.2 HEMS area deprivation score: Mean value of deprivation components by deprivation category for postcode sectors in England

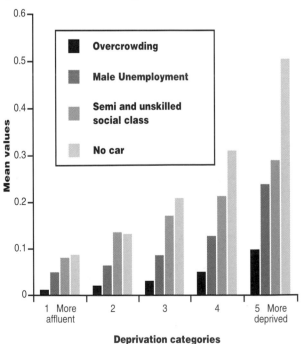

Deprivation categories

The categories ranged from 1 (most affluent areas) to 5 (most deprived areas). Table C.4.1 and Figure C.4.2 show the mean values of the component parts for each of the categories for the postcode sectors in England. The mean values for each component increase as the categories increase. In Table C.4.2, the distribution across deprivation categories is shown for all postcode sectors in England and for the HEMS responding sample. **(Figure C.4.2 and Tables C.4.1 to C.4.2).**

C.5 Measurement of neighbourhood social capital

The HEMS neighbourhood social capital score was derived from the following questions about respondents' neighbourhoods:

Would you say this neighbourhood…
* is a place you enjoy living in?
* is a place where you personally feel safe?
* is a place where the neighbours look after each other?
* has good facilities for young children?
* has good local transport?
* has good leisure facilities for people like yourself?

Answers to these questions were scored with +1 if the answer was 'yes' and –1 if the answer was 'no'. A "don't know" response was given a neutral score of zero. The score thus derived ranged from –6 to +6. This score was regrouped into the score used in many of the chapters in this report. The groupings were as follows:

Score 5 to 6   Very high social capital
Score 3 to 4   High social capital
Score 1 to 2   Medium social capital
Score –6 to 0   Low social capital

C.6 Measurement of levels of physical activity

C.6.1 The indicators of participation in physical activity

Physical activity as measured by the Health Education Monitoring Survey included:

* 'home' activities, (housework, gardening and DIY)
* walking
* sports and exercise activities including cycling
* activity at work

Stair climbing and caring activities were not included.

The summary measure used is based on occasions of 'moderate or vigorous' intensity activity, defined as having an energy cost of at least 5 kcals/min. This included:

* 'heavy' housework and 'heavy' gardening or DIY
* walks lasting 30 minutes or more, at a fast or brisk pace (see also Section C.6.4)

Table C.4.1   Mean value of deprivation components by deprivation category for postcode sectors in England

Deprivation components	Overcrowding	Male Unemployment	Semi & Unskilled Social Class	No Car
Deprivation category	Mean			
1 (More affluent)	0.01	0.05	0.08	0.09
2	0.02	0.07	0.14	0.13
3	0.03	0.09	0.17	0.21
4	0.05	0.13	0.21	0.31
5 (More deprived)	0.10	0.24	0.29	0.51
Total	*0.04*	*0.12*	*0.18*	*0.25*

Table C.4.2   Deprivation category by postcode sectors in England and HEMS 1998 responding cases and mean deprivation score

	England (postcode sectors)			HEMS 1998 (Cases)		
	Number	%	Mean deprivation score	Number	%	Mean deprivation score
Deprivation categories						
1 (More Affluent)	1451	20	-3.35	1060	20	-3.45
2	1451	20	-2.15	1098	19	-2.00
3	1530	21	-0.86	1460	25	-0.99
4	1373	19	1.08	1293	21	1.09
5 (More Deprived)	1450	20	5.39	905	15	4.68
Total	*7255*	*100*	*0.00*	*5816*	*100*	*-0.39*

- sports and exercise activities (including cycling) defined as having an energy cost of at least 5 kcal/min - see below
- occupational activity defined as involving at least moderate intensity activity - see below

A duration threshold of at least 30 minutes was applied to sports activities and walking. All other types of activity were included irrespective of duration.

C.6.2 Energy intensity categories and frequency measures by activity type

Home activities: Energy cost

Moderate   'Heavy' housework and 'heavy' gardening/DIY were both classified as moderate-intensity activities. Respondents were shown cards giving the following examples:

Walking with heavy shopping for more than 5 minutes, moving heavy furniture, spring cleaning, scrubbing floors with a scrubbing brush, cleaning windows, or other similar heavy housework.

Digging, clearing rough ground, building in stone/bricklaying, mowing large areas with a hand mower, felling trees, chopping wood, mixing/laying concrete, moving heavy loads, refitting a kitchen or bathroom or any similar heavy manual work.

Home activities: Frequency

Number of days in the past four weeks on which informant did 'heavy' housework plus number of days on which did 'heavy' gardening/DIY.

Occupational activity: Energy cost

Vigorous   Considers self 'very physically' active in job and is in one of the following occupations defined as involving heavy work, including:

fishermen/women, furnace operators, rollermen, smiths, forgers, faceworking coal-miners, construction workers, fire service officers, metal plate workers, shipwrights, riveters, steel erectors, benders, fitters, galvanisers, tin platers, dip platers, plasterers, roofers, glaziers, general building workers, road surfacers, stevedores, dockers, goods porters, refuse collectors.

Moderate	Considers self 'very physically' active in job and is not in occupation groups listed above
	OR
	considers self 'fairly physically' active in job and is in one of the occupations listed above.

Occupational activity: Frequency
Not collected for occupational activity.

Sports and exercise activities: Energy cost

Vigorous   a) All occasions of running/jogging, squash, boxing, kick boxing, skipping, trampolining.
b) Sports coded as vigorous intensity if they had made the respondent breathe heavily or sweat a lot, but otherwise coded as moderate intensity including: cycling, aerobics, keep fit, gymnastics, dance for fitness, weight training, football, rugby, swimming, tennis, badminton.

Moderate   (a) See 'vigorous' category (b), but where the activity did not make the respondent breathe heavily or sweat a lot.
(b) All occasions of a large number of sports including: basketball, canoeing, fencing, field athletics, hockey, ice skating, lacrosse, netball, roller skating, rowing, skiing, volleyball.
c) Sports coded as moderate intensity if they had made respondent breathe heavily or sweat a lot, but otherwise coded as light intensity, including: exercises (press-ups, sit-ups etc), dancing.

Sports and exercise activities: Frequency and duration
Number of days in past four weeks.
Time usually spent per day of activity.

Walking: Energy cost

Moderate   Walks of 30 minutes or more at a brisk or fast pace.

Walking: Frequency
Number of walks lasting 30 minutes or more in the past four weeks.

C.6.3 Reference period

A four-week reference period was used in the interview. Frequency of activity during the four-week period is expressed in the results as an average frequency per week, based on the following conversion:

Frequency of activity in past four weeks	Average frequency per week
0 3 occasions	Less than once a week
4-11 occasions	1-2 times a week
12-19 occasions	3-4 times a week
20+ occasions	5+ times a week

C.6.4 Changes to the physical activity questions in 1995, 1996 and 1998

Changes to the measure of 'walking'
There is always a dilemma in conducting repeated surveys as to whether it is more important to maintain total comparability from year to year or whether it is better to attempt to improve/modify the questions where necessary. The questions on walking have been modified in 1998.

The definition of minimum walking distance has been changed from a measure of *distance* to a measure of *time spent walking*. In 1995, HEMS analysis was based on walks of two miles or more. This was changed in 1996 to walks of 1–2 miles or more to be more closely aligned with the content of the HEA indicator based on participation in at least moderate-intensity activity. This indicator refers to 30 minutes of activity on five or more days a week. In 1998, the question was changed again, this time from a measure of distance to a measure of time, so that analyses was based on walks lasting 30 minutes or more, which, assuming a walking speed of at least three miles per hour, is equivalent to a walk of 1.5 miles or more.

The effect of the changes
A possible effect of this change would be to alter the numbers of respondents who reported such walks and therefore change the overall frequency of participation in activity.

The walking data for HEMS 98 was compared with those for HEMS 95 and HEMS 96 to investigate the effect of this change on the reported frequency of walking. Table C.6.1 shows that the proportion of men and women walking less than once a week (at the appropriate pace) was similar to 1995 and significantly lower than in 1996. The proportion of men and women who reported walking five times a week or more was higher in 1996 and similar to 1995. Although it is not possible to say conclusively that this does not represent a genuine population change in walking behaviour, it seems more likely that most of this difference is attributable to the change in definition. The size of the change would also serve to explain the apparent increase in the percentage, in 1996, of overall participation in at least moderate-intensity activity, shown in Chapter 6 (**Table 6.2**).

Table C.6.1   **Frequency of walking 2+ miles (1995 HEMS) compared with 1-2+ miles (1996 HEMS) and for 30+ minutes (1998 HEMS): all at a fast or brisk pace**

	Men			Women		
	HEMS 95	**HEMS 96**	**HEMS 98**	**HEMS 95**	**HEMS 96**	**HEMS 98**
	2+ miles	**1-2+ miles**	**30+ mins**	**2+ miles**	**1-2+ miles**	**30+ mins**
	%	%	%	%	%	%
Less than once per week	85	80	86	90	86	90
1-4 per week	12	13	12	7	9	8
5+ per week	3	7	3	3	5	2
Base	2122	2044	2308	2550	2601	2792

Figure C.7.1 Diet quality - derivation of the HEMS diet score

HEMS question	Score given to answers about each food item				
	-2	-1	0	+1	+2
Type of food usually eaten:					
Breads			Does not eat	White, Pitta, Other	Brown, Granary, Wheatmeal, Wholemeal, S. Asian
Spreads on bread	Butter, Hard or block margarine	Soft margarine, Reduced or low fat spread	Does not have usual type, Don't know		Does not use fat or spread on bread
Cooking fat or oil, for fried food	Solid cooking fat (inc. margarine)	Oil (inc. olive oil)	Does not have usual fat, Does not eat fried food, Don't know		
Milks in drinks, cereals, etc.			Whole milk, Other, Does not drink milk	Skimmed, Semi-skimmed	
Frequency of eating certain foods:					
Bread or rolls			Less than once a day	Once every day	More than once a day
Potatoes, rice or pasta			Less than once a day	Once every day	More than once a day
Fruit, vegetables or salad			Less than once a day	Once every day	More than once a day
Chips and other fried foods	More than once a day	Once every day	Less than once a day		
Biscuits, cakes, or confectionery (eg. sweets or chocolate)	More than once a day	Once every day	Less than once a day		

C.7 Measurement of diet quality – the HEMS diet score

The HEMS diet score, described in Chapter 7, was derived for each respondent based on their answers to nine of the survey questions: four about the types of foods that they said they usually ate, and five about how often they ate certain foods. (See Figure C.7.1 for details of the derivation of the score.) The diet scores derived in this way potentially range from –8 to +11. In practice, they ranged from -5 to +11 **(Figure C.7.1)**.

Notes and references

1   Office of Population Censuses and Surveys. *Standard Occupational Classification Volume 3.* HMSO (London: 1991).

2   The current definition of 'head of household' used by SSD is as follows:

    The member of the household in whose name the accommodation is owned or rented *except in the case of a married or cohabiting couple where the male partner takes precedence over the female.*

    If two people who are not a couple are jointly responsible for the accommodation, the oldest is taken if they are of the same sex, *but the male is taken if they are of different sex.*

    See McCrossan L. *A handbook for interviewers.* HMSO (London: 1991).

    SSD is continuing methodological work to investigate whether the concept of 'head of household' should be replaced by a 'household reference person'. *See* Martin J. Defining a household reference person, *Survey Methodology Bulletin* (1995), 37, 1–7, Martin J and Barton J. The effect of changes in the definition of the household reference person, *Survey Methodology Bulletin* (1996), 38, 1–8, and Martin J, Gill B and Lader D. A new definition for the household reference person, *Survey Methodology Bulletin* (1998), 43, 1–8.

3   Carstairs V and Morris R. *Deprivation and health in Scotland.* Aberdeen University Press (1991).

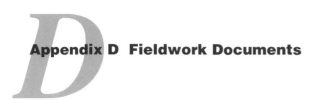

Appendix D Fieldwork Documents

The survey was carried out using computer-assisted interviewing. This is a copy of the questions.

HEALTH EDUCATION MONITORING SURVEY 1998

HOUSEHOLD BOX

Ask about everyone in the household

Whohere   Who normally lives at this address?

Name   RECORD THE NAME (OR A UNIQUE IDENTIFIER)
FOR HOH, THEN A NAME/ IDENTIFIER FOR
EACH MEMBER OF THE HOUSEHOLD.

    Name or other identifier

Sex   INTERVIEWER: CODE NAME's SEX.

    1   Male
    2   Female

Age   What was NAME's age last birthday?
    IF AGE NOT GIVEN, PROBE FOR AN ESTIMATE

Ask if household member is aged 16 or over

Marstat   Are you

    1   Single/never married
    2   Married and living with your husband/wife
    3   Married and separated from your husband/wife
    4   Divorced
    5   Widowed

**If more than one person in the household and Marstat =
single, separated or divorced**

Livewith   May I just check, are you living with someone in the
household as a couple?

    1   Yes
    2   No
    3   SPONTANEOUS ONLY - same sex couple

**If more than one person in the household and first person is
married or cohabiting**

Hhldr   In whose name is the accommodation owned or
rented?

    1   This person alone
    2   This person jointly
    3   NOT owner/renter

Ask all respondents

Relate   I would now like to ask how the other people in your
household are related to each other....

    1   Spouse
    2   Cohabitee
    3   Child son/daughter (incl. adopted)
    4   Stepchild (include step-son/daughter)
    5   Foster child
    6   Son-in-law/daughter-in-law
    7   Parent/guardian
    8   Step-parent
    9   Foster parent
    10   Parent-in-law
    11   Brother/sister (incl. adopted)
    12   Step-brother/sister
    13   Foster brother/sister
    14   Brother/sister-in-law
    15   Grand-child
    16   Grand-parent
    17   Other relative
    18   Other non-relative

HohNum   ENTER PERSON NUMBER OF HOH.

Respdnt   ENTER THE PERSON NUMBER OF
RESPONDENT

Ask respondents who are married, living as married, or living with a same sex partner

Livtgthr   How long have you and your husband/wife/partner been living together as a couple?

INCLUDE ANY TIME SPENT COHABITING BEFORE MARRIAGE.
ENTER TIME IN YEARS. IF LESS THAN ONE YEAR, ENTER 0

Ask respondents who are single, widowed, divorced or separated and aged 16-54

Partner   May I just check, do you have a regular partner who does not live in the household?

1   Yes
2   No

Ask all respondents

DoB   What is your date of birth?
INTERVIEWER: CODE NAME's DATE OF BIRTH

WorkLast   Did you do any paid work in the week ending last Sunday, either as an employee or as self-employed?

1   Yes
2   No

Ownorent   Does your household own or rent this accommodation?
CODE FIRST THAT APPLIES

1   Buying with a mortgage
2   Owned outright
3   Rented from Local Authority/New Town
4   Rented from Housing Association
5   Rented unfurnished
6   Rented furnished
7   Rented from employer
8   Other with payment
9   Rent-free

AccomTyp   INTERVIEWER CODE TYPE OF ACCOMMODATION

1   Detached house
2   Semi-detached house
3   Terraced/end of terrace house
4   Purpose-built flat
5   Flat in a converted house
6   Caravan, mobile home or houseboat
7   Other type of accommodation

Bedroom   How many bedrooms do you have available to your household?
A BEDROOM IS ANY ROOM USED FOR SLEEPING; THERE MUST BE ONE OR MORE. A ONE ROOM BEDSIT IS A BEDROOM.

0..20

Car   Is there a car or van normally available for use by you or any members of your household?

1   Yes
2   No

GENERAL HEALTH AND WELL-BEING

Ask all respondents

Genhlth   [*] Now I would like to ask you some questions about your health.
How is your health in general? Would you say it was..
RUNNING PROMPT

1   very good
2   good
3   fair
4   bad
5   or very bad?

Illness   [*] Do you have any long-standing illness, disability or infirmity? By long-standing I mean anything that has troubled you over a period of time or that is likely to affect you over a period of time?

1   Yes
2   No

Ask respondents who have a long-standing illness, disability or infirmity (Illness = Yes)

Lmatter   [*] What is the matter with you?

Limitact   [*] Does this illness or disability (Do any of these illnesses or disabilities) limit your activities in any way?

1   Yes
2   No

Ask of people aged 75+

Seventy   May I just check, have you had a '75 plus' Health Check?

1   Yes
2   No
3   Don't know

Ask all respondents

HlthIntr   Here are some things people have said about health. I'd like you to say how far you agree with each statement, choosing your answer from this card.

Hlthluck   [*] Generally health is a matter of luck.
SHOW CARD A

1   Strongly agree
2   Agree
3   Neither agree nor disagree
4   Disagree
5   Strongly disagree

Dontthnk   [*] I don't really have time to think about my health.
SHOW CARD A

1   Strongly agree
2   Agree
3   Neither agree nor disagree
4   Disagree
5   Strongly disagree

Stress   [*] Looking at this card, which of these statements best describes the amount of stress or pressure you experienced in the past 12 months, that is since (today's date) 1997.
SHOW CARD B

1   Completely free of stress
2   Small amount of stress
3   Moderate amount of stress
4   Large amount of stress
5   Don't know

Ask respondents who answered 2-4 to Stress

Copestr1   Which, if any, of the things on this card do you usually do to cope with stress or pressure?
SHOW CARD C
CODE ALL THAT APPLY

1   Try not to think about it
2   Discuss it with a close friend or relative
3   Work harder to occupy myself
4   Have a drink
5   Pray/meditate
6   Spend more time thinking about my problems
7   Spend more time going out with friends or relatives
8   None of these
9   Don't know

Copestr2   And which, if any, of the things on this card do you usually do to cope with stress or pressure?
SHOW CARD D
CODE ALL THAT APPLY

1   Take more exercise/more physical activity
2   Smoke more
3   Eat more
4   Get professional help or advice
5   Listen to/play music
6   Spend more time on hobbies
7   Other
8   None of these
9   Don't know

Harm   [*] How harmful would you say the amount of stress and pressure you have experienced in the last 12 months has been to your physical and mental health? Has it been...
RUNNING PROMPT

1   very harmful
2   harmful
3   or not harmful at all?
4   don't know

Ask all respondents

Hintr   Here is a list of issues which can affect people's health.

Badhelth   [*] Can you tell me which, if any, you feel have a bad effect on your health at the moment?
SHOW CARD E
CODE ALL THAT APPLY

1   The amount I smoke
2   Eating a poor diet
3   The quality of my housing
4   Stress
5   Living on my own
6   The amount of alcohol I drink
7   My weight
8   Environmental pollution
9   The quality of local health services
10 My sexual behaviour
11 Road traffic in this area
12 Being unemployed
13 Violent crime in this area
14 None of these

Futrill   [*] Can you look at this card and tell me which, if any, of these you are concerned might affect your health in the future?
SHOW CARD F
CODE ALL THAT APPLY

1   Violence/crime
2   Environmental pollution
3   Being unemployed
4   Cancer
5   The quality of local health services
6   The spread of HIV/AIDS
7   Stress
8   Heart disease
9   None of these

Futrill2   [*] And which, if any, of the things on this card, are you concerned might affect your health in the future?
SHOW CARD G
CODE ALL THAT APPLY

1   Road accidents
2   Health risks linked to smoking
3   My weight
4   Health risks linked to drugs
5   Eating a poor diet
6   The quality of my housing

7 Health risks linked to drinking alcohol
8 Being lonely
9 None of these

ENVIRONMENT

Ask all respondents

Howlong   How long have you lived in this area?

1 Less than 12 months
2 1 year
3 2 years
4 3 years
5 4 years
6 5-9 years
7 10-14 years
8 15-19 years
9 20 years or more
10 Don't know

Neighbr   I would like to ask you a few questions about your neighbourhood.

Enjyliv   [*] Would you say this neighbourhood is a place you enjoy living in?

1 Yes
2 No
3 Don't know

Feelsafe   [*] Would you say this neighbourhood is a place where you personally feel safe?

1 Yes
2 No
3 Don't know

Neighbhd   [*] Would you say this neighbourhood is a place where neighbours look after each other?

1 Yes
2 No
3 Don't know

Facilit   [*] Would you say this neighbourhood has good facilities for young children?

1 Yes
2 No
3 Don't know

Transprt   [*] Would you say this neighbourhood has good local transport?

1 Yes
2 No
3 Don't know

Leisure   [*] Would you say this neighbourhood has good leisure facilities for people like yourself?

1 Yes
2 No
3 Don't know

Neighlth   [*] Thinking about this neighbourhood, which, if any, of the items on this card do you think are a risk to your own health or well-being?
SHOW CARD H
CODE ALL THAT APPLY

1 The amount of road traffic
2 Industrial fumes and emissions
3 Litter and rubbish
4 The level of crime and vandalism
5 The level of noise
6 The amount of abuse or violence
7 Other risk
8 None of these
9 Don't know

Homehlth   [*] Thinking about your own home now, which, if any, of the items on this card do you think are a risk to your own health or well-being?
SHOW CARD I
CODE ALL THAT APPLY

1 Lack of heating
2 Dampness/condensation/mould
3 Cigarette smoke
4 The general maintenance of your home
5 Overcrowding
6 The quality of the drinking water
7 The level of noise
8 Other risk
9 None of these
10 Don't know

Workhlth   [*] Thinking about the work you do, which, if any, of the items on this card do you think are a risk to your own health or well-being?
SHOW CARD J
CODE ALL THAT APPLY

1 The materials you have to handle
2 The equipment you have to use
3 Industrial fumes and emissions
4 Cigarette smoke
5 The level of noise
6 Stress
7 The number of hours you work
8 Other risk
9 None of these
10 Don't know

SOCIAL SUPPORT

Ask all respondents

Socintro   The next few questions are about people you feel *close* to including relatives, friends and aquaintances.

Ask respondents who do not have another adult relative living with them

Closerel   [*] Do you have any close relatives whom you speak to or see regularly?

1 Yes
2 No

Ask all respondents

Closefri   [*] Do you have any close friends whom you speak to or see regularly?

1   Yes
2   No

Helpcomf   [*] If you had a serious personal crisis, how many people do you feel you could turn to for help and comfort?
ENTER NUMBER OF PEOPLE
IF MORE THAN 10 , ENTER 97.

0 .. 97

Sawlast   From this card, could you tell me which, if any, of these you have done in the past two weeks?
SHOW CARD K
CODE ALL THAT APPLY

1   Visited relatives/been visited by relatives
2   Spoke to relatives on the 'phone
3   Visited friends/been visited by friends
4   Spoke to friends on the 'phone
5   Spoke to neighbours
6   Spoke to a health professional (e.g. doctor, nurse, midwife, health visitor)
7   None of these

Donelast   And from this card, could you tell me which, if any, of these you have done in the past two weeks?
SHOW CARD L
CODE ALL THAT APPLY

1   Attended an adult education or night school class.
2   Participated in a voluntary group or local community group
3   Participated in community or religious activities
4   Went to a leisure centre
5   Went on a social outing
6   None of these

COMMUNITY INVOLVEMENT

Ask all respondents

Lifecont   For each of the following statements, please indicate how strongly you agree or disagree.

Satilife   [*] I am satisfied with the amount of control I have over decisions that affect my life.
SHOW CARD M

1   Strongly agree
2   Agree
3   Neither agree nor disagree
4   Disagree
5   Strongly disagree

Influenc   [*] I can influence decisions that affect my neighbourhood.
SHOW CARD M

1   Strongly agree
2   Agree
3   Neither agree nor disagree
4   Disagree
5   Strongly disagree

Ask all respondents

Thirdag   Have you heard of the term 'the third age'?

1   Yes
2   No

If has heard of 'third age'

WhatTage   What do you understand by this term?
DO NOT PROMPT

1   Older people/people over retirement age (no mention of active)
2   Active older people
3   Other answer
4   Don't know

OLDER PEOPLE

Ask all aged 65 or more

Wevent   Now I would like you to look at this card and say which, if any, of these things have happened to you in the past 12 months.
SHOW CARD N
CODE ALL THAT APPLY

1   Had a serious operation or illness
2   Had a serious injury
3   Death of close relative or friend
4   Personal experience of theft, mugging or other crime
5   Happy family event
6   Other event
7   None of these

Pubtrans   Do you use public transport at all nowadays?

1   Yes
2   No

If Pubtrans = Yes

Manage   Do you usually manage on your own or only with help from someone else?

1   On own
2   with help

If Pubtrans = No

Whynopub   [*] Why do you not use public transport?
(RUNNING PROMPT)
CODE ALL THAT APPLY

1   Health problem/ physical difficulty
2   Private transport is available/no need to use public transport
3   Public transport is not available/ not exist

	4	Public transport is too expensive
	5	Public transport is inconvenient
	6	Other reason

Taskintr   I would like to ask you about some tasks that some people may be able to do without any difficulty, while others may find them difficult or impossible. Please look at this card and tell me whether you find it not difficult, quite difficult, very difficult or impossible.
SHOW CARD O

Taskdiff   [*] How difficult is it for you to...
(RUNNING PROMPT)

Mobility   Get around the house, except for stairs, on your own?

	1	Not difficult
	2	Quite difficult
	3	Very difficult
	4	Impossible

Shopping   Do the household shopping on your own?

	1	Not difficult
	2	Quite difficult
	3	Very difficult
	4	Impossible

Persaffr   Deal with personal affairs (e.g. paying bills, writing letters, if you had to)?

IF DOES NOT DEAL WITH PERSONAL AFFAIRS, ASK COULD YOU IF YOU HAD TO

	1	Not difficult
	2	Quite difficult
	3	Very difficult
	4	Impossible

Service   I would now like to ask you about services you might make use of. Please look at this list and tell me which you have used in the last TWO WEEKS.
SHOW CARD P
CODE ALL THAT APPLY

	1	Local authority funded home help
	2	Local authority funded carer
	3	Private domestic help
	4	District nurse or health visitor
	5	Meals on wheels
	6	Lunch club run by council or voluntary body
	7	Day centre for older people run by council or voluntary body
	8	Helper from a voluntary organisation
	9	None of these

Acthelp   Do you act as a helper for any of the services listed on this card?
SHOW CARD Q

| | 1 | Yes |
| | 2 | No |

If Acthelp = Yes

Whchelp   Which of the services on this list do you help at?

	1	Meals on wheels
	2	Lunch club run by council or voluntary body
	3	Day centre for older people run by council or voluntary body
	4	Voluntary organisation
	5	Help at another service

SKIN CANCER

Ask all respondents

IntroSoc   There's been a lot of publicity recently about skin cancer. I would like to ask you a few questions about this.

Sunrisk   [*] What do you think are the main ways people can reduce their risk of developing skin cancer (DO NOT PROMPT)?
CODE ALL THAT APPLY

	1	Using sun cream
	2	Using high factor sun cream/ block
	3	Wearing a (wide brimmed) hat
	4	Staying in the shade
	5	Staying indoors
	6	Wearing cover-up clothing
	7	Staying out of the mid-day sun
	8	Don't use sunbeds
	9	Other
	10	None of these
	11	Don't know

Creamsun   Do you ever wear a suncream?

	1	Yes
	2	No
	3	Never go out in the sun

Ask if Creamsun = Yes

Whencrem   When do you use a suncream?
Please choose your answers from this card.
SHOW CARD R
CODE ALL THAT APPLY

	1	Sunbathing abroad
	2	Outdoors abroad, but not sunbathing
	3	Sunbathing in this country
	4	Outdoors in this country doing something else

Factor   Which factor level of suncream do you use most regularly?

	1	2-5
	2	6-8
	3	9-14
	4	15 or over
	5	Don't know

Ask all respondents

SunBurn   During the last 12 months, that is since (today's date) 1997, have you had sunburn causing redness and soreness of the skin lasting for at least 1-2 days?

1 Yes
2 No
3 Can't remember

Ask if Sunburn = Yes

FreqBurn   How many times?

1 Once
2 Twice
3 Three times
4 Four or more
5 Not in the last 12 months

Ask all respondents

SkinType   [*] Now I would like you to look at this card and say which of these statements best describes your **natural** skin type SHOW CARD S

1 White skin
2 Brown skin
3 Black skin
4 Olive skin
5 Other
6 Refused

Ask if answer 1 or 4 at SkinType

Sunbed   How many times have you used a sunbed in the last 12 months?

1 Not at all
2 1-10 times
3 11-20 times
4 More than 20 times

SunTan   [*] How important is having a suntan to you personally? Is it..
RUNNING PROMPT

1 very important
2 fairly important
3 or not important?
4 Don't know

SunIntr   How far do you agree with the following statement, choosing your answer from this card.

Sunhlth   [*] Having a suntan makes me feel healthier.
SHOW CARD T

1 Strongly agree
2 Agree
3 Neither agree nor disagree
4 Disagree
5 Strongly disagree

Ask all respondents

Spots   In the last year, have you checked your skin or asked a friend or relative or health professional to check your skin for spots that could be skin cancer?

1 Yes
2 No

SMOKING

Ask all respondents

Smokintr   The following questions are about smoking

SmokeSC   INTERVIEWER: 16 AND 17 YEAR-OLDS **MUST** SELF-COMPLETE. FOR INFORMANTS AGED 18 OR OVER THE QUESTIONS SHOULD BE ASKED BY YOU UNLESS YOU THINK THE INFORMANTS WOULD PREFER TO ANSWER THESE QUES-TIONS BY SELF-COMPLETION.

1 Completed by interviewer
2 Self-completion accepted and completed

Ask respondents who accepted self-completion

Smkintr2   I would like you to take the computer and answer the questions yourself. Instructions on how to answer the questions are given on the screen.

WORK THROUGH THE FIRST QUESTION WITH THE INFORMANT. IF THE INFORMANT MAKES A MISTAKE, TAKE THEM BACK TO THE QUESTION AND ALLOW THEM TO KEY IN THE RIGHT ANSWER.

Practice   This is the first time I have used a computer.

1 Yes
2 No
3 Don't want to answer

Ask all respondents

Cigever   Have you ever smoked a cigarette, a cigar or a pipe?

1 Yes
2 No

Ask respondents who have ever smoked a cigarette, cigar or a pipe (Cigever = Yes)

Cignow   Do you smoke cigarettes at all nowadays?

1 Yes
2 No

Ask current cigarette smokers (Cignow = Yes)

Qtywkend   About how many cigarettes a day do you usually smoke at weekends?
IF LESS THAN 1, ENTER 0.

Qtywkday   About how many cigarettes a day do you usually smoke on weekdays?
IF LESS THAN 1, ENTER 0.

Cigtype   Do you mainly smoke...
RUNNING PROMPT

1 filter-tipped cigarettes,
2 plain or untipped cigarettes,
3 or hand-rolled cigarettes?

Ask respondents who mainly smoke hand-rolled cigarettes (Cigtype = 3)

QtyTob   How much tobacco do you usually smoke per week? Would you prefer to give your answer in

1   quarter ounces
2   or in grammes?

Ask if QtyTob = Ounces

QtyTob1   ENTER NO. OF QUARTER OUNCES PER WEEK.
IF ANSWER GIVEN IN OUNCES, MULTIPLY BY FOUR.
IF LESS THAN QUARTER OF AN OUNCE, ENTER 0

0...20

Ask if QtyTob = Grammes

QtyTobM   ENTER NO. OF GRAMMES PER WEEK

0...150

Ask current cigarette smokers (Cignow = Yes)

Cigar   (May I just check) Do you smoke at least one cigar or cigarillo of any kind per month nowadays?

1   Yes
2   No

Trystop   Have you ever tried to give up smoking?

1   Yes
2   No

Ask respondents who have ever tried to give up smoking (Trystop = Yes)

Lasttime Thinking of the last time you tried to give up, how long was it for?

1   Less than a day
2   A day, less than a week
3   A week, less than a month
4   A month, less than 3 months
5   Three months, less than six months
6   Six months, less than a year
7   One year or more

WhenSt   And how long is it since you started smoking again?
1   Within last week
2   Within last month
3   Within last six months
4   Within last year
5   More than a year ago

Ask current cigarette smokers (Cignow = Yes)

Giveup   [*] Would you like to give up smoking altogether?

1   Yes
2   No
3   Don't know

Ask respondents who would like to give up smoking altogether (Giveup = Yes)

Stop1   [*] Now I would like you to look at this card, and say which of the statements best describes you.
SHOW CARD U

1   I intend to give up smoking within the next month
2   I intend to give up smoking within the next six months
3   I intend to give up smoking within the next year
4   I intend to give up smoking but not in the next year
5   I'm unlikely to give up smoking

Ask respondents who wouldn't like to give up smoking altogether (Giveup = No or don't know)

Stop2   [*] Now I would like you to look at this card, and say which of the statements best describes you.
SHOW CARD V

1   I'm unlikely to give up smoking
2   I intend to give up smoking within the next month
3   I intend to give up smoking within the next six months
4   I intend to give up smoking within the next year
5   I intend to give up smoking but not in the next year

Ask ex-cigarette smokers (Cignow = No)

CigReg   [*] Did you smoke cigarettes..
RUNNING PROMPT

1   regularly, that is at least one cigarette a day
2   or did you smoke them only occasionally?
3   SPONTANEOUS: Never really smoked cigarettes, just tried them once or twice

Ask ex-regular smokers, i.e. those who smoked at least one cigarette a day (CigReg = 1)

CigUsed   About how many cigarettes did you smoke in a day when you smoked them regularly?
IF LESS THAN 1, ENTER 0.

CigStop   How long ago did you stop smoking cigarettes regularly?
PROMPT AS NECESSARY

1   Less than 6 months ago
2   6 months but less than a year ago
3   1 year but less than 2 years ago
4   2 years but less than 5 years ago
5   5 years or more ago

WhyStop   [*] What was the main reason for giving up smoking?
DO NOT PROMPT

1   Health reasons
2   Cost
3   Family reasons
4   Pregnant

5   Advised to by health professional
6   Did not like it/enjoy it
7   Other: PLEASE SPECIFY

Ask respondents who answered 7 at Whystop

Xwhystop   Please specify other reasons for giving up.

DRINKING

Ask all respondents

DrnkIntr   I'd now like to ask you some questions about what you drink - that is, if you do drink.

DrinkNow   Do you ever drink alcohol nowadays, including drinks you brew at home?

1   Yes
2   No

Ask respondents who do not drink nowadays (DrinkNow = No)

DrinkAny   Could I just check, does that mean you never have an alcoholic drink nowadays, or do you have an alcoholic drink very occasionally, perhaps for medicinal purposes or on special occasions like Christmas or New Year?

1   Very occasionally
2   Never

Ask respondents who never drink alcohol (DrinkAny = Never)

TeeTotal   Have you always been a non-drinker, or did you stop drinking for some reason?

1   Always a non-drinker
2   Used to drink but stopped

Ask current drinkers (DrinkNow = Yes) or (Drinkany = occasionally)

Drtyintr   I'd like to ask you whether you have drunk different types of alcoholic drink in the last 12 months. I do not need to know about non-alcoholic or low alcohol drinks.

Shandy   How often have you had a drink of SHANDY (exclude bottles/cans) during the last 12 months, that is since (today's date) 1997
SHOW CARD W

1   Almost every day
2   5 or 6 days a week
3   3 or 4 days a week
4   once or twice a week
5   once or twice a month
6   once every couple of months
7   once or twice a year
8   not at all in the last 12 months

Ask respondents who have drunk shandy in the last 12 months (Shandy = 1-7)

ShandyAm   How much SHANDY (exclude bottles/cans) have

you usually drunk on any one day during the last 12 months, that is since (today's date) 1997?

ENTER NUMBER OF HALF PINTS.

Ask current drinkers (DrinkNow = Yes) or (Drinkany= occasionally)

Beer   How often have you had a drink of BEER, LAGER, STOUT, CIDER during the last 12 months, that is since (today's date) 1997?
SHOW CARD W

1   Almost every day
2   5 or 6 days a week
3   3 or 4 days a week
4   once or twice a week
5   once or twice a month
6   once every couple of months
7   once or twice a year
8   not at all in last 12 months

Ask respondents who have drunk beer in the last 12 months (Beer = 1-7)

BeerAm   How many HALF PINTS of .... BEER, LAGER, STOUT, CIDER have you usually drunk on any one day during the last 12 months, that is since (today's date) 1997? ENTER NUMBER OF HALF PINTS. IF YOU NORMALLY DRINK CANS OR BOTTLES, ENTER 97

Ask respondents who normally drink cans or bottles (Beeram = 97)

XBeeram   (Please write in) How many bottles or cans (do) you normally drink on one day. For example, 3 large cans or 2 small cans.

Ask current drinkers (DrinkNow = Yes) or (Drinkany= occasionally)

Spirits   How often have you had a drink of ... SPIRITS OR LIQUEURS (eg. gin, whisky, rum, brandy, vodka, advocaat, cocktails) during the last 12 months, that is since (today's date) 1997?
SHOW CARD W

1   Almost every day
2   5 or 6 days a week
3   3 or 4 days a week
4   once or twice a week
5   once or twice a month
6   once every couple of months
7   once or twice a year
8   not at all in last 12 months

Ask respondents who have drunk spirits in the last 12 months (Spirits = 1-7)

SpiritAm   How much .... SPIRITS OR LIQUEURS (eg. gin, whisky, rum, brandy, vodka, advocaat, cocktails) have you usually drunk on any one day during the last 12 months, that is since (today's date) 1997? ENTER NUMBER OF SINGLES (COUNT DOUBLES AS TWO SINGLES).

Ask current drinkers (DrinkNow = Yes) or (Drinkany = occasionally)

Sherry — How often have you had a drink of ... SHERRY OR MARTINI (including port, vermouth, cinzano, dubonnet) during the last 12 months, that is since (today's date) 1997?
SHOW CARD W

1 Almost every day
2 5 or 6 days a week
3 3 or 4 days a week
4 once or twice a week
5 once or twice a month
6 once every couple of months
7 once or twice a year
8 not at all in last 12 months

Ask respondents who have drunk sherry in the last 12 months (Sherry = 1-7)

SherryAm — How much .... SHERRY OR MARTINI (including port, vermouth, cinzano, dubonnet) have you usually drunk on any one day during the last 12 months, that is since (today's date) 1997?
ENTER NUMBER OF SMALL GLASSES

Ask current drinkers (DrinkNow = Yes) or (Drinkany= occasionally)

Wine — How often have you had a drink of ... WINE (including babycham, champagne) during the last 12 months, that is since (today's date) 1997?
SHOW CARD W

1 Almost every day
2 5 or 6 days a week
3 3 or 4 days a week
4 once or twice a week
5 once or twice a month
6 once every couple of months
7 once or twice a year
8 not at all in last 12 months

Ask respondents who have drunk wine in the last 12 months (Wine = 1-7)

WineAm — How much .... WINE (including babycham, champagne) have you usually drunk on any one day during the last 12 months, that is since (today's date) 1997?
ENTER NUMBER OF GLASSES

Ask current drinkers (DrinkNow = Yes) or (Drinkany= occasionally)

Lemon — How often have you had a drink of...ALCOHOLIC LEMONADE, ALCOHOLIC COLA OR OTHER ALCOHOLIC SOFT DRINKS during the last 12 months, that is since (today's date) 1997?
SHOW CARD W

1 Almost every day
2 5 or 6 days a week
3 3 or 4 days a week
4 once or twice a week

5 once or twice a month
6 once every couple of months
7 once or twice a year
8 not at all in last 12 months

Ask respondents who have drunk alcoholic lemonade/cola or other alcoholic soft drinks in the last 12 months

XlemonAm — How much ...ALCOHOLIC LEMONADE, ALCOHOLIC COLA OR OTHER ALCOHOLIC SOFT DRINKS have you usually drunk on any one day during the last 12 months, that is since (today's date) 1997?
ENTER AMOUNT

Ask current drinkers (DrinkNow = yes OR DrinkAny = occasionally)

Ifother — Have you had any other alcoholic drinks during the last 12 months, that is since (today's date) 1997?

1 Yes
2 No

Ask if Ifother = yes

XIfother — Please say which other kind of drink you have had

Otherd — How often have you had a drink of (other) during the last 12 months, that is since (today's date) 1997?
SHOW CARD W

1 Almost every day
2 5 or 6 days a week
3 3 or 4 days a week
4 once or twice a week
5 once or twice a month
6 once every couple of months
7 once or twice a year
8 not at all in last 12 months

Ask respondents who have drunk another type of drink in the last 12 months

OtherAm — How much of ....OTHER have you usually drunk on any one day during the last 12 months, that is since (today's date) 1997?
ENTER AMOUNT IN HALF PINTS, GLASSES OR SINGLES

Ask current drinkers (DrinkNow = Yes) or (Drinkany = occasionally)

Droften — Now I would like you to think about alcoholic drinks of all kinds. How often would you say you had an alcoholic drink of any kind?
SHOW CARD W

1 Almost every day
2 5 or 6 days a week
3 3 or 4 days a week
4 once or twice a week
5 once or twice a month
6 once every couple of months
7 once or twice a year
8 not at all in last 12 months

Ask all respondents

Units   As you may know, some drinks contain more alcohol than others. The amount is sometimes measured in terms of units of alcohol.

Unitalc   Have you heard about measuring alcohol in units?

     1   Yes
     2   No
     3   Don't know

Ask all who have heard of units

Unitglas   We are interested to know what people understand by a unit of alcohol.
How many units are there in a glass of wine?
IF LESS THAN ONE, CODE 0

Unitbeer   How many units are there in half a pint of normal strength beer?
IF LESS THAN ONE, CODE 0

Unitsprt   How many units are there in a single pub measure of spirits, for example, whisky or gin?
IF LESS THAN ONE, CODE 0

Ask all respondents

Drinkman   A unit of alcohol is equivalent to half a pint of beer, a glass of wine or a single measure of spirits.
[*] How many units of alcohol a day do you think a man can regularly drink without risking his health?
IF Don't Know ENTER 97

     0 .. 97

Drinkwom   [*] How many units of alcohol a day do you think a woman can regularly drink without risking her health?
IF Don't Know ENTER 97

     0 .. 97

Agredrnk   How much do you agree or disagree with each of the following statements?
SHOW CARD X

Drnkimp   [*] Drinking alcohol is an important part of having a good social life

     1   Strongly agree
     2   Agree
     3   Neither agree nor disagree
     4   Disagree
     5   Strongly disagree

Softdrnk   [*] I feel comfortable drinking soft drinks when my friends are drinking alcohol

     1   Strongly agree
     2   Agree
     3   Neither agree nor disagree
     4   Disagree
     5   Strongly disagree

Okdrunk   [*] It's OK to get drunk from time to time

     1   Strongly agree
     2   Agree
     3   Neither agree nor disagree
     4   Disagree
     5   Strongly disagree

Ask respondents who accepted self-completion (SmokeSC = 1)

Thankyou   That is the end of this section. Thank you for your help. Please now hand the computer back to the interviewer.

PHYSICAL ACTIVITY

Ask all respondents

ExerIntr   I'd like to ask you about some of the things you have done (at work or) in your free time that involve physical activity in the past 4 weeks.
SHOW THE LAST FOUR WEEKS ON THE CALENDAR

Ask respondents who did not have a job last week (WorkLast = No)

WrkLast4   Can I just check, have you done any paid work in the last four weeks either as an employee or as self-employed?

     1   Yes
     2   No

Ask respondents who had a job in last 4 weeks (Wrklast4 = Yes) OR (WorkLast = Yes)

Active   [*] Thinking about your job in general, (ASK ABOUT MAIN JOB ONLY) would you say that you are ....
RUNNING PROMPT

     1   very physically active
     2   fairly physically active
     3   not very physically active
     4   or not at all physically active in your job?

Ask all respondents

HouseWrk   I'd like you to think about physical activities you have done when you were not doing your paid job.
Have you done any housework in the past 4 weeks?

     1   Yes
     2   No

Ask respondents who have done housework in the past 4 weeks (HouseWrk = Yes)

HWrkList   Have you done any hoovering, dusting or ironing in the past 4 weeks?

     1   Yes
     2   No

Ask respondents who have done light housework in the past 4 weeks (HwrkList = Yes)

HevyHWrk   Some kinds of housework are heavier than others. This card gives examples of heavy housework, it does not include everything, these are just examples. Was any of the housework you did in the past 4 weeks this kind of heavy housework?
SHOW CARD Y

1   Yes
2   No

Ask respondents who have done heavy housework in the past 4 weeks (HevyHWrk = Yes)

HeavyDay   During the past 4 weeks on how many separate days have you done that kind of heavy housework?

Ask all respondents

Garden   (Apart from at work) Have you done any gardening, DIY or building in the past 4 weeks?

1   Yes
2   No

Ask respondents who have done some gardening, DIY, or building in the past 4 weeks (Garden = Yes)

GardList   Have you done any gardening, DIY or building work listed on this card?
SHOW CARD Z

1   Yes
2   No

Ask respondents who have done some light gardening, DIY, or building work (Gardlist = Yes)

ManWork   Have you done any gardening, DIY or building work from this card, or any similar heavy manual work?
SHOW CARD AA

1   Yes
2   No

Ask respondents who have done heavy gardening, DIY, or building work (Manwork = Yes)

ManDays   During the past 4 weeks, on how many days have you done this kind of heavy manual gardening or DIY?

Ask all respondents

WalkPre   I'd like you to think now about all the walking you've done in the past 4 weeks, either locally or away from here. Include any country walks and any walking to and from work, and any other walks that you have done.

WalkB   In the past four weeks have you done any walks that lasted between 5 and 10 minutes?

1   Yes

2   No
3   Can't walk at all/ housebound

Ask if WalkB = 1 or 2

MileWlkA   Did you do any walks that lasted for at least 15 minutes but less than 30 minutes?

1   Yes
2   No

Ask respondents who have done a walk of 15-29 minutes in the past 4 weeks (MileWlkA = Yes)

MileNumA   During the last 4 weeks, how many times have you done a walk that lasted for at least 15 minutes but less than 30 minutes?

1..97

MileWlkB   Did you do any walks that lasted for 30 minutes or more?

1   Yes
2   No

Ask respondents who have done any walks of 30+ minutes in the past 4 weeks (MileWlk B = Yes)

MileNumB   During the past 4 weeks how many times did you do any walks lasting for 30 minutes or more?

1..97

WalkPace   [*] Which of the following best describes your usual walking pace..
RUNNING PROMPT

1   a slow pace
2   a steady average pace
3   a fairly brisk pace
4   or a fast pace - at least 4 mph?

Ask all respondents

ActAny   Now I'd like you to think about any sports or exercise activities you do. Can you look at this card and tell me if you've done any of these types of activities during the past 4 weeks?
SHOW CARD BB

1   Yes
2   No

Ask if ActAny = Yes

WhchAc   Which of the activities did you do?
SHOW CARD BB
CODE ALL THAT APPLY

1   Aerobics/keep fit/gymnastics
2   Bowls/Crown bowls
3   Circuit training/weight training
4   Cycling
5   Exercises
6   Dancing

7	Football/rugby
8	Golf
9	Hiking
10	Hockey/netball/ice-skating
11	Jogging/running/athletics
12	Squash
13	Swimming
14	Tennis/badminton
15	Any other sport or exercise activity like these
16	Any other sport or exercise activity like these

Ask if WhchAc = Other 15 or 16

XWhchAc1/   SPECIFY OTHER ACTIVITY
XWhchAc2   (You can specify two extra types)

Ask about any activities which the informant has done

Occ   Can you tell me on how many separate days did you do (name of activity) during the past four weeks?

TimeAct   How much time did you usually spend (name of activity) on each day?
             ENTER TIME IN MINUTES IF MORE THAN ONE HOUR, CALCULATE TIME IN MINUTES

Effort   During the past four weeks, was the effort of (name of activity) usually enough to make you feel out of breath or sweaty?

             1   Yes
             2   No

Ask all respondents

EnufAct   [*] On the whole, do you think you get enough exercise at present to keep you fit?

             1   Yes
             2   No
             3   Can't take exercise

Ask if Enufact = Yes or No

LikeMore   [*] Would you like to take more exercise than you do at the moment?

             1   Yes
             2   No

Ask respondents who would like to take more exercise than at present (LikeMore = Yes)

Exermor1   [*] Now I would like you to look at this card, and say which of the statements best describes you.
             SHOW CARD CC

             1   I intend to take more exercise within the next month
             2   I intend to take more exercise within the next six months
             3   I intend to take more exercise within the next year
             4   I intend to take more exercise, but not in the next year
             5   I'm unlikely to take more exercise

Ask if Likemore = No or don't know

Exermor2   [*] Now I would like you to look at this card, and say which of the statements best describes you.
             SHOW CARD DD

             1   I'm unlikely to take more exercise
             2   I intend to take more exercise within the next month
             3   I intend to take more exercise within the next six months
             4   I intend to take more exercise within the next year
             5   I intend to take more exercise but not in the next year

NUTRITION

Ask all respondents

IntrDiet   Now I would like to ask you some questions about the foods you eat and buy.

Bread   What kind of bread do you usually eat?
             SHOW CARD EE
             CODE ONE ONLY

             1   white
             2   high fibre white
             3   brown, granary, wheatmeal
             4   wholemeal
             5   pitta bread
             6   South Asian breads (chapati, nan, roti, puri etc)
             7   or some other type of bread?
                  ESTABLISH TYPE AND CODE 1 TO 6 ABOVE IF APPROPRIATE OTHERWISE 7.
             8   does not eat any type of bread

Ask if eats bread

Spread   What do you usually spread on your bread?
             CODE ONE ONLY FROM CODING LIST

             1   Butter/hard margarine/block margarine
             2   Soft margarine
             3   Reduced fat spread
             4   Low fat spread
             5   **SPONTANEOUS**: Does not have usual type
             6   Don't know
             7   Does not use fat/spread on bread

Ask all respondents

CookOil   When you have fried foods, what kind of fat or oil are the foods usually cooked in? Is it ...
             RUNNING PROMPT
             CODE ONE ONLY

             1   solid cooking fat (i.e. is it in a packet or a tub)? INCLUDE MARGARINE
             2   or oil (i.e. is it in a bottle or a spray)? INCLUDE OLIVE OIL
             3   SPONTANEOUS: Does not have usual fat/oil
             4   Does not eat fried food
             5   Don't know

Milk	What kind of milk do you usually use for drinks, in tea or coffee or in cereals etc? Is it.. CODE ONE ONLY		1 More than once every day
			2 Once every day
			3 5-6 days a week
			4 3-4 days a week
	1 whole		5 1-2 days a week
	2 semi-skimmed		6 At least once a month
	3 skimmed		7 Less often than once a month
	4 or some other kind of milk?		8 Rarely or never
	5 SPONTANEOUS: Does not drink milk		

Milk

What kind of milk do you usually use for drinks, in tea or coffee or in cereals etc?
Is it..
CODE ONE ONLY

1 whole
2 semi-skimmed
3 skimmed
4 or some other kind of milk?
5 SPONTANEOUS: Does not drink milk

1 More than once every day
2 Once every day
3 5-6 days a week
4 3-4 days a week
5 1-2 days a week
6 At least once a month
7 Less often than once a month
8 Rarely or never

DietIntr

I would like to ask you about some foods which you may eat.
Can you tell me about how often on average you eat each of these foods by choosing your own answer from this card.
SHOW CARD FF

Ask all respondents

vHdiet

[*] In a few words, how would you describe a healthy diet?
ENTER VERBATIM AT THIS QUESTION AND CODE AT FOLLOWING QUESTION.
DO NOT PROMPT

Rolls

How often do you eat bread or rolls?

1 More than once every day
2 Once every day
3 5-6 days a week
4 3-4 days a week
5 1-2 days a week
6 At least once a month
7 Less often than once a month
8 Rarely or never

Hdiet

PLEASE CODE DESCRIPTION OF A HEALTHY DIET
CODE ALL THAT APPLY

1 Eat a balanced diet
2 Eat everything in moderation
3 Eat lots of fruit, vegetables or salad
4 Cut down on fatty or fried foods, eat grilled food
5 Eat lots of starch, carbohydrates, potatoes, pasta or rice
6 Cut down on sugar, cakes and confectionery
7 Eat lots of fibre, cereals, wholemeal food
8 Cut down on salt
9 Drink lots of water, fruit juice, liquid
10 Avoid red meat, eat white meat, fish
11 Eat lots of meat, eggs, cheese, drink lots of milk
12 Other

Starch

How often do you eat potatoes or rice or pasta?

1 More than once every day
2 Once every day
3 5-6 days a week
4 3-4 days a week
5 1-2 days a week
6 At least once a month
7 Less often than once a month
8 Rarely or never

If Hdiet = Other

SpHdiet   Please specify

Ask all respondents

Chips

How often do you eat chips and other fried foods? Please do not include oven chips

1 More than once every day
2 Once every day
3 5-6 days a week
4 3-4 days a week
5 1-2 days a week
6 At least once a month
7 Less often than once a month
8 Rarely or never

Agrehlth

Now I am going to read you a list of statements. I would like you to say whether you agree or disagree with them, choosing your answer from this card
SHOW CARD GG

HlthFood

[*] Eating healthy food is expensive.
SHOW CARD GG

1 Strongly agree
2 Agree
3 Neither agree nor disagree
4 Disagree
5 Strongly disagree

Veges

How often do you eat any fruit, vegetables or salad?

1 More than once every day
2 Once every day
3 5-6 days a week
4 3-4 days a week
5 1-2 days a week
6 At least once a month
7 Less often than once a month
8 Rarely or never

EnjyHlth

[*] Healthy foods are enjoyable.
SHOW CARD GG

1 Strongly agree
2 Agree
3 Neither agree nor disagree
4 Disagree
5 Strongly disagree

Sweets

How often do you eat biscuits, cakes or confectionery, eg. sweets or chocolate?

WhatHlth

[*] I get confused over what's supposed to be healthy and what isn't.
SHOW CARD GG

1 Strongly agree
2 Agree
3 Neither agree nor disagree
4 Disagree
5 Strongly disagree

DontCare   [*] I don't really care what I eat.
            SHOW CARD GG

1 Strongly agree
2 Agree
3 Neither agree nor disagree
4 Disagree
5 Strongly disagree

ExpertOp   [*] Experts never agree about what foods are good
            for you.
            SHOW CARD GG

1 Strongly agree
2 Agree
3 Neither agree nor disagree
4 Disagree
5 Strongly disagree

ExerEat   [*] As long as you take enough exercise you can eat
            whatever foods you like.
            SHOW CARD GG

1 Strongly agree
2 Agree
3 Neither agree nor disagree
4 Disagree
5 Strongly disagree

Ask all women aged 16 - 49

Folic   Have you heard of folic acid in connection with
            pregnancy?

1 Yes
2 No
3 Don't know

If heard of Folic acid

Folicimp   [*] Why do you think folic acid is important (DO NOT
            PROMPT)?
            CODE ALL THAT APPLY

1 Helps baby grow up properly
2 Protects against/helps prevent neural tube
  defects
3 Prevents Spina Bifida
4 Prevents mental handicap/disability
5 Prevents birth defects
6 Other
7 Don't know

CLASSIFICATION

Ask all respondents

Demintr   Now I would like to ask you a few more questions
            about yourself.

Quals1   May I just check, have you ever passed any exams?

1 Yes
2 No

Ask respondents who have passed any exams (Quals1 = Yes)

Quals2   Please look at this card and tell me the first exam
            you come to that you have passed.
            SHOW CARD HH

1 Degree or equivalent
2 Teaching or other higher qualification
3 A level or equivalent
4 GCSE, O level or equivalent
5 CSE or equivalent
6 CSE ungraded
7 Other qualifications

Ask all respondents

Origin   [*] To which of the groups on this card do you
            consider you belong?
            SHOW CARD II

1 White
2 Black Caribbean
3 Black African
4 Black Other
5 Indian
6 Pakistani
7 Bangladeshi
8 Chinese
9 SPONTANEOUS - Mixed Ethnic Group
10 None of these

Wrking   Did you do any paid work in the 7 days ending [last]
            Sunday, either as an employee or as self-employed?

1 Yes
2 No

**Ask if not in paid work in the last week and if female and aged
under 63 or male and aged under 65**

SchemeET   You said earlier that you were not in paid work last
            week, can I just check, were you on a government
            scheme for employment training?

1 Yes
2 No

**Ask if SchemeET = No OR female aged 63 or over or male
aged 65 or over (and not in paid work)**

JBAway   (You said earlier that you were not in paid work last
            week)
            Did you have a job or business you were away
            from?

1 Yes
2 No
3 SPONTANEOUS: Waiting to take up a new job/
  new business already obtained

Ask if JBAway = No

| OwnBus | Did you do any unpaid work in that week for any business that you own? | IndT | ENTER A TITLE FOR THE INDUSTRY |

OwnBus | Did you do any unpaid work in that week for any business that you own?

1 Yes
2 No

Ask if OwnBus = No

RelBus | ...or that a relative owns

1 Yes
2 No

Ask if RelBus = No

Looked | Thinking of the four weeks ending last Sunday were you looking for any kind of paid work or government training scheme at any time in those four weeks?

1 Yes
2 No

Ask if Looked = Yes

StartJ | If a job or a place on a government scheme had been available in the week ending last Sunday would you have been able to start work within two weeks?

1 Yes
2 No

Ask if Looked = No or StartJ = No

YInAct | What was the main reason you did not seek any work in the last four weeks/ would not be able to start in the next two weeks?

1 Student
2 Looking after family/home
3 Temporarily sick or injured
4 Long-term sick or disabled
5 Retired from paid work
6 Other reasons

Ask if not working last week, but not retired and not a student

Everwk | (Apart from the job you are waiting to take up) Have you ever been in paid employment?

1 Yes
2 No

Ask if working last week, has ever worked or retired or has a job he/she was away from or does unpaid work for a business owned by self or relative or is on a government scheme

IndD | What does/did the firm/organisation you work/ed for mainly make or do (at the place where you worked)?

DESCRIBE FULLY - PROBE MANUFACTURING or PROCESSING or DISTRIBUTION ETC. AND MAIN GOODS PRODUCED, MATERIALS USED, WHOLESALE OR RETAIL ETC.

IndT | ENTER A TITLE FOR THE INDUSTRY

OccT | What is/was your (main) job in the week ending last Sunday?
ENTER JOB TITLE

OccD | What did/do you mainly do in your job?
CHECK SPECIAL QUALIFICATIONS/TRAINING NEEDED TO DO THE JOB

Stat | Are/were you working as an employee or are/were you self-employed?

1 Employed
2 Self-employed

Ask respondents who are/were working as an employee (Stat = 1)

Manage | ASK OR RECORD
Did/do you have any managerial duties, or are/were you supervising any other employees?

1 Manager
2 Foreman/supervisor
3 Not manager/supervisor

EmpNo | How many employees are/were there at the place where you work/ed?

1 1-24
2 25 or over

Ask respondents who are/were self-employed at any time in the last 4 weeks (Stat = 2)

Solo | ASK OR RECORD
Are/were you working on your own or did you have employees?

1 On own/with partner(s) but no employees
2 With employees

Ask if has employees (Solo=2)

SENo | How many people did/do you employ at the place where you work/ed?

1 1-24
2 25 or over

Ftptwk | In your (main or last) job, were you working?

1 Full-time
2 Part-time

Ask if informant is not HOH

HOHIntro | I would now like to talk about HOH's employment

Hworking | May I just check, did HOH do any paid work in the week ending last Sunday, either as an employee or as self-employed?

1 Yes
2 No

Ask if HOH not in paid work in the last week and if female and aged under 63 or male and aged under 65

Hscheme   Was HOH on a government scheme for employment training?

     1   Yes
     2   No

Ask if HScheme = No OR female and aged 63 or over or male and aged 65 or over (and not in paid work)

HJBAway   Did HOH have a job or business he/she was away from?

     1   Yes
     2   No
     3   **SPONTANEOUS**: Waiting to take up a new job/ new business already obtained

Ask if HJBAway = No

HOwnBus   Did HOH do any unpaid work in that week for any business that he/she owns?

     1   Yes
     2   No

Ask if HOwnBus = No

Hrelbus   or that a relative owns?

     1   Yes
     2   No

Ask if HRelbus = No

HLooked   Thinking of the four weeks ending last Sunday was HOH looking for any kind of paid work or government training scheme at any time in those four weeks?

     1   Yes
     2   No

Ask if HLooked = Yes

HStartJ   If a job or a place on a government scheme had been available in the week ending last Sunday would HOH have been able to start work within two weeks?

     1   Yes
     2   No

Ask if HLooked = No or HStartJ = No

HYInAct   What was the main reason HOH did not seek any work in the last four weeks/ would not be able to start in the next two weeks?

     1   Student
     2   Looking after family/home
     3   Temporarily sick or injured
     4   Long-term sick or disabled
     5   Retired from paid work
     6   Other reasons

Ask if HOH was not working last week or was not retired or not a student

HEverwk   (Apart from the job he/she is waiting to take up) Has HOH ever been in paid employment?

     1   Yes
     2   No

Ask if HOH was working last week or has ever had a job or has a job he/she was away from last week or does unpaid work for a business owned by self or a relative or if on a government scheme

HIndD   What does/did the firm/organisation HOH work/ed for mainly make or do (at the place where HOH worked)?
DESCRIBE FULLY - PROBE MANUFACTURING or PROCESSING or DISTRIBUTION ETC. AND MAIN GOODS PRODUCED, MATERIALS USED, WHOLESALE OR RETAIL ETC

HIndT   ENTER A TITLE FOR THE INDUSTRY

HOccT   What is/was HOH's (main) job (in the week ending last Sunday?
ENTER JOB TITLE

HOccD   What does HOH mainly do in his/her job?
CHECK SPECIAL QUALIFICATIONS/ TRAINING NEEDED TO DO THE JOB

HStat   Was HOH working as an employee or was he/she self-employed?

     1   Employed
     2   Self-employed

Ask respondents who are/were working as an employee (HStat = 1)

HManage   ASK OR RECORD
Did HOH have any managerial duties, or was he/she supervising any other employees?

     1   Manager
     2   Foreman/supervisor
     3   Not manager/supervisor

HEmpNo   How many employees are/were there at the place where HOH work/ed?

     1   1-24
     2   25 or over

Ask respondents who are/were self-employed (HStat = 2)

HSolo   ASK OR RECORD
Is/was HOH working on his/her own or did he/she have employees?

     1   On own/with partner(s) but no employees
     2   With employees

Ask if (HSolo=2)

HSENo — How many people does/did HOH employ at the place where he/she works/ed?

1. 1-24
2. 25 or over

Hftptwk — In your (main or last) job, were you working?

1. Full-time
2. Part-time

INCOME

Ask all respondents

Benefits — Are you or anyone else in your household receiving any of the following state benefits?
SHOW CARD JJ
CODE ALL THAT APPLY

1. Income support
2. State Retirement Pension
3. Family credit
4. Housing benefit
5. Disability benefits/attendance allowance
6. Carer's allowance
7. None of these
8. Don't know

TotHhInc — The next question is on income. Choose the number from this card which represents the group in which you would place your TOTAL HOUSEHOLD INCOME from all sources BEFORE tax and other deductions. (EXPLAIN IF NECESSARY: INCOME FOR LAST TWELVE MONTHS)
SHOW CARD KK

	Per Year	Per Week
1	Under £2,500	Under £50
2	£2,500 - £4,999	£50-£99
3	£5,000 - £9,999	£100-£199
4	£10,000 - £14,999	£200-£299
5	£15,000 - £19,999	£300-£399
6	£20,000 - £29,999	£400-£599
7	£30,000 or more	£600 or more
8	Don't know	
9	SPONTANEOUS: Nothing	
10	SPONTANEOUS: Refused	

Ask if answer 2 at Benefits

Penplus — So may I just check, apart from the state retirement pension, does your household regularly receive any income from a pension from a previous employer?

1. Yes
2. No
3. Don't know

SEXUAL HEALTH

Ask respondents aged 16-54

Nonresp — The following section is self-completion. I would like you to take the computer and answer the questions

yourself. Instructions on how to answer the questions are given on the screen.
WORK THROUGH THE FIRST QUESTION WITH THE RESPONDENT.
IF THE RESPONDENT MAKES A MISTAKE, TAKE THEM BACK TO THE QUESTION AND ALLOW THEM TO KEY IN THE RIGHT ANSWER.
HAS THE RESPONDENT ACCEPTED THE SELF-COMPLETION?

1. Self-completion accepted and completed
2. Self-completion started, but not completed
3. Completed by interviewer
4. Self-completion refused

Ask respondents who refused to accept self-completion (Nonresp = 4)

Whyrefd — INTERVIEWER - CODE REASON WHY RESPONDENT REFUSED

1. Didn't like computer
2. Eyesight problems
3. Other disability
4. Objected to subject
5. Worried about confidentiality
6. Could not read or write
7. Ran out of time
8. Language problems
9. Couldn't be bothered
10. Other - Specify at next question

Ask respondents who answered 'Other' at Whyrefd

XWhyrefd — Specify reasons for refusal.

Ask respondents who started but did not complete (Nonresp = 2)

Whystopt — INTERVIEWER - CODE REASON WHY RESPONDENT STOPPED.

1. Objected to subject
2. Worried about confidentiality
3. Q on no of sexual partners
4. Ran out of time
5. Couldn't be bothered
6. Other - Specify at next question

Ask respondents who answered 'Other' at Whystopt

XWhystopt — Specify reasons for stopping.

Ask respondents aged 16-54 who answered 1 or 3 at Nonresp - do not ask if respondent did smoking and drinking self-completion

Intro2 — The next few questions require an answer which is either YES or NO. If your answer is YES, please press 1. If your answer is NO, please press 2. After each answer, either YES or NO, PRESS THE ENTER BUTTONRED BUTTON and this will take you to the next question. If you make a mistake ask the interviewer for help. To go to the next question now, PRESS 1 for YES and PRESS THE ENTER BUTTONRED BUTTON.

Practice	This is the first time I have used a computer.

1 Yes
2 No
3 Don't want to answer

Ask respondents aged 16-54 who answered 1 or 3 at Nonresp

Sexpart	The following questions are about sexual behaviour. Please answer them honestly. THE ANSWERS YOU GIVE ARE COMPLETELY CONFIDENTIAL. Have you ever had sexual intercourse? **Don't forget to include your husband/wife/ partner**

1 Yes
2 No
3 Don't want to answer

Ask respondents who have had at least one sexual partner (Sexpart = Yes)

Ask Men

TPart	Now I would like you to think about sexual partners you have had during your life. Which one of the following statements applies to you ..? SHOW CARD LL

1 I have had sex with women only
2 I have had sex mainly with women, but with some men as well
3 I have had sex with both men and women
4 I have had sex with men only
5 I have had sex with men, but with some women as well

Ask Women

TPart	Now I would like you to think about sexual partners you have had during your life. Which one of the following statements applies to you ..? SHOW CARD MM

1 I have had sex with men only
2 I have had sex mainly with men, but with some women as well
3 I have had sex with both men and women
4 I have had sex with women only
5 I have had sex mainly with women, but with some men as well

Firstsex	How old were you on the first occasion that you had sexual intercourse? PLEASE TYPE IN THE NUMBER THEN PRESS THE ENTER BUTTON RED BUTTON

Ask respondents who first had intercourse in the last five years

Frstuse	Now we would like you to think about the very first occasion that you had sexual intercourse. Did you or your partner use any of the following? PLEASE TYPE IN THE NUMBER OF ANY OF THE ANSWERS THAT APPLY. WHEN YOU HAVE

FINISHED PRESS THE ENTER BUTTON
SHOW CARD NN

1 The contraceptive pill
2 Emergency ('morning after') contraception
3 Male condom/sheath/durex
4 The female condom
5 Other method of protection (including sterilisation)
6 None of these
7 Can't remember

Ask respondents who have had at least one sexual partner (Sexpart = Yes)

Numparts	Now I would like you to think about the last 12 months, that is since (today's date) 1997. How many sexual partners, in total, have you had intercourse with during that time? Please remember to include your husband/wife/ present partner. PRESS 0 IF YOU HAVE NOT HAD ANY SEXUAL PARTNERS IN THE LAST 12 MONTHS TYPE IN THE NUMBER THEN PRESS THE ENTER BUTTON

Ask respondents who have had one sexual partner in the last 12 months (Numparts = 1)

Newpart	Did you have sexual intercourse with this person for the first time in the last 12 months? PRESS 1 FOR YES, PRESS 2 FOR NO THEN PRESS THE ENTER BUTTON

1 Yes
2 No
3 Don't want to answer

Ask respondents who have had one or more sexual partners in the last 12 months (Numparts = 1 or more)

Lastsex	On the last occasion that you had sexual intercourse, was that with ...

1 your husband/wife/partner
2 a regular partner you were not living with
3 a new partner
4 a casual partner
5 or can't you remember?

Ask respondents who have had partners of both sexes and at least one partner in the last year

Whichsex	And on that last occasion that you had sexual intercourse, was that..

1 with an (opposite sex) partner
2 or with a (same sex) partner?
3 Don't want to answer

Ask respondents who have had at least one partner in the last year (Numparts = 1 or more)

Lastuse	Thinking (again) about the last occasion on which you had sexual intercourse, which of the following, if any, were used? PRESS THE NUMBER OF ANY OF THE ANSWERS THAT APPLY.

WHEN YOU HAVE FINISHED PRESS THE ENTER
BUTTON
SHOW CARD NN

1   The contraceptive pill
2   Emergency ('morning after') contraception
3   Male condom/sheath/durex
4   The female condom
5   Other method of protection (including
    sterilisation)
6   None of these
7   Can't remember

**Ask respondents who used a condom on the last occasion
they had sexual intercourse (Lastuse = 3-4)**

Lastcon   What were your reasons for using a condom on that
            last occasion?
            PRESS THE NUMBER OF ANY OF THE REASONS
            THAT APPLY.
            WHEN YOU HAVE FINISHED PRESS THE ENTER
            BUTTON
            SHOW CARD OO

1   For contraception
2   For protection against HIV/AIDS
3   For protection against other sexually transmitted
    infections (STIs)
4   Other reason
5   Can't remember/Don't know

**Ask respondents who gave more than one reason for using a
condom on that occasion**

Mainrea   What was the main reason for using a condom?
            SHOW CARD OO

1   For contraception
2   For protection against HIV/AIDS
3   For protection against other other sexually
    transmitted infections (STIs)STIs
4   Other reason
5   Can't remember/Don't know

**Ask respondents who have had at least two sexual partners in
the last 12 months (Numparts = 2 or more)**

Newpart2   Have you had a new sexual partner within the last
            12 months? Please include any partner, even if you
            only had sexual intercourse on one occasion.

1   Yes
2   No
3   Don't want to answer

**Ask respondents who have had a new partner in the last 12
months (Newpart = Yes or Newpart2 = Yes)**

Condnew   Now we would like you to think of the last occasion
            that you **first** had sexual intercourse with someone
            new. Did you/your partner use a condom on that first
            time?

1   Yes
2   No
3   Can't remember

**Ask respondents who used a condom on that occasion
(Condnew = Yes)**

Whycon   Why did you use a condom on that occasion?
            PRESS THE NUMBER OF ANY OF THE REASONS
            THAT APPLY. WHEN YOU HAVE FINISHED
            PRESS THE ENTER BUTTON
            SHOW CARD OO

1   For contraception
2   For protection against HIV/AIDS
3   For protection against other sexually transmitted
    infections (STIs)
4   Other reason
5   Can't remember/Don't know

Whosugst   Who suggested using a condom?

1   Me
2   My partner
3   Both of us
4   We didn't talk about it
5   I can't remember

**Ask respondents who did not use a condom on that occasion
(Condnew = No)**

Whynoc   Here are some of the reasons people give for not
            using a condom with a new partner. Which of them
            applies to you?
            PRESS THE NUMBER OF ANY OF THE REASONS
            THAT APPLY.
            WHEN YOU HAVE FINISHED PRESS THE ENTER
            BUTTON
            SHOW CARD PP

1   You didn't discuss the question
2   You were very much in love
3   You knew your partner well enough
4   Partner didn't want to use one
5   You did not think at all about HIV risk
6   You and your partner didn't have one
7   You were afraid to lose your partner
8   Problems of impotence with a condom
9   Found it difficult to raise the subject
10   Using another method of contraception
11   Other

**Ask respondents who did not use a condom with a new
partner, on the last occasion of intercourse or on the first
occasion of intercourse**

Evercond   Have you (your partner) ever used a condom?

1   Yes
2   No
3   Don't want to answer

Ask all respondents

Aids   Have you changed your own sexual lifestyle or
            made any decisions about sex, because of concern
            about catching HIV/AIDS?

1   Yes
2   No
3   My lifestyle has changed but not because of AIDS

Ask respondents who have changed their sexual lifestyle because of HIV/AIDS (Aids = Yes)

Howchge   In which of these ways have you changed? What decisions have you made? PRESS THE NUMBER OF ANY ANSWERS THAT APPLY. WHEN YOU HAVE FINISHED PRESS THE ENTER BUTTON SHOW CARD QQ

1   Not having sex
2   Having fewer partners
3   Finding more out about a person before having sex
4   Using a condom
5   Keeping to one partner
6   Using sexual practices other than intercourse
7   Other changes

Ask all respondents

IntrAIDS   The following questions are about the risks of getting HIV/AIDS and other sexually transmitted infections. PRESS THE ENTER BUTTON TO CONTINUE

Aidsrisk   On the whole, compared to other people in this country, I have..

1   a greater risk of getting HIV/AIDS
2   the same risk of getting HIV/AIDS
3   less risk of getting HIV/AIDS
4   Don't know

Stdrisk   On the whole, the risk of someone like me getting another sexually transmitted infection (STI) is ..

1   very high
2   quite high
3   low
4   or is there no risk at all?
5   Don't know

CondIntr   Listed below are some of the things people have said about using condoms. Please say how much you agree with each of the following statements. To go to the next question now, PRESS 1 for YES and PRESS THE ENTER BUTTON.

Embarass   I would find it difficult to raise the subject of using a condom with a new partner. SHOW CARD RR

1   Strongly agree
2   Agree
3   Neither agree nor disagree
4   Disagree
5   Strongly disagree

CondHiv   Using condoms would protect against being infected with HIV/AIDS. SHOW CARD RR

1   Strongly agree
2   Agree
3   Neither agree nor disagree
4   Disagree
5   Strongly disagree

CondSTI   Using condoms would protect against being infected with other sexually transmitted infections (STIs). SHOW CARD RR

1   Strongly agree
2   Agree
3   Neither agree nor disagree
4   Disagree
5   Strongly disagree

Newcond   If in the near future you did have sex with a new partner do you think you would ...

1   always use a condom
2   it would depend
3   never use a condom
4   or wouldn't you contemplate having sex?

Vaccine   Do you think a vaccine against HIV/AIDS is Ö

1   available right now
2   will be available in the next 5 years
3   will be available in the next 10 years
4   will be available at some time in the future but more than 10 years away
5 4   will never be available

HeardTr   Have you heard of any new treatments for HIV/ AIDS?

1   Yes
2   No
3   Not sure

Ask if HeardTr = Yes or not sure

AidsIntr   Listed below are some of the things people have said about a treatment for HIV/AIDS. Please say how much you agree with each of the following statements. To go to the next question now, PRESS 1 for YES and PRESS THE ENTER BUTTON

Newtreat   With the new treatments, it is possible to be cured of HIV/AIDS. SHOW CARD RR

1   Strongly agree
2   Agree
3   Neither agree nor disagree
4   Disagree
5   Strongly disagree

Transmit   With the new treatments, it is possible for HIV positive people not to transmit the virus. SHOW CARD RR

1   Strongly agree
2   Agree
3   Neither agree nor disagree
4   Disagree
5   Strongly disagree

Ask respondents who have had a new partner in the last 12 months (Newpart2 = Yes or Newpart = Yes)

Lastintr   The following questions are about the person you had sexual intercourse with for the first time in the

last 12 months. Please answer them honestly. THE
ANSWERS YOU GIVE ARE COMPLETELY
CONFIDENTIAL .
To go to the first question, PRESS THE ENTER
BUTTON.

Ask if Newpart= Yes

Frstpart   Were they your first sexual partner?

    1   Yes
    2   No

Ask if Newpart = Yes or Newpart2 = Yes

AgeNPart   (Thinking of the last occasion when you first had
sexual intercourse with someone new) What was
his/her age?
PLEASE TYPE IN THE NUMBER THEN PRESS
THE ENTER BUTTON
IF YOU DO NOT KNOW THEIR AGE PLEASE
MAKE A GUESS AND ENTER THAT NUMBER

**Ask if had sexual intercourse with a member of the opposite
sex**

Whchsex1   And on that occasion, was that...

    1   with an (opposite) sex partner
    2   or with a (same sex) partner
    3   Don't want to answer

Partfrst   Was it the first time this person had had sexual
intercourse?

    1   Yes
    2   No
    3   Don't know

Ask if Newpart = Yes or Newpart2 = Yes

WellNPrt   How well would you say you knew him/her

    1   Very well
    2   Fairly well
    3   Not very well
    4   Not at all

WherNPrt   In which country was this partner normally living?

    1   United Kingdom
    2   Abroad
    3   Don't know

IF WherNPrt = Abroad

XWherPrt   Please specify this partner's country

YouPart   On the occasion of your first intercourse with this
partner were you in another relationship with another
partner?

    1   Yes, with one other partner
    2   Yes, with more than one other partner
    3   No
    4   Don't know

ThemPart   On the occasion of your first intercourse with
partner, was she/he in a sexual relationship with
another partner?

    1   Yes, with one other partner
    2   Yes, with more than one other partner
    3   No
    4   Don't know

Howmeet   How did you meet this partner?

    1   Studies
    2   Work
    3   Recreation/sports club
    4   On holiday in the UK
    5   On holiday abroad
    6   Public place/on public transport
    7   Nightclub/pub
    8   Prostitution/massage parlour/escort agency
    9   Other (specify)

Whointro   Who introduced you to this partner?

    1   Friends
    2   Family member
    3   Colleague/fellow student
    4   Dating agency/advertisement
    5   Nobody
    6   Other (specify)

Xwhointr   Please specify

Thinkprt   When you first had sexual intercourse with this
partner, which of the following statements best
describes how you thought of them?

    1   Possible spouse, fiancée or steady partner
    2   Casual partner
    3   One-night stand
    4   Holiday affair
    5   Paid sex
    6   Not sure

HIVNPrt   When you first had sexual intercourse with this
partner, did you think about HIV risk?

    1   Yes
    2   No

StillRel   Is the relationship with this partner still going on?

    1   Yes
    2   No

If No

Numsex   Did you have sex with this partner on more than
one occasion?

    1   Yes
    2   No

**Ask if (StillRel = Yes) or (Numsex = Yes) and Condnew = Yes
or Can't remember**

Stillcon	Which of the following best describes your use of condoms (during this relationship)? SHOW CARD SS 1 You discussed the risks and (have) stopped using condoms 2 You and/or your partner (have) had an HIV test and then you stopped using condoms 3 You just stopped using condoms without discussing the risks or taking an HIV test 4 You still (continued to) use condoms 5 Can't remember	Paidsex	Have you ever paid for sex, either with money, goods, services or drugs? 1 Yes 2 No

Ask if (StillRel = Yes) or (Numsex=Yes) and Condnew = No or Can't remember

Evercon	During this relationship, did (have) you ever use(d) a condom ? 1 Yes, used a condom 2 No, not used a condom 3 Can't remember		

If yes

		Whenpaid	When did you last pay for sex? 1 During the past 12 months 2 Between 1 and 5 years ago 3 More than 5 years ago 4 More than 15 years ago

Ask if Sexpart = Yes

STIever	Have you ever been diagnosed by a medical doctor as having a sexually transmitted infection? 1 Yes 2 No 3 Don't know	Whopaid	What was the sex of this person? 1 Male 2 Female
		Paidcon	Did you use a condom with that person? 1 Yes 2 No

Ask all respondents

If STIever = Yes

WhenSTI	When did you have a sexually transmitted infection for the last time? 1 During the past 12 months 2 Between 1 and 5 years ago 3 More than 5 years ago	Safesex	There has been a lot of publicity about 'safer sex' in recent years. Have you heard of 'safer sex' or 'safe sex'? 1 Yes 2 No 3 Don't know

Ask respondents who have heard of 'safer sex' or'safe sex' (Safesex = Yes)

STItreat	On this occasion, where did you go first for treatment? 1 G.P. 2 GUM/Sexual health clinic 3 Other	Safesex2	Please say what you mean by 'safer sex' or 'safe sex'. YOU CAN EITHER TYPE IN THE ANSWER YOURSELF OR, IF YOU PREFER, WRITE YOUR ANSWER ON PAPER FOR THE INTERVIEWER TO TYPE IN LATER
WhchSTI	Which sexually transmitted infection was it? 1 Chlamydia 2 Gonorrhea, clap 3 Syphilis 4 Trichomonas 5 Herpes 6 Gonalitis 7 Genital warts 8 Mycosis/candidiasis/thrush 9 Hepatitis 10 Other sexually transmitted infection/don't know name	ThankYou	That is the end of the self-completion. Thank you for your help. To finish the interview, PRESS 1 for YES and PRESS THE ENTER BUTTON.
		Laptop	NOW HAND THE COMPUTER BACK TO THE INTERVIEWER.

Ask if Sexpart = Yes

The survey was carried out using computer assisted interviewing. These are copies of the showcards.

HEALTH EDUCATION MONITORING SURVEY 1998

B	
1	Completely free of stress
2	Small amount of stress
3	Moderate amount of stress
4	Large amount of stress

A	
1	Strongly agree
2	Agree
3	Neither agree nor disagree
4	Disagree
5	Strongly disagree

D	
1	Take more exercise/more physical ativity
2	Smoke more
3	Eat more
4	Get professional help or advice
5	Listen to/play music
6	Spend more time on hobbies
7	Other
8	None of these

C	
1	Try not to think about it
2	Discuss it with a close friend or relative
3	Work harder to occupy myself
4	Have a drink
5	Pray/meditate
6	Spend more time thinking about my problems
7	Spend more time going out with friends or relatives
8	None of these

E

1. The amount I smoke
2. Eating a poor diet
3. The quality of my housing
4. Stress
5. Living on my own
6. The amount of alcohol I drink
7. My weight
8. Environmental pollution
9. The quality of local health services
10. My sexual behaviour
11. Road traffic in this area
12. Being unemployed
13. Violent crime in this area
14. None of these

F

1. Violence/crime
2. Environmental pollution
3. Being unemployed
4. Cancer
5. The quality of local health services
6. The spread of HIV/AIDS
7. Stress
8. Heart disease
9. None of these

G

1 Road accidents

2 Health risks linked to smoking

3 My weight

4 Health risks linked to drugs

5 Eating a poor diet

6 The quality of my housing

7 Health risks linked to drinking alcohol

8 Being lonely

9 None of these

H

1 The amount of road traffic

2 Industrial fumes and emissions

3 Litter and rubbish

4 The level of crime and vandalism

5 The level of noise

6 The amount of abuse or violence

7 Other risk

8 None of these

I	
1	Lack of heating
2	Dampness/condensation/mould
3	Cigarette smoke
4	The general maintenance of your home
5	Overcrowding
6	The quality of drinking water
7	The level of noise
8	Other risk
9	None of these

J	
1	The materials you have to handle
2	The equipment you have to use
3	Industrial fumes and emissions
4	Cigarette smoke
5	The level of noise
6	Stress
7	The number of hours you work
8	Other risk
9	None of these

L

1   Attended an adult education or night school class

2   Parcipated in a voluntary group or local Community group

3   Parcipated in community or religious activities

4   Went to a leisure centre

5   Went on social outing

6   None of these

K

1   Visited relatives Been visited by relatives

2   Spoke to relatives on the 'phone

3   Visited friends Been visited by friends

4   Spoke to friends on the 'phone

5   Spoke to neighbours

6   Spoke to a health professional (e.g. doctor, nurse, midwife, health visitor)

7   None of these

M

1	Strongly agree
2	Agree
3	Neither agree nor disagree
4	Disagree
5	Strongly disagree

N

1	Had a serious operation or illness
2	Had a serious injury
3	Death of close relative or friend
4	Personal experience of theft, mugging or other crime
5	Happy family event
6	Other event
7	None of these

P

1. Local authority funded home help
2. Local authority funded carer
3. Private domestic help
4. District nurse or health visitor
5. Meals on wheels
6. Lunch club run by council or Voluntary body
7. Day centre for older people run by council or voluntary body
8. Helper from a voluntary organisation
9. None of these

O

0. Not difficult
1. Quite difficult
2. Very difficult
3. Impossible
4.

R	
1	Sunbathing abroad
2	Outdoors abroad, but not sunbathing
3	Sunbathing in this country
4	Outdoors in this country doing something else

Q	
1	Meals on wheels
2	Lunch club run by council or voluntary Body
3	Day centre for older people run by council or voluntary body
4	Voluntary organisation
5	Help at another service

T	
1	Strongly agree
2	Agree
3	Neither agree nor disagree
4	Disagree
5	Strongly disagree

S	
1	White skin
2	Brown skin
3	Black skin
4	Olive skin
5	Other

U

1 I intend to give up smoking within the next month

2 I intend to give up smoking within the next six months

3 I intend to give up smoking within the next year

4 I intend to give up smoking but not in the next year

5 I'm unlikely to give up smoking

V

1 I'm unlikely to give up smoking

2 I intend to give up smoking within the next month

3 I intend to give up smoking within the next six months

4 I intend to give up smoking within the next year

5 I intend to give up smoking but not in the next year

X

Strongly agree	1
Agree	2
Neither agree nor disagree	3
Disagree	4
Strongly disagree	5

W

Almost every day	1
5 or 6 days a week	2
3 or 4 days a week	3
Once or twice a week	4
Once or twice a month	5
Once every couple of months	6
Once or twice a year	7
Not at all in the last 12 months	8

Y

HEAVY HOUSEWORK

1   **Moving heavy furniture**

2   **Spring cleaning**

3   **Walking with heavy shopping (for more than 5 minutes)**

4   **Cleaning windows**

5   **Scrubbing floors with a scrubbing brush**

Z

GARDENING, DIY AND BUILDING WORK

1   **Hoeing, weeding, pruning**

2   **Mowing with a power mower**

3   **Planting flowers/seeds**

4   **Decorating**

5   **Minor household repairs**

6   **Car washing and polishing**

7   **Car repairs and maintenance**

BB

1 Aerobics/keep fit/gymnastics
2 Bowls/Crown bowls
3 Circuit training/ weight training
4 Cycling
5 Exercises
6 Dancing
7 Football/rugby
8 Golf
9 Hiking
10 Hockey/netball/ice-skating
11 Jogging/running/athletics
12 Squash
13 Swimming
14 Tennis/badminton
15 Any other sport or exercise activity like these

AA

HEAVY MANUAL WORK

1 Digging, clearing rough ground
2 Building in stone/bricklaying
3 Mowing large areas with a hand mower
4 Felling trees/chopping wood
5 Mixing/laying concrete
6 Moving heavy loads
7 Refitting a kitchen or bathroom

CC

1   I intend to take more exercise within the next month

2   I intend to take more exercise within the next six months

3   I intend to take more exercise within the next year

4   I intend to take more exercise, but not in the next year

5   I'm unlikely to take more exercise

DD

1   I'm unlikely to take more exercise

2   I intend to take more exercise within the next month

3   I intend to take more exercise within the next six months

4   I intend to take more exercise within the next year

5   I intend to take more exercise, but not in the next year

EE	
White	1
High fibre white	2
Brown, granary, wheatmeal	3
Wholemeal	4
Pitta bread	5
South Asian breads (chapati, nan, roti, puri etc)	6
Some other type of bread	7
Do not eat any type of bread	8

FF	
More than once every day	1
Once every day	2
5-6 days a week	3
3-4 days a week	4
1-2 days a week	5
At least once a month	6
Less often than once a month	7
Rarely or never	8

HH

Degree (or degree level qualification) level 5 NVQ/SVQ — 1

Teaching qualification HNC/HND, BRC/TEC Higher, BTEC Higher, City and Guilds Full Technological Certificate, Nursing Qualifications (SRN, SCM, RGN, RM, RHV, Midwife) Level 4 NVQ/SVQ — 2

A levels, SCE Higher ONC/OND/BTEC/TEC/BTEC not higher City and Guilds Advanced/Final level Level 3 NVQ/SVQ/Advanced GNVQ/GSVQ — 3

O level passes (Grade A-C if after 1975) GCSE (Grades A-C) CSE Grade 1 SCE Ordinary (Bands A-C) Standard Grade (Level 1-3) SLC Lower/SUPE Lower or Ordinary School Certificate or Matric City and Guilds Craft/Ordinary Level Level 2 NVQ/SVQ/Intermediate GNVQ/GSVQ — 4

CSE ungraded — 6

Other qualifications — 7

GG

Strongly agree — 1

Agree — 2

Neither agree nor disagree — 3

Disagree — 4

Strongly disagree — 5

JJ

1 Income support
2 State Retirement Pension
3 Family credit
4 Housing benefit
5 Disability benefits/attendance allowance
6 Carers allowance
7 None of these

II

1 White
2 Black Caribbean
3 Black African
4 Black Other
5 Indian
6 Pakistani
7 Bangladeshi
8 Chinese
9 None of these

LL

I have had sex with women only   1

I have had sex mainly with women but with some men as well   2

I have had sex with both men and women   3

I have had sex with men only   4

I have had sex mainly with men but with some women as well   5

KK

PER WEEK	
Under £50	1
£50 - £99	2
£100 - £199	3
£200 - £299	4
£300 - £399	5
£400 - £599	6
£600 or more	7

PER YEAR
Under £2,500
£2,500 - £4,999
£5,000 - £9,999
£10,000 - £14,999
£15,000 - £19,999
£20,000 - 29,999
£30,000 or more

MM

I have had sex with men only	1
I have had sex mainly with men but with some women as well	2
I have had sex with both men and women	3
I have had sex with women only	4
I have had sex mainly with women but with some men as well	5

NN

The contraceptive pill	1
Emergency ('morning after') contraception	2
Male condom/sheath/durex	3
The female condom	4
Other method of protection (including sterilisation)	5
None of these	6
Can't remember	7

OO

1   For contraception

2   For protection against HIV/AIDS

3   For protection against other sexually transmitted infections (STIs)

4   Other reason

5   Can't remember

PP

1   You didn't discuss the question

2   You were very much in love

3   You knew your partner well enough

4   Your partner didn't want to use one

5   You did not think at all about HIV risk

6   You and your partner didn't have one

7   You were afraid to lose your partner

8   Problems of impotence with a condom

9   Found it difficult to raise the subject

10   Using another method of contraception

11   Other reason

QQ

1 Not having sex

2 Having fewer partners

3 Finding more out about a person before having sex

4 Using a condom

5 Keeping to one partner

6 Using sexual practices other than intercourse

7 Other changes

RR

1 Strongly agree

2 Agree

3 Neither agree nor disagree

4 Disagree

5 Strongly agree

SS

You have discussed the risks
and (have) stopped using
condoms   1

You and/or your partner (have)
had an HIV test and then you
stopped using condoms   2

You just stopped using condoms
without discussing the risks or
taking an HIV test   3

You still (continued to) use
condoms   4

List of figures

List of tables

Appendix A

Appendix C